Praise for Jan Bondeson's Books

The Two-Headed Boy

W9-BUB-856

"Bondeson takes another look at those whom some call freaks and medical monstrosities. He examines these strange persons sympathetically, with concern for how they lived, drawing on original, often contemporary descriptions to understand them. . . . Good reading for anyone with a strong stomach, sufficient curiosity, and appreciation for the odd touch of wry humor." —*Booklist*

The Feejee Mermaid and Other Essays in Natural and Unnatural History

"Jan Bondeson has poked about in dusty seaside museum stores for lost stuffed mermaids and moth-eaten garments made of vegetable lambswool; he has unearthed mummified toads . . . has uncovered the perils, sorrows, and achievements of pet elephants and prophetic pigs, and recorded showers of toads and eels and bricks (and frying pans)." —*Times Literary Supplement*

A Cabinet of Medical Curiosities

"Folklore, literature, cultural history, and medicine are all brought together, to set the curiosity in a broad background. Each chapter ends with the modern medical explanation of how the abnormality might have occurred genetically or what the disease really was. . . . This is a book for a wide audience, not just for medical people. . . . The broad setting and many illustrations add greatly to its appeal." —*The Lancet*

The Feejee Mermaid and Other Essays in Natural and Unnatural History

"Presented here are ten investigations into natural history at its most odd and occasionally macabre: barnacle geese purported to grow from trees, lambs born of plants in the wilds of Tartary, toads-in-the-hole blinking back the sunlight after being unlocked from centuries encased in solid stone. . . . Bondeson doesn't seek important truths behind the grotesqueries, nor trenchant social criticisms. If he educates, it's as a broadly inquisitive and keen naturalist; that he amuses is not a point for debate." —*Kirkus Reviews*

"In the finest tradition of the bestiaries of old, Bondeson presents tales of amazing animals. . . . He successfully couples a wealth of historical material with the latest biological information. In doing so, he demonstrates winsomely that science has solved some long-standing mysteries, but that others remain beyond its reach." —*Publishers Weekly*

"Bondeson illustrates the unusual in natural history with his collection of essays describing scientific hoaxes, misconceptions, and other assorted oddities of the natural world. The 'strange but true' nature of these pieces is immediately appealing." —*Library Journal*

"Bondeson has a consummate skill in finding and presenting [his] material, producing a rare and entertaining package for the curious reader." — *The Bloomsbury Review*

"Bondeson . . . has done a masterful job . . . Liberal doses of wit and humor are hallmarks of this book . . . Highly recommended for all levels." — *Choice*

"A wonderful book about a wonderful subject . . . Richly illustrated." —*Virginia Quarterly Review*

"Jan Bondeson has poked about in dusty seaside museum stores for lost stuffed mermaids and moth-eaten garments made of vegetable lambswool; he has unearthed mummified toads . . . has uncovered the perils, sorrows, and achievements of pet elephants and prophetic pigs, and recorded showers of toads and eels and bricks (and frying pans)." — *Times Literary Supplement*

The Two-headed Boy,
and Other Medical Marvels

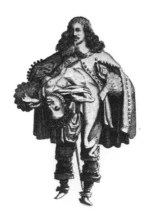

The Two-headed Boy,

and Other Medical Marvels

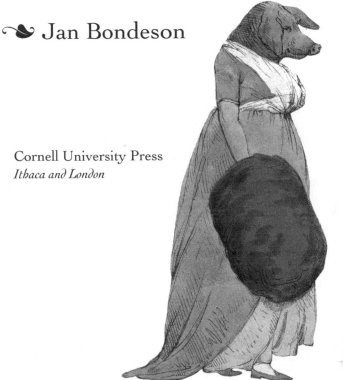

❧ Jan Bondeson

Cornell University Press
Ithaca and London

First published 2000 by Cornell University Press
First printing, Cornell Paperbacks, 2004
Printed in the United States of America

Library of Congress Cataloging-in-Publication Data
Bondeson, Jan.
    The two-headed boy, and other medical marvels / Jan Bondeson.
        p. cm.
    Includes bibliographical references.
    ISBN 0-8014-3767-9 (cloth: alk. paper)
    ISBN 0-8014-8958-X (pbk.: alk. paper)
    1. Abnormalities, Human.   I. Title.

QM690 .B66 2000
610—dc21   00-020902

Cornell University Press strives to use environmentally responsible suppliers and materials to the fullest extent possible in the publishing of its books. Such materials include vegetable-based, low-VOC inks and acid-free papers that are recycled, totally chlorine-free, or partly composed of nonwood fibers. Books that bear the logo of the FSC (Forest Stewardship Council) use paper taken from forests that have been inspected and certified as meeting the highest standards for environmental and social responsibility. For further information, visit our website at www.cornell-press.cornell.edu.

Cloth printing   10 9 8 7 6 5 4 3 2 1
Paperback printing 10 9 8 7 6 5 4 3 2 1

Contents

The Two Inseparable Brothers; and a Preface   vii

The Hairy Maid at the Harpsichord   1

The Stone-child   39

The Woman Who Laid an Egg   51

The Strangest Miracle in the World   64

Some Words about Hog-faced Gentlewomen   95

Horned Humans   120

The Biddenden Maids   141

The Tocci Brothers, and Other Dicephali   160

The King of Poland's Court Dwarf   189

Daniel Cajanus, the Swedish Giant   217

Daniel Lambert, the Human Colossus   237

Cat-eating Englishmen and French Frog Swallowers   261

Notes on Sources   285

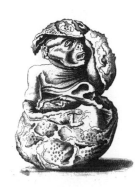

Lavinia
Fontana's
painting of
Tognina
Gonzales.
Reproduced
by permission,
© Château et
Musée de
Blois, France.

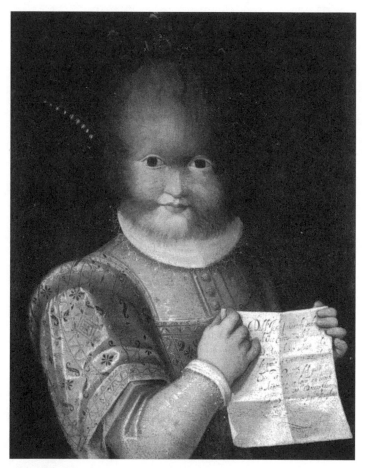

The Two Inseparable Brothers; and a Preface

I many Prodigies have seene,
Creatures that have preposterous beene,
to nature in their birth,
But such a thing as this my theame,
Makes all the rest seeme but a dreame,
the like was nere on earth.

Thus begins the ballad "The Two Inseparable Brothers," written by Martin Parker, one of London's most prolific authors of valedictory poems, songs, and ballads of the 1630s and 1640s. On November 23, 1637, a certain Robert Milbourne registered this ballad as "a Picture of the Italian yong man with his brother growing out of his side with some verses thereunto." The admittedly coarse illustration shows exactly that: a man with a much smaller conjoined twin brother growing out of his body. This was the famous Lazarus Colloredo, who had already toured Italy, Germany, Spain, and France and who was now ready to make his bow before King Charles I and his liege subjects in London. On November 4, 1637, Sir Henry Herbert, master of the rolls, had granted "Lazaras, an Italian" permission to "shew his brother Baptista, that grows out of his navell, and carryes him at his syde."

A Gentleman well qualifide,
Doth beare his brother at his side,
inseparably knit,
As in this figure you may see,
And both together living be,
the world admires at it.

Throughout his career, Lazarus Colloredo was described as a "gentleman," and it is likely that he was of above-average breeding. A later handbill about him actually stated that he was an Italian count, but this is unlikely to have been the truth. A letter from Dr. Augustin Pincet, of Genoa, to the celebrated Fortunio Liceti, revealed that the two inseparable brothers were born on March 20, 1617; their parents were Baptista and Pellegrina Colloredo, living in the parish of Saint Bartholomeus de Costa in Genua. Both twins were baptized at the font: the larger one was named Lazarus and his tiny brother, Joannes Baptista. Their parents were healthy and had previously had several healthy children. Dr. Pincet examined the twins and found that while Lazarus's body was healthy and complete in every respect, Joannes Baptista had a malformed body, lacked one leg, and did not open his eyes. He was amazed that Lazarus was the only one to suckle his mother and to emit excrement and urine. When his tiny brother got some droplets of milk on his lips, his lips moved as if he tried to swallow them. Dr. Pincet was astonished that this "monstrum novissimum"—this novel species of monster— actually seemed fully capable of life. So was Dr. Paulus Zacchias, who described the inseparable brothers in his *Questionum Medico-Legalium*. He had seen them in Rome in 1617 and later in 1623. Their mother had died in 1620. Lazarus had a handsome face and curly golden hair. From his belly, near the cartilages of his rib cage, grew another child. Joannes Baptista was devoid of any sense, wrote Zacchias, except that of sensation. He moved his arms, and frothy saliva dribbled from his mouth.

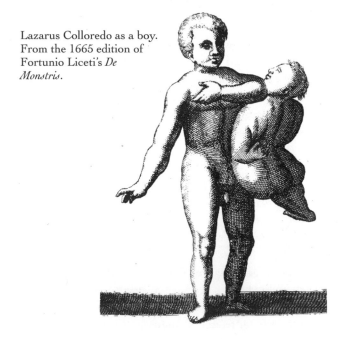

Lazarus Colloredo as a boy.
From the 1665 edition of
Fortunio Liceti's *De
Monstris*.

> *But that to ratifie this truth,*
> *Now in the Strand this wondrous youth*
>   *is present to be seene,*
> *And he with his strange burden, hath*
> *Bin shewne (with maruaile) as he saith*
>   *to our good King and Queene.*

Lazarus Colloredo's stay in London appears to have been quite success-ful. He was received in an audience by King Charles I and Queen Henrietta, and there exists a curious old engraving of him, with the somewhat confus-ing caption "Israel and his twin brother exhibited to King Charles II," that I have seen. I am convinced that it really portrays Lazarus Colloredo, how-ever, since the position of the twin is almost exactly the same as on the other engravings of him. Other confusing circumstances are that the individual on this engraving is rather youthful looking and that the engraving is marked "aet. 17"; it is reasonable to propose that this was an older engraving of him, perhaps made at the onset of his career, that Lazarus himself or some other person had brought to London.

> *This yong-man doth completely walke,*
> *He can both read, write, sing, or talke,*
>   *without paine or detraction,*
> *And when he speaks the other head,*
> *Doth moue the lips both ruby red,*
>   *not speaking but in action.*

In 1638, Lazarus Colloredo toured France. When in Paris, he was seen by M. Henri Sauval, who spoke to him at length and recorded some extra-ordinary facts in his *Histoire et antiquités de la ville de Paris*. Both Lazarus and his brother had blond hair, and they did not look like Italians. Lazarus told him that when they were young, Joannes Baptista's head had been much smaller; now, it was twice as big as his own. The imperfect twin's open mouth, dribbling with saliva, showed some large teeth and had appalling hal-itosis. Lazarus also said that they had been ill three times and that the doc-tors had bled him twenty times for various ailments; the learned medics had never hazarded purgation, however, since they feared that this might have been too much for a digestive system shared between two human beings. M. Sauval was greatly impressed when Lazarus accepted his challenge to play handball at the Paris ball-house; the Italian played with skill and vigor, with his brother tightly tied to his own body. After the game, Lazarus told M.

x   Sauval that he had once been in big trouble. A man had teased him at a public house, and Lazarus had struck him a mighty blow on the head and killed
him. He had been sentenced to death, but was reprieved after he had shown,
to the court's satisfaction, that if he was killed, his brother, who was innocent
of the deadly assault, would be unjustly murdered!

> *One arme's about his brother cast,*
> *That doth embrace his body fast,*
>   *the other hangeth by,*
> *These armes haue hands with fingers all,*
> *Yet as a childs they are but small,*
>   *pinch any part hee'l cry.*

The print depicting
the Colloredo
brothers in 1634,
as they set out on
their travels.

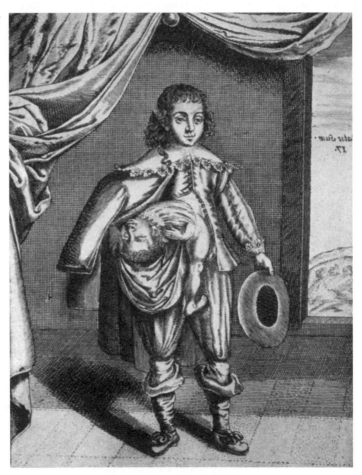

Lazarus later made another tour of the British Isles, and went to Nor-
wich, as shown by a record in the mayor's court book for December 21,
1639: "This daie Larzeus Colloretto have leave to shewe a monster until the
day after twelve, he shewing to the Court a lysence signed with his Maties
owne hand." In 1640, he was in Gdansk in Poland, where he told an English
traveler that he was going to Turkey next. In 1642, Lazarus returned to the
British Isles. A day or two before Easter, he visited Aberdeen, as evidenced
by John Spalding's curious *Memorialls of the Trubles in Scotland and in England*.
He had two servants with him, who like himself were well dressed. He also
brought with him a large portrait of himself, which he hung out at his lodg-
ing, to advertise himself. When the show was to begin, one of the servants
blew a trumpet and called out that Colloredo was now receiving visitors; the
other servant stood by the door and collected money from the curious Scots
who flocked to see this marvel. According to Spalding, "this gryte wark of
God was admired of be many in Abirdene and throw the countries as he
trauellit." Spalding himself was among the visitors and could confirm the
earlier observations of their anatomy: Lazarus was perfectly formed, but the
twin's malformed head was drooping backward and downward, and the eyes
were closed. The twin had three fingers on each hand, six toes on the sole
foot, and "the prik of ane man, bot no balcod." He also confirmed that the
twin "had a kind of lyf, and feilling," but that he ate nothing and was fed
from the nourishment taken by Lazarus. When Colloredo was traveling, he
carried his brother within a fold of his great cloak and cape, and no person
could guess his unique deformity.

> *Th'imperfect once the small poxe had,*
> *Which made the perfect brother sad,*
>   *but he had neuer any,*
> *And if you nip it by the arme,*
> *Or doe it any little harme,*
>   *(this hath been tried by many,)*
>
> *It like an infant (with voyce weake)*
> *Will cry out though it cannot speake,*
>   *as sensible of paine . . .*

Lazarus Colloredo and his brother left Scotland in 1642, after which
there are fewer observations of them, but the best description of him is that
by the celebrated Danish anatomist Thomas Bartholin, who saw him being
exhibited in 1645. It is worth quoting verbatim:

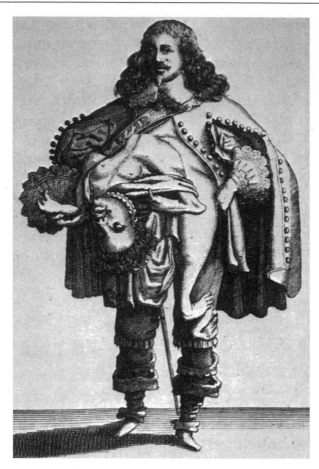

Thomas Bartholin's engraving of the brothers, as reissued as a plate in *Gentleman's Magazine* of 1777.

Twice I saw with astonishment Lazarus Colloredo, a Genoese, aged about twenty-eight; first in Copenhagen and later in Basle in Switzerland. This Lazarus had a little brother born with him, growing out of his breast and adhering to him at the level of the xiphoid cartilage of the breastbone. The little brother had a left leg and foot; he had two arms, but just three fingers on each hand. If pressure was made against his chest, he moved his hands, ears and lips. He received no food or nourishment but through the body of his greater brother Lazarus. Their vital

and animal parts appeared to be distinct, as the little brother
might sleep when Lazarus was awake, stir whilst Lazarus was
sleeping, and sweat when Lazarus was without perspiration.
They had both been baptized, the greater one named Lazarus at
the font, the smaller John Baptist. The head of the little brother
was well formed and covered with hair. His respiration was
weak, since I could hold a feather to his mouth and nostrils, and
it moved but slightly. His mouth was always open and gaping,
and had no lack of teeth. No part of him seemed to increase in
size except the head, which was larger than that of Lazarus, deformed and with long dangling hair. They both had beards, but
whilst that of Lazarus was well combed and kept clean, that of
the other was neglected.

Yet nothing doth the lesser eate,
He's onely nourish'd with the meate
  wherewith the other feeds,
By which it seemes though outward parts
They haue for two, yet not two hearts,
  this admiration breeds.

A handbill issued in Strasbourg where Lazarus Colloredo exhibited
himself in August 1645 repeated the usual facts about him. Interestingly, it
also stated that although Joannes Baptista was without understanding,
voice, and speech, the brothers could actually *communicate* with each other.
There is no record of Lazarus Colloredo and his strange twin brother after
they toured Italy in 1646; it is likely that Colloredo either died or retired
from show business shortly after this year. The fame of these inseparable
brothers survived them, however. In 1777, the *Gentleman's Magazine* reproduced an engraving of Colloredo, copied from Bartholin's work, with an ex-
planatory text by Dr. J. Greene giving a true account of "a Man with a Child
growing out of his Body." The same engraving was reissued as a plate in
1815 and later was reproduced in several nineteenth-century works of popular "biographia curiosa," with more or less confused commentary. Both G.
M. Gould and W. Pyle's *Anomalies and Curiosities of Medicine* and C. J. S.
Thompson's *The Mystery and Lore of Monsters* quote Bartholin's description of
Colloredo. Some later commentators doubted, from the extraordinary nature
of his deformity and the fact that no similar case of parasitic conjoined twinning has been observed in the nineteenth or twentieth century, that Colloredo
ever existed. Others suspected that Bartholin was exaggerating. The discov-

xiv ery of several independent descriptions of Colloredo and his brother, like
those by Paulus Zaccias, Henri Sauval, and John Spalding, as well as the
handbills issued in Strasbourg in 1645 and Verona in 1646, proves without
doubt not only that they definitely existed, but also that Bartholin's description contained no exaggeration.

> *Through Germany, through Spain & France,*
> *(Devoyd of danger or mischance)*
> *and other Christian Lands*
> *They travell'd haue, nay rather one*
> *For both, so many miles hath gone,*
> *to shew th' work of Gods hands.*

It would have been fashionable just to dismiss the inseparable brothers
as a unique freak of nature and just another "curiosity" that impedes the se-

The German handbill
about Lazarus
Colloredo and his
brother, from
Strasbourg, dated
August 1645.

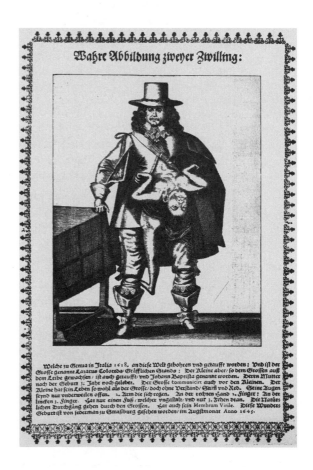

rious study of the history of medicine. A more constructive approach is to examine more closely the many aspects of their influence on contemporary culture, as well as to study, in an interdisciplinary manner, how they have influenced the history of teratology and how they have made appearances in literature and popular culture.

❧

Having surveyed Lazarus Colloredo and his strange brother, how can we explain this strange deformity? Conjoined, or Siamese, twins can be divided into several subgroups. Among these are craniopagus twins, who are joined by the skulls; thoracopagus twins joined by the rib cage; omphalopagus twins joined by the belly; pygopagus twins joined by the hips; and ischiopagus twins joined by the sacrum. Another, parallel classification represents the difference between symmetrical conjoined twins, with two complete individuals, and asymmetrical ones, where one of the twins is an incompletely developed parasite. The German teratologists Friedrich Ahlfeld, Ernst Schwalbe, and Hans Hübner independently considered the case of the Colloredo brothers and diagnosed them as *thoracopagus parasiticus* conjoined twins. The modern definition of thoracopagi entails that the twins should have joined thoraxes, however, and this was not the case with the Colloredo twins; in modern terminology, they should be classified as *omphalopagus parasiticus* conjoined twins, since they were joined near the umbilicus.

It is also possible to establish the exact mechanism behind this form of parasitic conjoined twinning. Conjoined twins are the result of imperfect splitting of a fertilized ovum, and the site of conjunction depends on in which part the splitting has not occurred. Lazarus and Joannes Baptista Colloredo began their intrauterine life as two equally sized omphalopagus conjoined twins, but Joannes Baptista's body lost at least part of its contact with the umbilical vesicle. The parts of his body that were not in contact with this vesicle, and not supplied with blood from the body of Lazarus, began to atrophy. The inner organs did not develop normally either, and it is unlikely that the parasitic twin had a functional heart and lungs or any functional gut or urinary system. There must have been a gradual development of a collateral circulation, enabling Joannes Baptista to survive on the oxygen-rich blood and the nutrients digested by his brother. The contemporary accounts agree that Joannes Baptista was capable of movement and reflex actions, and that his lungs and larynx were sufficiently well developed for him to cry out. The fact that his head increased in size can only have been due to the development of hydrocephalus caused by insufficient drainage of cerebrospinal fluid.

Lazarus and Joannes Baptista Colloredo represent one of the very few convincing cases of viable omphalopagus parasiticus twins. The German teratologist Hans Hübner described two cases of stillborn twins, both from the nineteenth century, and the old monster medicine records describe several more or less fabulous instances. The famous Ambroise Paré described, in his *Des monstres et prodiges*, a man with a parasitic head extending from the epigastric region. This man lived to an adult age and took nourishment using both heads; this latter, rather unlikely, circumstance led to the case being (probably erroneously) considered doubtful. While visiting Genua (!) in 1699, a certain Dr. Walther saw a fourteen-year-old boy who was carrying from the abdomen a parasitic twin with a head, neck, shoulders, and chest. The celebrated anatomist Jacques-Bénigne Winslow made a similar observation at about the same time. This may well be a reference to the celebrated James Poro, born in Genua in 1686, who later exhibited himself in London. He was described by Mr. James Paris du Plessis in his manuscript *History of Prodigies*, and none less than Sir Hans Sloane, secretary to the Royal Society of London, commissioned his portrait to be painted. James Poro had a second head growing from just below the chest. The parasitic head was well shaped, du Plessis wrote, although an engraving of Poro does not support this; it had some kind of independent life, although it could not speak or open its eyes. James Paris du Plessis had also seen a twenty-year-old German, born near Ratisbon in 1678, who had a parasitic twin growing from his waist on the right side. This twin had a chest, arms, and a well-developed head and face, with a downy beard and two long locks of hair on the head. He took nourishment with a good appetite and *could speak as distinctly as his brother*. All these individuals would also be classified as omphalopagus parasiticus conjoined twins, with variable degrees of resorption of the lower body.

There is no hint in the contemporary sources of any discussion to separate Lazarus Colloredo from his brother by means of a surgical operation. The extent of the junction between their bodies is not immediately apparent from the illustrations, but from the descriptions of Pincet and Zacchias, it appears to have been of considerable thickness. It may well be that they had a common liver, and it is certain that the conjoined area contained several large arteries. Thus, an attempt to separate Lazarus Colloredo from his brother with seventeenth-century techniques would have ended fatally. With modern surgical techniques, such an operation would have been a relatively simple matter: Lazarus and his brother would have been separated at an early age, and this would probably have restored Lazarus to a normal life. Joannes Baptista would of course have lost his lingering half-life once he was removed from his brother and host.

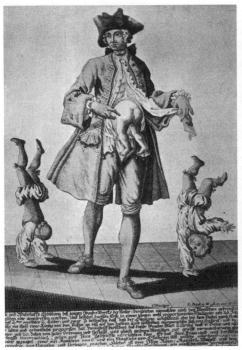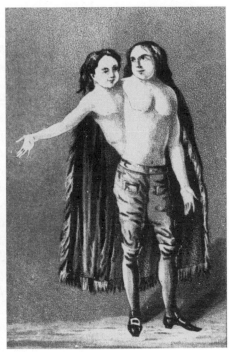

Two other instances of parasitic conjoined twinning: a German print of a dancer with a parasitic twin (left) (from the author's collection) and an early-eighteenth-century print of the very strange boy seen by James Paris du Plessis (right). Reproduced by permission of the Wellcome Institute Library, London.

If Lazarus Colloredo had been born today, would his parasitic twin have been cut away as if he had been a wart or mole, or would ethical arguments have been raised about deliberately killing a creature that was definitely a human being and definitely showed signs of independent life? The latter is unlikely, however, as this book later shows that "sacrifice" surgery of extensively conjoined twins, in which one twin is deliberately killed to serve as an organ donor to the one best fit for survival, has been practiced several times in the 1980s and 1990s.

Even disregarding Martin Parker's long ballad about them, Lazarus Colloredo and his brother made an impact on seventeenth-century poetry. They were mentioned in several contemporary poems and pamphlets; these allusions have proved obscure to present-day literary historians and even prompted speculation that the authors had had a very weird view of the relation between the biblical Lazarus and John the Baptist. The poet Alexander Brome wrote, in a poem about a close friend of his:

My self am from myself, but here and there I
Suppose my self grown an Ubiquitary;
We are a miracle, and tis with us
As with John Baptist and his Lazarus.

The cavalier poet John Cleveland also knew about Lazarus Colloredo and his brother, although he made the same mistake as Alexander Brome and mixed them up. His satirical poem *Smectymnuus* was inspired by a clerical club of that name, consisting of five divines who had written a tract about the merits of bishops and presbyters, which was published in 1641. John Cleveland, who was always ready to attack the roundhead clergy with cutting satire, took affront at the contents of this pamphlet and the outrageous pen name of the five authors, which had been formed by adding their initials together. In the poem *Smectymnuus, or the Club Divine*, he blasted all five faces of this "Monstrous Brotherhood of Five" with the words:

So the vaine satyrists stand all a row
As hallow teeth upon a Lute-string show.
Th' Italian Monster pregnant with his Brother,
Natures Dyræresis, halfe one another,
He, with his little Sides-man Lazarus,
Must both give way unto Smectymnuus.

Next Strubridge Faire is Smec's; for loe his side
Into a five fold Lazar's multipli'd,
Under each arme there's tuckt a double Gyssard,
Five faces lurke under one single vizzard.

The literary influence of Lazarus Colloredo and his brother appears to have survived them, as evidenced by "Unheavenly Twin," one of the short stories by Robert Bloch, the author of *Psycho* and one of the heirs of H. P. Lovecraft in the American tradition of macabre fiction. This story takes place in Malone's Boarding House, which is the winter home, in between tours, for a party of sideshow "freaks." The narrator is an "armless wonder," and there is also a giant, a dwarf, a human skeleton, a fat lady, and Ordo the Dog-faced Man, among others. The weirdest of all is Count Vomar, who never joined in the poker and bridge games of the others and always ate alone. The reason for this is that he is unique even among his peers. Out of his waist grows a malformed twin, and although Vomar hides it in a wide dressing gown, just as Colloredo had used a cloak for the same purpose, the others are disconcerted to see the twin's beady eyes glare at them from underneath his dress. During the shows, Vomar is disgusted by the people exclaiming with horror at the "thing" squirming on his stomach, and these experiences have embittered him and made him a loner. The twin has an independent life and intelligence; it lives off the bloodstream of its host, and while Vomar himself grows leaner, the twin increases in size. Vomar confides to the narrator that his situation is a desperate one. The twin has a superior intelligence and wishes to dominate, or even destroy, its host. The ending of the story is that the hideous, bloated body of the evil twin is discovered feeding on the body of the lifeless Vomar. Robert Bloch wrote several stories and film scripts using sideshow interiors, and it is likely that he found an illustration and a brief description of Lazarus Colloredo in one of his source books; his imagination did the rest.

The most obvious point of approach to Lazarus Colloredo and his brother is that of simple human interest, however. Like in many of the chapters of this book, one is drawn into admiration for a man born with the most fearful physical deformity, but who nevertheless not only survived in a time not noted for kindness or compassion for the disabled and deformed, but actually managed to create a tolerable existence for himself by turning his unique deformity into profit. He spoke with kings, queens, and nobles; saw the larger part of Europe; earned much money; and lived in relative comfort. One unverified account told that Lazarus Colloredo actually married and that he was the father of several children. It is telling that Lazarus Colloredo is often described as a gentleman, with the polite, affable manners of a courtier. The Scottish history of 1642 specifically stated that he was the master of two servants and that he had no showman or impresario to direct him. Many of the people we encounter in this book were not so lucky, but were the victims of human vampires in the shape of showmen who exploited and humiliated them in a most dismal and degrading way. In a way, Colloredo combined the roles of freak and showman: he applied for a license to show his monster, advertised it well, and spoke courteously to the audience. In turn, the audience treated him well and made him a wealthy man, but they pinched and slapped his semiconscious brother to make him give his shrill cry.

❧

My structuring of the tale of the two inseparable brothers serves as a blueprint for the remainder of this book, which can be seen as a companion volume to my earlier book, *A Cabinet of Medical Curiosities*. This book was first published in 1997 and appeared in paperback and in multiple foreign translations in 1999. It was a bit of a "mixed bag" of medical oddities, with some sections on folk medicine and popular beliefs. In contrast, the present book deals almost entirely with various aspects of the history of teratology, the science of monstrous births. Its scope and general layout somewhat resemble that of Dr. Charles J. S. Thompson's book *The Mystery and Lore of Monsters*, a collection of essays on "some giants, dwarfs, and prodigies" that was first published in 1930. C. J. S. Thompson was honorary curator of the historical collection of the Royal College of Surgeons of London, and a gentleman of great erudition. A both stylish and prolific writer, he published books on black magic, perfume, astrology, historical mysteries, and the development of surgical instruments. The bestseller by far is *The Mystery and Lore of Monsters*, which was first published in the United States in 1931 and reissued in 1958, 1968, and 1994, long after Thompson's death; apparently, it found interested buyers on each of these occasions.

One does not have to be a politically correct zealot to object to the title of Thompson's book: to refer to a pair of conjoined twins or an individual with pituitary gigantism as a "monster" was a thing of the past among most educated people in the 1930s. Today, such individuals are alternately referred to as "freaks" or "very special people," among other more or less inspired neologisms. The term *freak* is actually of some interest, as it originates in the expression "freak of nature," implying that the malformed child was a unique, unclassifiable phenomenon, the result of some strange "maternal impression," a witch's curse, or divine displeasure. From the early seventeenth century onward, medical science struggled to understand and classify these freaks of nature, and to incorporate all kinds of human congenital malformations in a system of teratology. By the late nineteenth century, it had succeeded: impressive standard works, such as those by the Frenchman Geoffroy Saint-Hilaire, the Germans Förster, Ahlfeld, and Schwalbe, and the American George Jackson Fisher, left no variety of human malformation undescribed. The late nineteenth and early twentieth centuries also saw great advances in the study of inherited diseases. The early popular accounts, like those by Gould and Pyle and Thompson already mentioned, took these advances in teratology and clinical genetics into account, and in spite of their age, they are often quite sophisticated, medically speaking, compared with more recent works in the same genre. The vast majority of these modern books have been written by social scientists, and while they are strong on sociological speculation and cautiously "politically correct" banter adhering to whatever school of historiography is currently in favor, they are weak on historical scholarship and even weaker with regard to medical insights. This impedes any attempt of an interdisciplinary approach.

The modern sociological treatises are also responsible for the re-emergence of the notion of a multitude of freaks of nature with no rational explanation even within the realm of modern medicine, and certainly do nothing to diminish the public ignorance and bigotry about these matters. Indeed, correct medical information on freaks and human deformities is difficult to come by, except in the form of highly advanced textbooks aimed at professionals within this area, and the gap has been filled by other, more sinister forces. Religious movements claiming that a deformed child is the punishment of God, or the result of sins in a previous life, have no lack of adherents in the United States as well as in Europe. The notion of inexplicable freaks of nature that are outside the boundary of medicine has even led to a resurfacing of the old doctrine of "maternal impressions"—that the mother's experiences during pregnancy determines the shape of her child. This age-old doctrine, which I described at length in *A Cabinet of Medical Curiosities*, still has supporters on the Internet, and also with certain Christian fundamentalists. Indeed, the cyberspace domain is a mine of misinformation and bigoted nonsense on these matters. Various oddballs and political extremists do their best to supply explanations—from their own warped minds—of the freaks of nature. A recent search on the Internet about Julia Pastrana, a Mexican woman unfortunate enough to be born with a rare genetic syndrome of excessive hairiness, illustrates this in a vivid manner. One "hit" was a racist magazine claiming that she was a baboon-human hybrid; another was a Bigfoot homepage that speculated that she might well be a distant relation of this elusive creature; the third claimed, in no uncertain terms, that she was Darwin's missing link.

The main theme of this book is the human interest, however. Rather than dismiss people like Nicolas Ferry, the King of Poland's court dwarf, and the dicephalous Tocci brothers, as freaks, I have regarded them as human beings, born with sometimes appalling congenital deformities, and tried to chronicle their lives and vicissitudes as closely as possible. A remarkable feature of many modern books on freaks is their tendency to concentrate on only one (American) cultural context. Being fortunate enough to possess a decent knowledge of several European languages, I have introduced some other aspects into the story, making the full use of various French, German, Dutch, and Scandinavian sources. It was sometimes amazing to see how much valuable original material, particularly from non-English sources, had been overlooked by the late twentieth-century writers, and what shallow and derivative research had been presented even in books issued from respectable university presses. Another aim was not to limit the discussion only to the medical point of view, but to bring in aspects of ethnology, literature, and cultural history as well. During the course of writing this book, I was sometimes amazed to see how the modern world related to the medical wonders of old. When writing about the hairy people, I was annoyed to notice an American television "documentary" uncouthly and erroneously suggesting that they had actually influenced the werewolf myth; and the news that an artificially inseminated woman gave birth to octuplets is made into nothing by the prodigious birth of Countess Margaret of Henneberg, who gave birth to 365 infants on Good Friday 1276. As I was writing about the stone-child of Sens, there was a great uproar in the London *Sun* newspaper, among others, about such a unique medical freak accident just having taken place; the commentary of the sixteenth-century writers seems rather more adequate than the flippant harangues of the silly hack journalist of the present time. The debate, in the mid-1990s, about whether radical surgery should be performed on extensively conjoined twins should be rekindled by the spectacle of the Tocci brothers, who lived joined together for 63 years. As I was writing about Daniel Lambert, the first drug for the treatment of obesity became available.

I am very pleased to see this paperback edition of my *Two-headed Boy*, which first appeared in print early in the year 2000. Care has been taken to correct some minor errors and to add references to some valuable recent scholarship. Two new illustrations have also been added. One of them may be unique: a cabinet card of the Tocci brothers, signed on the reverse by both twins, which I purchased on eBay in 2003.

JAN BONDESON

Cardiff

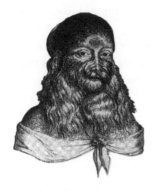

The Hairy Maid
at the Harpsichord

HER NAME WAS BARBARA URSLERIN AND SHE
really did play the harpsichord. John Evelyn saw her being exhibited in London in 1657. He was amazed by her strange appearance and described her thoroughly in his diary:

> The Hairy Maid, or Woman whom twenty years before I had
> also seene as a child: her very Eyebrowes were combed upwards & all her forehead as thick & even as growes on any
> woman's head, neatly dress'd: There comes also two locks very
> long out of Each Eare: she had also a most prolix beard & *moustachios*, with long locks of haire growing on the very middle of
> her nose, exactly like an Iceland Dog: the rest of her body not
> so hairy, yet exceedingly long in comparison, armes, neck,
> breast and back; the colour of light browne, & fine as well
> dressed flax.

Barbara Urslerin was born near the village of Kempten, not far from Augsburg in Germany, in February 1629 (some sources say 1633). As she told John Evelyn (and probably many other visitors), none of her family, neither parents nor relations, had been hairy. She was now married, she said, and had one normal child, of which she was very proud. John Evelyn approvingly stated that the Hairy Maid was "for the rest very well shaped, plaied well on the Harpsichord &c." John Evelyn is likely to have seen Barbara in London twenty years earlier, as early as 1637, when she was just eight years old, as all records agree that she was exhibited for money since a very early age. In 1639, she was seen in Copenhagen, and later in Belgium, by the celebrated anatomist Thomas Bartholin. Her parents were taking her all around Europe, he wrote, to show her for money. Bartholin examined the lively little girl and found that her entire body was covered with soft, blond hair. She had a luxuriant beard, and even from the ears themselves grew long, beautiful curls of hair, all handsomely dressed.

In 1646, the Frenchman Elie Brackenhoffer visited a fair in Paris. In his diary, he described its various attractions: a lioness, a five-footed cow, a monstrous dolphin, an Italian water-spouter, a man without hands, a rope dancer, and a dromedary. He had come across similar animal and human curiosities quite a few times before and gave them scant attention; he had never seen anything like the Hairy Maid, however, and described her in detail. She was eighteen years old, she said, and of German ancestry. Her hair was luxuriant and soft as silk, with the long curls beautifully dressed. M. Brackenhoffer, who was apparently either a lecher or a determined lover of curiosities, then proceeded to undress her, after the payment of an additional fee. Her back was covered with thick, soft hair like a coat of fur. Her breasts, he noted approvingly, were round and white and less hairy than the rest of the skin. M. Brackenhoffer ended his account by stating that he had ascertained that she was a true woman and not a hermaphrodite.

Barbara Urslerin lived during the heyday of the old monster medicine, when scholars and medical men were always on the hunt for marvels and curiosities; she had the honor of being mentioned in almost every chronicle of medical rarities of the time. The learned Hieronymus Welsch saw her in Rome in 1647, and later in Mailand in 1648, and described her in his *Observationes Medicarum Episagma*. In November 1653, she passed through her home town, Augsburg. An artist drew a beautiful portrait of her, which was later purchased by a physician in Basel; in the late nineteenth century, it was still kept in a collection in that city. Barbara Urslerin visited Frankfurt in 1655, and later the same year, she was seen in Copenhagen by the physician

Georg Seger. Her entire body, including the face, was covered with soft, blond, curly hair. Her luxuriant beard reached down to her waist. She told Seger that she had married a year ago, but that she did not have any children. On the exhibition handbill, which Seger used as a figure to his paper, she was depicted seated at the harpsichord; this was an engraving from a portrait by Isaac Brunn, which has remained the best-known illustration of her. The text told that her father and mother were Balthasar and Anna Ursler from Augsburg, and that she was "hairy all over with beautiful yellow curls growing from the face, and large curls growing from each ear."

In 1655, Barbara Urslerin came to London for the first time. According to an old note quoted by James Caulfield in his *Portraits, Memoirs and Characters of Remarkable Persons*, she was twenty-two years old at the time. A man named Vanbeck (or van Beck) had married "this frightful creature" only to

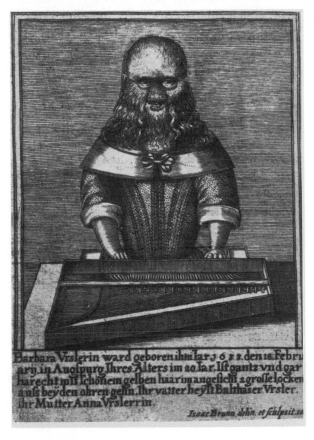

A German drawing of Barbara Urslerin at the harpsichord, by Isaac Brunn. From print in the author's collection.

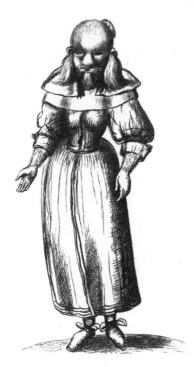

Another German drawing of Barbara Urslerin, made in 1653. From an article by Dr. Ecker in the *Archiv für Anthropologie* of 1879.

make money by putting her on show. They had toured many parts of Europe. In 1656, a fine portrait of her was engraved by Gaywood.

In 1660, Barbara toured France. When they came to Beauvais, her husband, the German Johann Michael van Beck, applied to the local bailiff for permission to exhibit a strange prodigy of nature, a woman with a hairy, bearded face and moustachio. He did not mention that this monstrous woman was actually his wife, but instead pointed out that she had already received much attention from the curious in Paris and other French cities. An engraving of Gaywood's portrait was now used as the exhibition handbill, and a copy was enclosed with van Beck's letter. The local police were pleased to allow van Beck to show his hairy wife for money and to advertise her by striking a tambourine in the marketplace if he promised that the exhibition was a decent one and that it was closed down in good time in the afternoon.

The last thing we know about Barbara Urslerin is that in 1668, she was seen in London by the Dane Holger Jacobsen, who left a description of her in Thomas Bartholin's *Acta Medica et Philosophica Hafnensis*. Jacobsen boldly suggested that the Hairy Maid must be the loathsome result of a copulation between a woman and a humanoid ape, a hypothesis that was outdated already in his time. Jacobsen had seen a large ape called Mammonett that was kept as a pet in the king of Denmark's gardens, and could well remember that this creature often "tried to take lascivious liberties with women" who visited the royal gardens. He ended his brief description of this "Monstrous hairy girl" by emphasizing that the length and softness of her hair was excessive all over the body and that he had thoroughly examined her genitals to see if they had any similarity with those of a monkey.

Anatole F. Le Double and François Houssay, two French anthropologists and zoologists who wrote the book *Les velus*, a valuable early treatise on excessive hairiness, are not the only people who asked themselves what fi-

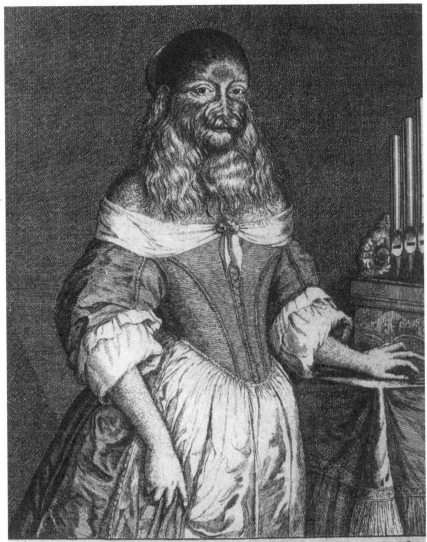

Vera Effigies Barbara, vxor Iohannis Michaelis Van Beck, nata Augustæ
Vindelicorm in Germania Superiori (vulgo Auspourge) ex parentibus
Balthazaro et Annæ Vrsler. Anno Christi. 1629. februæ 18:

R. Gaywood fecit Londini .1656

A portrait of Barbara Urslerin, engraved by Gaywood when she was in London in
1656. This is probably the best likeness of her. From the author's collection.

6   nally happened to Barbara Urslerin. It is possible to follow her travels all around Europe from 1637 to 1668 in some detail, but after the latter year, mention of her completely disappears. It may be that she retired from the monster shows, but this does not seem very likely: her husband had been relentless in exploiting her and showed no sign of letting his most valuable possession go to waste. If her husband had died, there were many other showmen ready to take over the management of this hairy celebrity. The most likely explanation is that Barbara herself died in or about 1668. The many either coy or lewd allusions to visitors to the exhibition undressing and fondling the Hairy Maid prompted Le Double and Houssay to query whether prostitution had played any part in the exploitation of her. This is possible, but by no means necessary. At this time, it was the custom that any person paying to see a human or animal curiosity also had the right to thoroughly examine the creature on show, to make sure there was no imposition. A six-legged calf had its extra legs pulled, a giant's trousers were pulled up so that it could be ascertained that he did not wear stilts, and Lazarus Colloredo's parasitic twin was pinched until he uttered a cry. None of Barbara Urslerin's visitors had seen anything like her before, and those who wanted to make sure she really was a true woman, from motives of lechery, curiosity, or scientific inquiry, were free to do so, after paying an additional fee.

The Isaac Brunn engraving of Barbara Urslerin has appeared in many European works on monstrosities and "biographia curiosa." It was later reproduced in a queer French magazine, appropriately named *Bizarre*. Today it is posted on an Internet site aimed to titillate those belonging to weird "sexual minorities." The French author Jean Boullet instead reproduced the remarkable Gaywood engraving, which is a far better likeness of her, as well as artistically superior, with the telling caption "Belle et Bête"; in one body, the personified characteristics of both.

The Wild Man from the Canaries

It is almost a relief to turn the attention from the Hairy Maid at the Harpsichord to another, slightly more edifying story of an individual affected with inherited excessive hairiness. Petrus Gonzales, the hero of this strange tale, was born in the Canary Islands in the year 1556. At this time, there was widespread belief in a particular race of hairy savages or "wild men." The belief that monstrous races of cynocephali, sciapods, and troglodytes inhabited parts of Asia and Africa was a time-honored part of medieval mythology that had been originated by the writings of Pliny. The wild men, fierce, hairy, carrying a club, and always ready to carry off women into the deep woods, represented another medieval stereotype, implying a violent nature, lack of civilization, and want for a moral sense. According to legend, wild men existed not only in the African and Asian backwoods, but small remnants of these savages were still hiding in the deep forests of Germany, France, and Scandinavia. Some of the early observations of Asian or African wild men were definitely misinterpretations of encounters between early explorers and anthropoid apes. In the fifteenth and sixteenth centuries, the wild man was much used in heraldry: the symbol of the urge to civilize and dominate what appeared rude and wild was a wild man, club in hand, as upholder of the arms of some noble family.

The discovery of an infant in the Canary Islands whose face and body were just as hairy as that of a wild man or a great ape was quite a sensation. Little Petrus Gonzales, of whose parents we know nothing, was lucky to escape being killed as a monster or demon by the superstitious country people; instead, he was taken to Paris by the express order of King Henri II of France, who wanted to study this prodigy closer. Petrus Gonzales's entire body, particularly his head and face, was covered with long, soft, wavy hair, and already at an early age, his face resembled that of a terrier dog. In 1557, the savant Julius Caesar Scaliger wrote that Paris had just obtained a novel curiosity: a young boy from Spain, taken from the Indian Isles, who was entirely covered with hair. The Frenchmen called this boy Barbet, the same name used to signify a race of shaggy Belgian dogs, which the people of Flanders called *Watterhund*. Another observer, a certain Dr. Boschius, told Count Ulysses Aldrovandi that King Henri had recently received a young boy, hairy all over like a dog. Probably astounded that this extraordinary "wild boy" seemed intelligent and alert, Henri II ordered that he should be taught Latin and given a good education, since the king wanted to find out whether such a wild boy was at all educable. In addition, little Petrus should be kept at the royal court as a curiosity, and his progress carefully monitored. Henri II's successors honored this agreement scrupulously, and Petrus Gonzales spent his entire youth at the French court. Many visiting princes and noblemen were introduced to this prodigy, whose hairy face, resembling that of a shaggy dog, looked even more extraordinary when he was dressed in his richly embroidered court costume. Even more astonishingly to the visitor who had read about the savagery of the race of wild men, the king's hairy "savage" was intelligent and well informed and spoke excellent

8   Latin. In 1573, the seventeen-year-old Petrus Gonzales was given permission to marry a young French lady. Whether this match was made according to his own choice or arranged as some court festivity is not known, but Gonzales and his wife remained united by wedlock for several decades and had at least four children. Allegedly to prevent the "wild" Petrus Gonzales from feeling homesick, he was given a cave to dwell in with his entire family, like some bizarre ornamental hermit, in one of the royal parks. Most of the time, he resided at the court in Fountainebleau, however, where the king showed him to visiting dignitaries like some trained dog or monkey.

By 1581, Petrus Gonzales was the father of two children. Although his wife was perfectly normal, both children were as hairy as their father. This marvelous hairy family was Europe's greatest curiosity of their time. Many princes and noblemen wanted to see them, and later in 1581, the entire family was sent for an extended tour all over Europe. Firstly, they visited Duchess Margaret of Parma's court in Flanders. In early 1582, they went to Munich, where their life-sized portraits were painted at the order of Duke Albrecht IV of Bavaria, who was known as a lover of curiosities. These portraits were later given to Archduke Ferdinand of Tyrol, who installed them in his famous Kunst-kammer at Schloss Ambras outside Innsbruck. The children—a daughter of five to six years and a son of three to four years—are dressed in rich, costly garments, which increase the startling contrast to their hairy faces. They look like little animal dolls dressed up in human clothes by their childish owner. The wife is pretty and demure, and her clothes are Dutch looking in style. Petrus Gonzales himself is dressed in a rich ankle-length garment like a cassock. His face is as hairy as ever, and at the age of twenty-six he has a venerable-looking beard, but the expressive look in his brown eyes seems to say, "I am not what you think I am."

Two other paintings of the Gonzales family were also made during their stay in Bavaria, by Albrecht IV's court artist Joris Hoefnagel. One of these depicts Petrus Gonzales and his wife; the other, the two children. Hoefnagel included these two portraits in a volume of his *The Four Elements*, entitled *Animalia Rationalia et Insecta*; they are the only humans to be portrayed. Petrus Gonzales was found at Tenerife in the Canaries, Hoefnagel wrote, and later received a superior education at the French court. He was a scholar and a man of letters, and a sonorous speaker of Latin. Not long after their visit to Munich, the Gonzales family went to Vienna, at the order of Emperor Rudolf II. Here, a group portrait was painted, in oil on parchment, by court painter Dirck van Ravensteyn; it was later kept in one of the emperor's large folders of zoological drawings. In this portrait, Petrus Gonzales is standing up and his wife is seated, and their two children are standing in front of them. The little boy is leaning on his mother's lap. The girl is holding a tame owl, or rather owlet, that is facing the artist just like the four people.

In 1583, Petrus Gonzales and his family came to Basel, where they were seen by the celebrated anatomist Felix Plater. In a valuable note, published posthumously in his *Observationum*, Plater affirmed that the adult Petrus Gonzales seen by him was certainly the same person as the young wild boy who was taken from the Canaries to the court of Henri II many years earlier. The king and his successors valued Gonzales greatly and took good care of him. He was now on his way to Italy, where several princes desired to make his acquaintance. Petrus Gonzales's abundant facial hair was excessively soft, and the eyebrows were so long and bushy that he had to trim them to be able to see. According to Felix Plater, he had two children, a boy aged nine and a girl aged seven. Both had hairy faces, the boy more than the girl; the skin of both children was also covered with long, soft hair along the spine of the back.

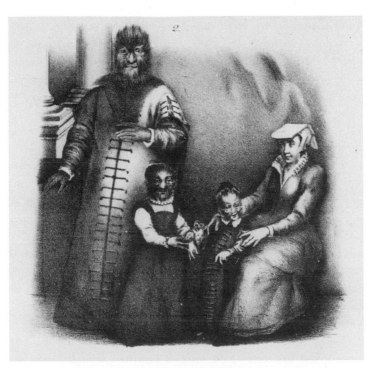

An engraving of a group portrait of the Gonzales family. From an article by Dr. Bartels in the *Zeitschrift für Ethnologie* of 1879.

The next account of the Gonzales family is that of Count Ulysses Ald-rovandi. He was one of the leading natural scientists of the sixteenth century, and his vast collections of anatomical, zoological, and botanical specimens were justly famous. In the mid-1590s. Count Aldrovandi met and examined, by permission of the marchioness of Sorania, the eight-year-old daughter of Petrus Gonzales. This little girl, whose face was covered with thick, soft hair just like her father's, was introduced to Count Aldrovandi by the marchioness herself, when on a trip to Bologna. Count Aldrovandi then ordered an artist to draw a picture of the entire Gonzales family: the forty-year-old father, the twenty-year-old son, and the two daughters, twelve and eight years old. It is very likely that this twenty-year-old son was the same little boy depicted on the Ambras and Hoefnagel pictures. What had happened to his elder sister is left unsaid, nor is it known whether the wife of Petrus Gonzales was still alive, but their absence from Aldrovandi's portraits would indicate that they were both dead. The two young girls in Aldrovandi's drawings indicate that during his stay in Italy, Gonzales had fathered two more children, both of them girls and both sharing his excessive hairiness.

Another remarkable memorial of the Gonzales family is an engraving of the Medusa-like head of a hairy young girl, by the artist and engraver Giacomo Franco. The caption states that this is the portrait of Tognina, the young daughter of the hairy man from the Canary Islands. Her brother, who was just as hairy as herself, was given as a present to Signor Farnesi, a wealthy nobleman. Tognina herself resided at the ducal court of Parma. Another remarkable portrait of a hairy girl residing at the court of the duchess of Parma was painted at about the same time, by Paulo Cagliari; it may well be another painting of Tognina Gonzales. This portrait is in the collection of the earl of Haddo, at Haddo House. A third drawing of one of Petrus Gonzales's daughters, probably Tognina, is now at the Pierpont Morgan Library in New York; it was the work of the celebrated portrait painter Lavinia Fontana. It appears in the Hood Museum of Art's catalogue *The Age of the Marvelous* and is dated around 1583. This date implies that Tognina was the oldest daughter of Petrus Gonzales. The girl looks about eight years old, indicating that Tognina was born around 1575. The New York drawing is probably one of Lavinia Fontana's sketches for this fine portrait. A note in Ulysses Aldrovandi's *Historia Monstrorum* revealed that Tognina later married during her stay at Farnesi's court in Parma, and that she lived there for many years and had several children of her own, at least some of whom were as hairy as herself.

A few years later, another portrait of a hairy man, most likely a member

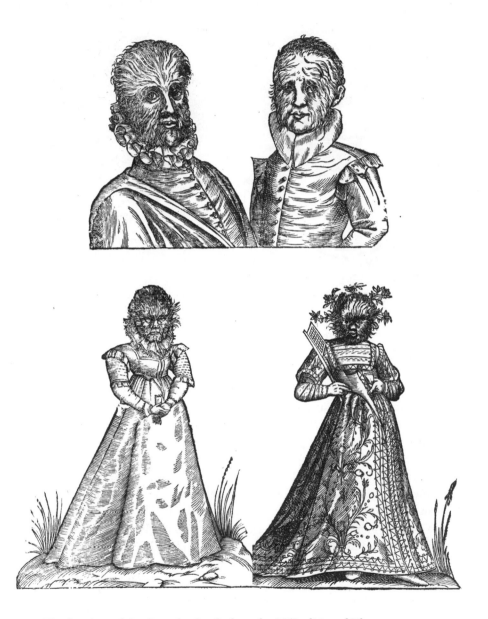

The drawings of the Gonzales family from the 1642 edition of Ulysses Aldrovandi's *Monstrorum Historia*.

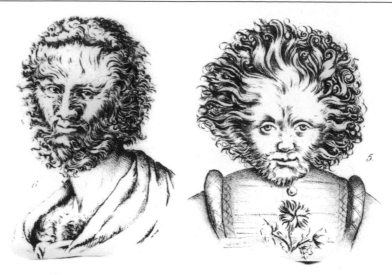

The later Italian engravings of Horatio and Tognina Gonzales. From an article by Dr. Bartels in the *Zeitschrift für Ethnologie* of 1879.

of the Gonzales family, was painted by Agostino Carraci. It depicted Arrigo the Hairy, Pietro the Fool, Amon the Dwarf, and a group of "other animals": the animals were two dogs, two apes, and a parrot, all belonging to Cardinal Odoarda Farnese just like the humans. An *Avis de Rome* of July 1, 1595, tells us that the duke of Parma had given Cardinal Farnese a costly present: a savage man, 18 years old, whose face and brow were covered with long blond hair. It is likely that this Arrigo was the same individual as the twenty-year-old son of Petrus Gonzales depicted by Aldrovandi. Arrigo Gonzales stayed at Cardinal Farnese's establishment for many years and was included in an inventory of his house staff made in 1626. The final memorial of the Gonzales family is an engraving given to a certain Mercurio Ferrari after the death of his particular friend, the hairy man Horatio Gonzales, in 1635. It is accompanied by a Latin poem, which can be translated as:

> *Here you see Gonzales, once famous in the court of Rome,*
> *Whose human face was covered with hair like an animal's.*
> *He lived for you, Ferrari, joined to you in love.*
> *And in this portrait he lives on, still breathing although he is dead.*

This engraving is dated 1635, and it is not known whether this Horatio was another son of Petrus Gonzales or maybe a son of Arrigo.

The Hairy Family of Burma

It was a long time before the world saw another hairy phenomenon like Barbara Urslerin or Petrus Gonzales and his family; indeed, from the 1630s to the 1820s, no novel instance of excessive hairiness was described either by scientists or by lovers of curiosities. Had these two famous sixteenth- and seventeenth-century cases not been detailed by the leading medical scientists of the world, and painted from life by several celebrated artists, they would have been considered yet another figment of imagination of the old monster medicine. Even so, many were confused by these extraordinary descriptions of hairy "wild people." In Everhard Happel's *Relationes Curiosae*, published in 1729, the Forest People from the Canaries are depicted in a remarkable illustration. Standing in a sylvan glade, they are listening, in rapt attention, to a *concerto* played by the Hairy Maid at the Harpsichord. Two other hairy savages come crawling out of the undergrowth, enchanted by her music. In the *Eccentric Magazine*, published in London 1813, there is an engraved portrait of Barbara Urslerin taken from an old print. According to the caption to this illustration, great doubts were entertained as to whether she was really human. The editor of *Eccentric Magazine* managed to resolve this controversy, however. He had seen an old print of Barbara Urslerin, which was formerly in the collection of Mr. Frederich, a bookseller in Bath. It had the following brief but telling note written on it: "This woman I saw in Ratcliffe Highway, in the year 1668, and was satisfied she was a woman. John Bulfinch."

In 1826, a mission of the governor-general of India, led by John Crawfurd, visited the court of the king of Ava, a province in Burma. In a published account of this mission, Crawfurd described meeting a thirty-year-old hairy man named Shwe-Maong. At the age of five, he had been given to the king by the local chief of his district and since then, had lived within the palace as a curiosity and court entertainer. He was very clever in acting the buffoon, dancing, and making the most terrible grimaces. Shwe-Maong stated that his parents were perfectly normal and that none of his tribesmen were hairy. When aged twenty-two years, having attained puberty only two years previously, the king chose a wife for him from the beautiful women in his retinue. There were four children, all girls, of this union. Two of them died at an early age, and a third was the very image of her mother; only one was abnormal, a girl named Maphoon, who was covered with hair just like her father and resembled an elderly bearded man. Crawfurd stated that the father never had more than two incisors and two canines in the upper jaw, and four incisors and one canine in the lower jaw. Importantly, because it

14   seems to eliminate the possibility that the other teeth simply failed to erupt, he says that where teeth were missing, the alveolar process was missing also.

In 1855, a second mission visited Ava, this time reported by Captain Henry Yule, who described the thirty-one-year-old Maphoon, who was now married to a normal Burmese and mother of two boys. Her father had been murdered by robbers, and she had been brought up in the king's household. The story told of her marriage was that the king had offered a reward to any man who was willing to marry her. Finally, an individual who was bold enough or avaricious enough ventured forth. Yule's description of Maphoon deserves to be quoted more or less verbatim:

> The whole of Maphoon's face was more or less covered with hair. On a part of the cheek, and between the nose and mouth, this was confined to short down, but over all the rest of the face was a thick silky hair of a brown colour, paling about the nose and chin, four or five inches long. At the alae of the nose, under the eye, and on the cheekbone, this was very fully developed, but it was in and on the ear that it was most extraordinary. . . . The hair over her forehead was brushed so as to blend with the hair of the head, the latter being dressed (as usual with her countrywomen), *à la Chinoise*. It was not so thick as to conceal altogether the forehead. The nose, densely covered with hair as no animal's is that I know of, and with long fine locks curving out and pendent like the wisps of a fine Skye terrier's coat, had a most strange appearance. The beard was pale in colour, and about four inches in length, seemingly very soft and silky.

Maphoon's manners were modest, her voice soft and feminine, and her expression not unpleasing. Captain Yule thought her more like a pleasant-looking woman at a masquerade than a brutal, horrible monstrosity. Her dentition consisted of a few incisors only; the canine teeth and grinders were absent, and the back parts of the gum merely a hard ridge. Maphoon's oldest son, about four to five years old, was not abnormal, although it is notable that by the age of fourteen years, he seemed to have become more hairy than his younger brother. This brother, aged fourteen months, had tufts of long silky hair growing from his ears, a description that corresponds closely to the childhood state of the grandfather who later became so hairy. It is interesting that Yule commented that had the great Barnum heard of Maphoon, he would surely have wished to bring her to Europe.

In 1875, when the hairy family of Burma was discussed before the Anthropological Society of Paris, a photographic record of them appeared in the French journal *La Nature*. The French teratologist Boullet identified the hairy Burmese as Maphoon, her son Moung-Phoset, and her daughter Mah-Mé. Moung-Phoset would have been about twenty-one to twenty-five years old at this time, depending on which of Maphoon's two sons he was. No other account of this time refers to more than one son; it seems likely that one of them died between 1867 and 1875. According to Yule and others, Maphoon did not have a living daughter. Instead, there is good evidence that Moung-Phoset had a daughter named Mah-Mé, who would have been seven years old at the time of the photograph. It thus seems highly probable that the members of the family depicted in this photograph are Maphoon, her son Moung-Phoset, and her granddaughter Mah-Mé. Several other photographs of Maphoon, alone or in a family group, were taken by L. Allen Goss in 1872. One of them, showing Maphoon, two other hairy people, and a normal Burmese, resembles the 1875 picture. Goss referred to the lively little girl in this picture, thus adding further evidence that Mah-Mé was really the daughter of Moung-Phoset. Two other excellent photographs in the Goss collection depict Maphoon and Moung-Phoset in detail.

In 1885, there was a revolution in Burma, leading to the so-called Third Burmese War; the king's palace was set on fire, and its inhabitants were driven away or killed. The hairy family managed to escape into a forest, Moung-Phoset carrying his fragile mother Maphoon on his back, followed by his wife and children. An Italian officer, Captain Paperno, who had been a military advisor to the Burmese court, was sent out to rescue them. When the Italian found them, he was astounded by their extraordinary appearance. He suggested that the hairy Burmese should make a tour of Europe, to be exhibited for money. Together with a fellow countryman, Mr. Farini, the captain, who was himself without employment after the gutting of the Burmese court, decided to act as their impresario. Before the hairy Burmese left for Europe, Moung-Phoset's daughter Mah-Mé died at the age of eighteen. During the summer of 1886, the family appeared at the Egyptian Hall, Piccadilly, where they were seen by Mr. J. J. Weir. He described Maphoon as a blind old woman, but lively and full of fun, and an inveterate chewer of betel in spite of her few teeth. He suspected that her hairy growth had thinned somewhat due to age, as Moung-Phoset had much more hair on the face and ears. Moung-Phoset certainly presented a grotesque appearance, his entire features being hidden by the hair, which he combed over his face. His entire body was clothed with soft hair some inches in length, which he

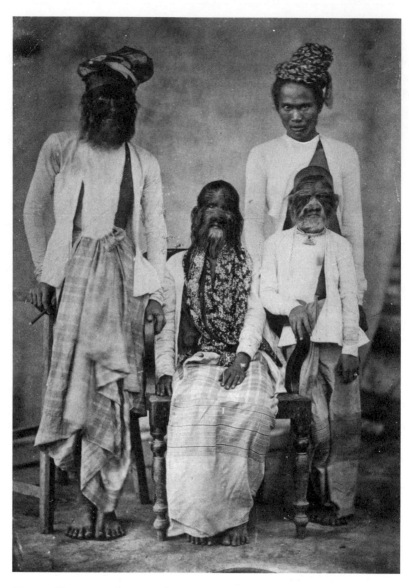

Moung-Phoset, Maphoon, Mah-Mé, and a nonhairy relative in 1872. From the collection of Professor A. E. W. Miles, reproduced by permission.

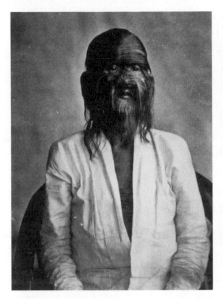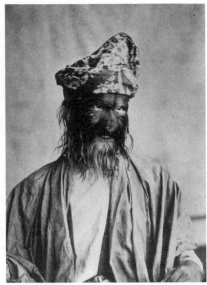

Close-ups of Maphoon (left) and Moung-Phoset (right) from the Goss photographs. From the collection of Professor A. E. W. Miles, reproduced by permission.

cut from time to time; furthermore, he was tattooed from below the waist to above the knees. In spite of his bizarre exterior, Weir described Moung-Phoset as a well-educated and decent man. Importantly, he also stated that the hair of both Maphoon and Moung-Phoset was soft, wavy, and of a brownish color, quite unlike the hair of an ordinary Burmese. Captain Paperno, the family's impresario, informed Weir that although the dentition of all the hairy people was deficient, their nonhairy relatives all had perfect teeth. Mr. Weir examined a cast of Moung-Phoset's mouth, finding in the upper jaw two canines and two large incisors, and in the lower jaw two canines and four small incisors; the molar and premolar teeth were all absent.

From London, the Burmese went on to Paris, where they appeared at the Folies Bergère. The French anthropologist M. Guyot-Daubès saw them there in 1887 and obtained an interview with their impresario, who told a remarkable story about Shwe-Maong's marriage. A beautiful young Burmese lady of high birth, a lady in waiting to the queen, had committed a crime against religion and was sentenced to be tortured to death in the most horrible way, at the churchyard of her dead ancestors. Just when the dreadful ceremony was about to start, a courtier rode up to offer her a pardon if she

18 agreed to marry the court buffoon. After due consideration, she accepted the offer. The marriage ceremony was a ludicrous and degrading spectacle, as Shwe-Maong was joined by a veritable congress of dwarfs, albinos, idiots, and jesters. It is odd that Crawfurd's original account did not mention this remarkable occurrence; it might have been a figment of Captain Paperno's imagination in order to make his hairy charges' life stories even more interesting. Like his grandfather, Moung-Phoset married one of the maids of honor at the court, this time one who chose him of her own free will. Mah-Mé was their only daughter. In 1888 or 1889, the hairy Burmese went to the United States during their world tour, and their stage name was the "Sacred Hairy Family of Burma." The ultimate fate of Maphoon and Moung-Phoset is unknown; probably they went back to Burma and died in obscurity there.

Jo-Jo, the Dog-faced Boy

From 1856 until 1860, the famous Julia Pastrana was exhibited in the United States and Europe. She was a Mexican Indian woman with excessive hairiness over large parts of the body, as well as an overdevelopment of the gums that gave her an apelike visage. She had a luxuriant beard and whiskers. Her husband, the American Theodore Lent, who was also her impresario, exploited her mercilessly and milked her considerable fame for all it was worth. When their tour reached Moscow in early 1860, Julia gave birth to a son, who was as hairy as his mother. Both mother and child died, but the resourceful impresario had their bodies mummified and continued the tours all over Europe, together with his second wife, who was also a bearded lady. Julia Pastrana's career coincided with the advent of Darwinism. Actually, Charles Darwin himself described her in one of his books, but he made no attempt to link her strange appearance with the theories about the descent of humankind. Some of his more radical followers went much further than that and postulated that Julia Pastrana and other hairy people shared primitive characteristics with mankind's early ancestors. According to the so-called recapitulation theory of embryology, advanced creatures like humans repeated the adult stages of their ancestors during their embryonic development. The study of anatomy and teratology was, according to this theory, a useful tool to unravel the secrets of the evolution of mankind. Thus, a tailed or hairy child was considered to have reverted to a lower stage of development, and these characteristics were relics of the primate ancestors of human beings. The great majority of people in the 1860s and 1870s knew very little about these embryological theories; their definition of Darwinism was that they themselves were the descendants of an ape. This inferior level of understanding, shared by many people of low intellect even today, certainly did not impede them from visiting Julia Pastrana and other hairy phenomena on show, particularly if these human curiosities were ostentatiously advertised as "The Missing Link" and lurid parallels were made about their various apelike or beastlike characteristics.

In 1873, thirteen years after the death of Julia Pastrana, the European public had an opportunity to make the acquaintance of two other hairy "missing links": the Russian Adrian Jeftichejev and his son Fedor. The public attitude toward a hairy man or woman had not changed much since the sixteenth century; if anything it had become even more saturated with superstition and fanaticism. After all, Joris Hoefnagel and others treated Petrus Gonzales with some respect and acknowledged him as a learned man. In 1857, Julia Pastrana was advertised as a hybrid between baboon and human; in 1873, Adrian was presented by the showman as "The Wild Man from the Kostroma Forest," the loathsome product of a short-lived and illicit *amour* between a bear and a Russian peasant woman. The French anthropologist Mme Clémence Royer saw Adrian and Fedor Jeftichejev being exhibited in Bruxelles in 1873. This learned lady told Adrian's impresario, in no uncertain terms, that she did not believe for a moment that a woman could give birth to a child fathered by a bear; the shameless showman replied that nor did he, but that it was good advertisement! He then gave Mme Royer and her friends a private showing of the Russian phenomenon.

At the time he was exhibited, Adrian Jeftichejev was fifty-five years old. He was a native of the Kostroma province of Russia. His memory of his parents was somewhat hazy, but he believed that his father had been a soldier; he could not recollect that either parent had any peculiarity of the hair. Adrian also had two normal siblings, a brother and a sister, both of whom were alive when he left Russia. Adrian had married in his youth, he said, and had sired two children in this marriage: a normal boy who died young and a girl, also deceased, who was hairy just like her father. Young Fedor, who was on show with him, was actually Adrian's illegitimate son, the impresario said, although many of the female visitors to the exhibition must have experienced a *frisson* of horror that even a sex-starved Russian peasant woman had once consented to copulate with such a monster. Adrian was like a man half changed into an animal, a spectacle destined to strike horror into nineteenth-century people. His face was entirely covered with hair, like that of a Skye terrier. A French doctor likened him to a Griffon dog of Flanders; exactly the same simile had been made about little Petrus Gonzales more than three hundred years earlier. On Adrian's body were isolated patches of hairy growth, with hair between 1½ and 2 inches in length. The hair was said to be a dirty yellow, but this was probably influenced by Adrian's reluctance to wash. Just as with Petrus Gonzales, Barbara Urslerin, and the hairy Burmese, Adrian's hair was very soft and fine. The celebrated Dr. Bertillon, who had taken some hair samples from the Russian phenomenon, found that a hair from Adrian's chin was three times as thin as a very fine hair from a man's beard, and that a hair from Adrian's head was half as thick as an ordinary man's head hair. The hairy-faced man was of medium height, strongly built, and dressed in not very clean-looking Russian garments. His eyes were a curious yellow, and his skin an unhealthy gray.

The showman said that as a young man, Adrian had fled into the woods to escape the derision and rough usage of his fellow villagers. For a time, he had lived in a cave and eaten the nuts and berries of the Kostroma woods. He also developed a taste for drunkenness during this period of solitary life and consumed strong vodka in quantities considered excessive even by his fellow Russian peasants. A German journal stated that even when surrounded by all the delicacies of Berlin, Adrian lived chiefly on sauerkraut and schnapps. A doctor was impressed to see Adrian drink a pint of undi-

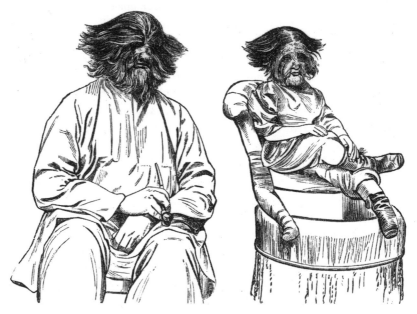

A drawing of Adrian and Fedor. From an article in *Lancet* in 1873.

luted vodka with relish, as he carved his beefsteak at the exhibition. A German authority told that Adrian was kindly and affectionate, in spite of his degraded intellect. He was incapable of learning any foreign language, and even his Russian dialect was difficult to understand. He showed little affection for his son Fedor, and Mme Royer and her friends saw that he much resented it when some visitors to the exhibition spoke to the lively young Fedor and tipped him handsomely, and then passed by the smelly, unprepossessing father with horror. After observing Adrian, and speaking to him through an interpreter, Mme Royer concluded that he was by no means idiotic, and certainly a human being; he was in fact a good representative of the moral and intellectual development among the inferior tribes of Russia. The showman said that ever since he had first put Adrian on show before the curious in St. Petersburg the year before, the hairy man had vowed to return to his native village as soon as his tour of the European capitals was over, and to spend all the money he had earned entirely on strong drink. According to another, slightly more prepossessing version, Adrian was a devout member of the Russo-Greek Church. Others in that faith had told him that he must surely have been cursed by the Devil, and poor Adrian spent all his money on the purchase of prayers from a devout community of monks near Kostroma, "hoping one day to be able to introduce his frightful countenance in the court of heaven," as the exhibition pamphlet flippantly expressed it.

If many visitors to the exhibition were disgusted or horrified by the debauched, unkempt spectacle of Adrian, all were charmed by his little son Fedor. Although just three years and four months old, he was more intelligent and much more sprightly and vigorous than his wretched father. The growth of down on his face was not yet so heavy as to conceal his features, but the medical men who saw him did not doubt that he would one day become just as hairy as his father. Fedor's hair was white and as thick as that of an Angora cat, and he had long whiskers and a tuft of long hair at the outer angle of either eye. He liked to travel and to meet new people, and was already getting spoiled and petulant. He spoke French, and in spite of his tender age, gave rational replies to questions from the audience. He did not share his father's bestial and vicious facial expression, wrote Mme Royer, but otherwise the two were as alike as a young orangutan and an adult orangutan. After surveying Adrian and Fedor, she believed them to be the product of some strange atavism, or reversion to characteristics of a long-lost ancient race of man. Fedor's higher intelligence and less thick hairy coat were explained by the fact that he was a crossbreed between a hairy savage and an ordinary Russian woman, she wrote, just like a crossbreed between a white man and an American Indian woman showed some of the superior characteristics of the white race.

During their tour of Europe, Adrian and Fedor were examined by some of the leading anthropologists and medical scientists of the time. In Berlin, they were seen by Professor Rudolf Virchow, who left a thorough description of them. In Paris, they were more popular than ever, and Adrian was billed as "L'Homme-Chien du Tivoli Vaux-Hall." He was examined there by Dr. E.-B. Perrin in 1873. For some time Adrian had been feeling weak and nauseated, and had been troubled by persistent diarrhea. The doctor found a considerable swelling in the gastrohepatic region, the origin of which he did not hazard to guess. But considering the yellow discoloration of Adrian's eyes and his habit of drinking several pints of vodka every day, it is reasonable to suggest that the wretched man was suffering from quite advanced alcoholic cirrhosis of the liver. If the story of his purchase of prayers was true, these prayers were not wasted, and Adrian may well have guessed his fate. According to Dr. Perrin, he still drank pints of vodka with every meal, breakfast included. While impervious to other European customs, he embraced that of using tobacco and was never without a length of coarse chewing tobacco. Perhaps as a result of Mme Royer's objections, Adrian was no longer exhibited as a hideous product of bestiality, but instead it was alleged, before the cultured French nation, that the two hairy men were members of a tribe of savage "missing links" living in the Kostroma region.

In March 1874, Adrian and Fedor came to London. Their exhibition pamphlet was entitled *The Story of Adrian and Fedor, the Hirsute or Hairy-Faced People, found in the woods of Kostroma in Russia. The First of their Kind ever discovered. The Darwin Theory established*. They were seen by Professor C. S. Tomes and Mr. Oakley Coles, two noted dental practitioners, who examined them closely and took casts of their teeth. The reason for this was that as Rudolf Virchow and others had already discovered, the dentition of both Adrian and Fedor was very defective. Adrian had only the stump of a tooth in the upper jaw and four rotten teeth in the lower jaw. Fedor had a perfectly edentulous upper jaw, with no alveolar processes, and only four incisors in the lower jaw.

After their triumphal tour of Europe from 1872 to 1874, Adrian and Fedor completely disappeared, and some authors have presumed that they either died or returned to obscurity in Russia. It is notable, however, that just a few years later, a Russian boy billed as Theodore Petroff, and later as "Jo-Jo, the Dog-faced Boy," or "The Human Skye Terrier," began his career in show business. He was active for many years and probably one of the most successful human curiosities ever. With a singularly unapposite comparison, the French teratologist Jean Boullet, who was writing in the 1960s, called him "la Brigitte Bardot des merveilles de la Nature"! Another French source, the book *Les velus* by Le Double and Houssay, stated that at the age of eight, Jo-Jo was engaged by an impresario named Forster and later exhibited all over the world. The story of Jo-Jo's origin, repeated many times in the exhibition pamphlets, was that he had been found at a tender age by huntsmen in the Kostroma forest of Russia. He was accompanied by some kind of strange monster, hairy just like himself, who served as his father. The huntsmen took these two hairy savages with them to the civilized world, where the "father" soon died. The boy was named Jo-Jo from some sounds he first made when he was found, and the huntsmen took care of him. He was sent to school, where he learned to read and speak both Russian and English. He then set out to tour the world. All these circumstances hint that Fedor and Jo-Jo were one and the same, but what clinches the matter is that, in 1884, when Jo-Jo was exhibited in Berlin, he allowed Dr. Max Bartels and Professor Rudolf Virchow to demonstrate him before the Anthropological Society of Berlin. He was introduced as Fedor Jeftichejev! Many of the Berlin anthropologists were delighted to see him again, since they had made his acquaintance eleven years earlier. Fedor, alias Jo-Jo, was now fourteen years old. He was a sturdily built, clever lad, completely normal except for his extraordinary hairy growth and his defective dentition. His impresario, the Russian Nicholas Forster, said that Adrian had returned to Kostroma after the successful tour of 1872–1874, and that he had rapidly drunk himself to death there. Fedor had then been taken to St. Petersburg, where he was exhibited at a waxworks museum owned by Mr. Theodore Lent, the former husband of Julia Pastrana, who was now married to Zenora Pastrana, another bearded celebrity. The German dentist Julius Parreidt took new casts of Fedor's teeth and found that he had only two canine teeth in the upper jaw and two incisors and a canine in the lower one; the discrepancy between this observation and that by Coles and Tomes in 1874 is accounted for by the replacement, in the intervening years, of the deciduous by the permanent dentition.

Later in 1884, Jo-Jo was exhibited in Liverpool by his Russian agent, and plans were made to take him to London. One of P. T. Barnum's agents spotted him there, however, and invited him to came to the United States for the first time, and to join Barnum & Bailey's Circus. Nicholas Forster was

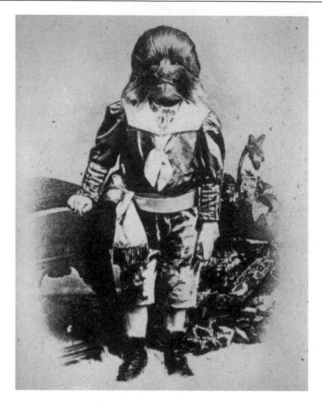

Fedor, alias Jo-Jo, as a boy. From the author's collection.

soon persuaded that far greater profit could be gained on the other side of the Atlantic. They all boarded the steamer *City of Chicago*, which arrived in New York on October 12, 1884. Nicholas Forster, his young wife, and Barnum's agents immediately set up a press conference for Jo-Jo at Astor House. He was advertised as "the most prodigious paragon of all prodigies secured by P. T. Barnum in over 50 years," and billed as the ward of the Russian government who had come to the United States by the express desire of the czar; Forster and his wife acted the part of a noble Russian couple, to whom the czar had entrusted the guardianship over this valuable *lusus naturae*. The assembled newspaper men looked on aghast when the dog-faced boy came to greet them; never, in their entire lives, had they seen anything like him. Barnum's reputation as a hoaxer meant that no human or animal specimen exhibited by him could be taken at its face value, however. After a polite question to the impresario whether the dog-faced boy might bite was answered in the negative, the entire press corps took turns to pull his facial hair to make sure it was not fastened by artificial means, and to examine his four teeth like a farmer surveyed the mouth of a horse on exhibition. In spite of this ludicrous treatment, Jo-Jo remained polite and affable, and the press did much to help advertise him. He was as full of play as a puppy, they wrote, and although he could speak both Russian and German, they thought that his voice resembled the barking and growling of a dog. The *New York Herald* described him as "the most extraordinary and absorbingly interesting curiosity that has ever reached these shores."

In the 1880s, Jo-Jo was widely famous, and he was photographed many times. For some reason, he used to wear the clothes of a trapper and carry a long rifle. Other photographs depict him dressed in Russian garb or wearing a cavalry uniform. In 1885, the fifteen-year-old Fedor, alias Jo-Jo, was examined by a certain Dr. G. T. Jackson in New York, as Barnum & Bailey's Greatest Show on Earth was passing through this city. In 1887, an advertisement in the *Avant Courier* newspaper depicted him with the head of a dog, but claimed that behind this canine visage there was a prodigious intellect, and that Jo-Jo could speak four languages. He later toured the world and went to Australia and Europe, and then back to the United States again, to rejoin Barnum & Bailey's circus. In their *Book of Marvels*, issued in 1899, he is advertised as "The Human Skye Terrier." He was an intelligent man and an avid reader, but according to some historians of the American sideshow, Jo-Jo sometimes used to act the part of a dog on stage and to snap, growl, bark, and chew bones.

In 1901 and 1902, Barnum & Bailey's Greatest Show on Earth toured Europe, and Jo-Jo was one of the star performers. In Paris, he was billed as L'Homme-Caniche, or the Poodle-Man. It was said on the handbill that he seemed to represent all that was shocking and repulsive: the soul of a man in the guise of a woolly poodle . . . the mouth of a dog speaking four languages. Jo-Jo did his usual act in front of the astonished Frenchmen, and the circus was as successful as ever. He died from pneumonia during a tour of Greece in early 1904 and was mourned by many American sideshow enthusiasts. He was a particular favorite also of the French nation, and the paper *L'Illustration* published a photograph of him on his deathbed, as if he had been a prominent statesman or magnate. According to various Internet sources, he subsequently made his mark on twentieth-century popular culture: a song entitled "Jo-Jo the Dog-faced Boy" was recorded by Annette Funicello in

26   A photograph of Jo-Jo as an
       adult, taken in the late 1880s.
       From the author's collection.

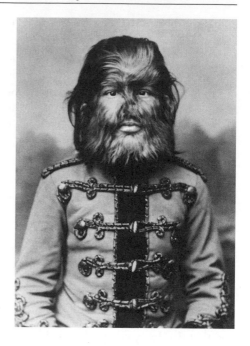

the 1960s, and the character Jo-Jo later appeared in the television series
"Buffy the Vampire Slayer."

Krao, the Human Monkey

The record of the memorable sitting of the Berlin Anthropological Society in
1884, when Max Bartels and Rudolf Virchow demonstrated Fedor
Jeftichejev, alias Jo-Jo, was entitled "den Affenmenschen und den Bären-
menschen"—The Ape-people and the Bear-people. Adrian and Fedor belonged to the latter category; the former was represented by Julia Pastrana
and another hairy celebrity of the time, the little girl Krao, who had been
taken from her home in Siam by the German explorer Carl Bock. In 1884, at
the age of eight, she was exhibited in the Berlin Aquarium as the Ape-girl;
Rudolf Virchow briefly mentioned that the German police did not allow her
manager to put her in the same cage as four anthropoid apes, as was the
original plan.

     In January 1883, Krao first appeared before the curious, at the Royal
Aquarium in London. Mr. Farini, her manager, presented her as the missing
link between human and ape and the living proof of Darwin's theory of evo-

lution. He claimed that the explorer Bock had also captured Krao's parents, and that all three belonged to a hairy tribe of people living in the interior of Laos. Her father's body was completely covered with a thick hairy coat, exactly like that of an anthropoid ape. His long arms and rounded belly added further to his simian appearance. He was incapable of speech when caught, but before his death from cholera, before Herr Bock could get him on board ship, he was able to utter a few words in Malay. For reasons unexplained, the mother was detained at Bangkok by the Siamese government, but these authorities apparently had no objections to little Krao being taken from her parents and transported to the other side of the globe.

In no less a publication than *Nature* magazine, Krao was described by the anthropologist Dr. A. H. Keane, who was one of the many Darwinists searching for the missing link between human and ape. Both Africa and Asia were given attention by the zealous evolutionists, who were searching for atavistic signs, like tails or abnormal hairiness, in what they termed inferior races of mankind. Dr. Keane had previously published a paper on the Ainu tribe in Yesso and Sakhalin, and postulated the existence of a primitive hairy race in Further India. These preconceived notions made him a willing dupe to the showman's spiel. With rapt attention, he examined little Krao, who had then been in London for ten weeks. She had already acquired several English words, which she used intelligently, and Dr. Keane had to conclude that her intellect was that of a normal human child. Her entire body had a coat of rather thick, black hair, but its growth was nowhere close enough to conceal the skin. She was remarkably supple and agile; Dr. Keane was interested to note that her feet had particularly long toes, with which she could actually grasp objects, and that her hands were so flexible that they could bend back over the wrists. He could detect no simian characteristics in the shape of her face, although the showman assured him that she used to stuff food into her cheeks just like a monkey, and that her lips could protrude so far as to give her "quite a chimpanzee look." She was given to terrible outbursts of rage when denied something, Mr. Farini said, and the only thing that could suppress her unruly behavior was the threat that she would be sent back to her own people. With these observations in mind, Dr. Keane concluded that Krao was the living proof of a hairy race in Laos, and thus a phenomenon of exceptional scientific importance.

In 1884 and 1885, Krao toured Germany and Austria. She was exhibited at the Frankfurt Zoological Gardens, and the usual ostentatious advertising ensured a record audience: The zoo was so crowded that a twentieth-century German writer pronounced these shows the most memo-

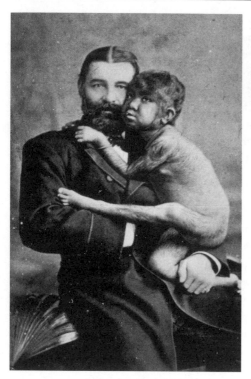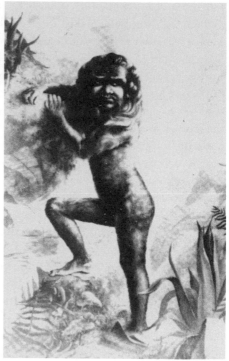

An early photograph of Krao (left), along with one of her exhibition posters.

rable in its 150-year history. On the handbills and posters, a distinctly simian-looking Krao was portrayed dressed in a loincloth only; her hairy growth was exaggerated, and she stood grasping the branch of a tree in front of a jungle background. Several medical men examined her, among them the German dentist Julius Parreidt. He was interested to note that unlike the hairy Burmese and Adrian and Fedor, Krao did not have a diminished number of teeth. In 1885, a certain Herr Bastian announced that the explorer Bock's dramatic account of how Krao had been captured with her "wild" family was nothing but a pack of lies; in fact, she had been born in Bangkok, the child of two normal parents, both of whom were still living.

In 1886, Krao and Mr. Farini came to Paris. Here, she was examined by the French anthropologist Dr. Fauvelle, who was as eager as Dr. Keane in his search for her supposed primitive and apelike characteristics. Krao was lively and agreeable throughout the interview and did not object to being examined. Apart from her hairy growth, Dr. Fauvelle noted that her ears were rather large, her nose was flat, and her joints very supple and flexible; all these observations were given a sinister interpretation. The impresario, always eager to make his charge appear even more interesting, assured him that she had thirteen ribs and the same number of thoracic vertebrae, that she had double rows of teeth, and that her behavior was often quite apelike. In all earnestness, Dr. Fauvelle wrote that unfortunately, he had been unable to assess the intelligence of this strange "ape-girl," since her command of the English language was far superior to his own! When Dr. Fauvelle's paper was read before the Société d'Anthropologie de Paris, Mme Royer, the forthright French lady anthropologist whose observations on Fedor and Adrian have been quoted previously, commented on it. She began a lengthy lecture of her own, reviewing her observations of the hairy Russian father and son and also drawing parallels between Krao and Julia Pastrana. Independently from the German dentist Parreidt quoted earlier, Mme Royer had examined some casts of Julia Pastrana's teeth taken by the Frenchman Magitot in 1857. She was clever enough to make the correct deduction, from a study of these, that Pastrana certainly did not have double rows of teeth, but instead a considerable overgrowth of the gums, which had led to some parakeratinized nodules of gum being mistaken for extra teeth. Krao had exactly the same disorder, but to a much lesser degree. Mme Royer then reverted to her own pet theories of anthropology, with the startling conclusion that poor Adrian, "L'Homme-Chien de Kostroma," may well be the image of the Precursor of Mankind, the missing link between civilized man and the Neanderthals. Probably dismayed that Mme Royer had completely dominated the meeting, and that his own observations had been somewhat overshadowed, Dr. Fauvelle's only retort was that "Le terrain sur lequel Mme Royer vient de s'aventurer est le champ des conjectures"!

Krao spent all her life in show business. Throughout the 1890s, she toured Europe with her manager, Mr. Farini, who had become her adopted father, and her English governess. In 1893, a certain Herr Maass saw the now seventeen-year-old Krao being exhibited in Berlin. The prudish German considered her short dress somewhat lewd, although not unbecoming. She was quite a young lady, he wrote, and her manner was decent and friendly. It was clear to him that all the stories about her supposed apelike characteristics were just inventions to make her even more interesting to the gullible public. Krao later became one of the stars of Ringling Bros. and Barnum & Bailey's circus in the United States. One would not have supposed that a young girl who spent her adolescent years being exhibited as "The Human Monkey" in various zoos and monster museums would grow up to be a harmonic and and well-adjusted individual, but it is claimed that Krao became one of the most popular "old troupers" of the circus. She was an educated, well-read woman who spoke many languages. Krao died in New York in 1926.

According to D. P. Mannix's book, *Freaks: We Are Not as Others*, Krao was later succeeded by another hairy celebrity who looked remarkably like her. In the true tradition of the American sideshow, she was billed as Percilla the Monkey Girl, and exhibited together with her pet chimpanzee Johanna. Her showman, Carl Lauther, was also her adopted father. The French writer Martin Monestier added a remarkable story about her in his *Human Oddities*. When the sideshow came to Havana, a very wealthy lady was quite taken with the seventeen-year-old Percilla and offered to adopt her as her own child and give her a superior education. Lauther was quite tempted to accept this offer, but he became somewhat worried when he found out that the Cuban lady lived in a large, high-walled estate with no other companions than a flock of apes and monkeys. Surely, this lady had an unhealthy fascination for the simian tribe, and Lauther was somewhat uneasy with what would become of poor Percilla if he accepted her offer. The stalemate was broken by Emmett the Alligator Man, another of the sideshow performers, who offered to marry Percilla, and was accepted by her. The newlyweds were billed as The World's Strangest Married Couple; they both became old troupers within the sideshow business and were still active in the late 1970s. Percilla died in 2001, aged more than 80. Emmett had predeceased her some years earlier.

Lionel, the Lion-man

Stephan Bibrowski, later to be known as Lionel the Lion-man, was born near Warsaw in 1891. Even at birth, he was covered with fine, soft hair about one inch long. His mother was so upset and frightened by his appearance that at first she wanted to get rid of him. He grew up to be a lively, intelligent boy, however. His parents and six sisters had no abnormality of the hair whatsoever. Already as a four-year-old child, Stephan entered the world of show business. He was "discovered" by a German impresario named Meyer, and appears to have been on permanent display at a large German amusement arcade, the Panoptikum in Berlin, for some years. A certain Professor Minakow examined him in Moscow at the age of five. His face and body were covered with fine blond hair, up to 8 inches long on his face and

2–3 inches long all over the rest of his body. His dentition consisted of a solitary canine tooth in the lower jaw.

In 1901, the ten-year-old Stephan was taken to the United States, to succeed Jo-Jo at Barnum & Bailey's Greatest Show on Earth. Stephan's mother had probably never even seen a lion, but the exhibition posters claimed that the boy's father had been torn to pieces by an escaped circus lion before her very eyes; this horrid sight had of course "marked" her unborn child in this sinister way. In 1904, he toured large parts of the world with the circus. After this tour, he returned to the Panoptikum in Berlin. The German anthropologist von Luschan saw him there in 1907, at the age of thirteen. With his tremendously long facial hair like a mane down his neck, he had a distinct resemblance to a big cat; at the Panoptikum, he was known as Der Löwenknabe — The Lion-boy. In 1910, when he was seen by Dr. Paul Sarasin in Basel, his artist's name had been changed to Lionel the Lion-man.

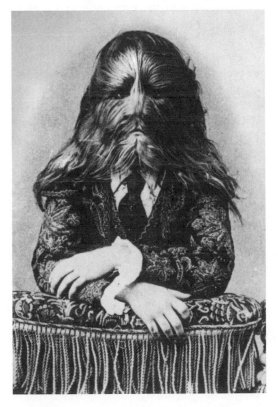

An old photograph of Lionel, as a young boy. From the author's collection.

He was exhibited at the Spring Fair in Basel and was immensely popular. This was as much due to his merry and jovial nature, and his impressive grasp of languages, as to his hairy face and long mane. The next record of him is that in 1921, when the German pathologists Aschoff and Mense examined him thoroughly. They took hair samples from various parts of his body, and X-rayed his jaws.

In 1923, Lionel went back to the United States. He received a very good offer from the Coney Island amusement park: the authorities there had agreed to pay him five hundred dollars a week for taking up permanent residence at the park during the summer seasons. He liked living in the United States and remained at Coney Island for quite a few years; millions of Americans must have seen him there. Several accounts agree that his shows were far removed from the degrading spectacles around Julia Pastrana and Adrian: Lionel spoke five languages, was a well-read and intelligent man, and was quite an entertainer. He was something of a body-builder and very strong; he sometimes gave demonstrations of his gymnastic and athletic skills. One ribald newspaper account reported that he was also something of

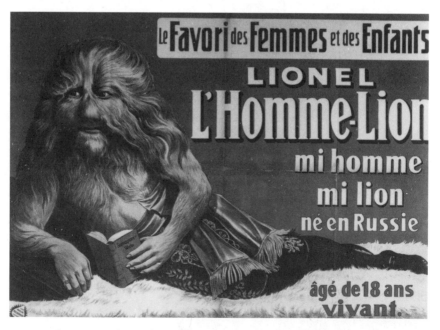

A poster from 1909 of Lionel, the favorite of women and children. From the author's collection.

a ladies' man: in spite, or perhaps rather because, of his extraordinary hairy face and body, he never had any difficulty getting admirers among the female visitors. After his successful stay in the United States, Lionel went back to Germany; in 1931, he died at a hospital in Berlin.

From the Annals of Congenital Hypertrichosis

In his famous essay "The Elephant Man," Sir Frederick Treves described how he had first come across, in the Mile End Road near the London Hospital where he worked, a canvas poster depicting John Merrick, the original Elephant Man. On the poster, his transformation into an elephant was by no means complete; it had only just begun, and there was still much more of the man than of the beast, only "the loathsome fascination of a man being changed into an animal." The perpetual popular fascination of hairy people has the same rather sinister explanation. Singled out by their extraordinary appearance and enhanced by their extreme rarity, they were exhibited as "wild men," man-animal hybrids, or "missing links." Interestingly, the oldest case, Petrus Gonzales, fared reasonably well and likely had a far more interesting life touring Europe with his family, and reading Latin to kings and princes, than if he had been a nonhairy peasant in the Canaries. The callous exploitation of Barbara Urslerin and Julia Pastrana is sad to contemplate. Their lives had many parallels, but the macabre tours with Pastrana's mummy for many years, even 110 years after her death, is fortunately without precedent in the annals of human deformities. The exhibition of little Krao as "The Human Monkey," which occurred as late as the 1880s under the most degrading forms, is an equally unsavory phenomenon.

The exhibition of the chronically ill, debauched Adrian Jeftichejev before the unfeeling crowds must also have been a repulsive spectacle. In contrast, his son Fedor, alias Jo-Jo, who had spent all his life in show business, was an extrovert character, and intelligent enough to take advantage of his abnormal condition to make an almost unprecedented success in international sideshows. He willingly played the buffoon and both frightened and amused the spectators by barking, snapping, and growling in the ring. Some advertisements actually depicted him with the head of a dog, standing on stage with a number of Skye terriers, before an admiring audience. According to one account, the novelty of his act finally palled, and after thirty years on the road, Jo-Jo died a bitter and disillusioned man. Perhaps his spirit was broken the one-thousandth time some rapier wit among the American sideshow "rubes" asked him where he had mislaid his razor, or inquired whether he had paid the dog tax. Lionel the Lion-man appears to have had a rather more pleasant existence. In his heyday, he was almost as famous as Jo-Jo and earned considerable sums of money; he was a celebrated star of the American sideshow and the favorite of many emancipated American ladies who visited Coney Island. It is not unlikely that a photograph of Lionel might have inspired an American television series from the 1980s, entitled "Beauty and the Beast." The hero of this odd, sentimental melodrama is a leonine-looking, hairy man who lives in an underground community in the sewers of New York.

Some parts of nineteenth-century anthropology are today categorized as pseudoscience, particularly the race theory with the white man at the top of the pyramid, and the sometimes ludicrous by-products of early Darwinism. One of the more fruitful consequences of the great interest in anthropology in nineteenth-century Germany was that many of the cases of congenital hypertrichosis (inherited excessive hairiness) were well described. The anthropologists not only attended the exhibitions of Julia Pastrana, Krao, and Jo-Jo and left valuable descriptions of them, but also carried out considerable research, which has been largely ignored by later writers, to find sources of the historical cases, like Barbara Urslerin and the Gonzales family. The more gifted anthropologists, like Rudolf Virchow and Max Bartels, were fully aware that individuals like Jo-Jo and Krao really had no sinister apelike or primitive characteristics, as more ostentatious commentators had claimed. They knew that this kind of excessive hairiness was an inherited disorder, and although they discussed that it might be an atavism, the reappearance of a lost character typical of the remote ancestors of mankind, they remained undecided on this issue. It was they who gave this disease its name: congenital hypertrichosis lanuginosa (inherited excessive hairiness with lanugo hair).

During the next one hundred years, from 1890 until 1990, very little advance was made, however. Few novel cases of congenital hypertrichosis were described, and the commentary around the older ones was often confused and muddled. Several influential dermatologists and geneticists, like the Englishman Cockayne and the German Salaman, divided the individuals with congenital hypertrichosis lanuginosa into one "dog-faced" and one "monkey-faced" group: the former containing the Gonzales family, Barbara Urslerin, Adrian and Fedor, and Stephan Bibrowsky, alias Lionel; the latter consisting only of Julia Pastrana and Krao. As even the scientists were faltering to explain, or even classify, the hairy people of yesteryear, it is not at all surprising that the popular opinion about them was as much steeped in ignorance and bigotry as it was one hundred years earlier. When Julia Pastrana's mummy was exhibited in the United States and in Scandinavia in 1971–1973, she was still advertised as a hybrid between baboon and human. A similar message was repeated by the Ku Klux Klan in the 1970s; this venerable body published photographs of Julia Pastrana in their loathsome pamphlets, with the caption that she was a hybrid between Negro and ape. At least one other American racist organization followed suit, and another used the lurid nineteenth-century photographs of Krao for a similar purpose. An Internet search on Pastrana and Krao turned up a racist publication called *The Liberty Bell*, in which a scholar named Professor Revilo P. Oliver claims that Pastrana was a baboon-human hybrid. Another homepage, concentrating on the elusive Bigfoot, suggested that both Krao and Pastrana may well have been hybrids between Bigfoot and humans. Similarly ludicrous is the suggestion that the hairy people may have inspired the werewolf legend; there is no evidence for this whatsoever in the original sources. The recent books on human malformations provide little support for those wishing to dispel these silly fantasies and racist lies. In Barry Humphrey's *Bizarre*, Julia Pastrana is referred to as the Gorilla Woman, a unique freak of nature and the most hideous creature of all times; in Martin Monestier's *Human Oddities*, Krao is accepted as a unique missing link with simian characteristics.

In 1990, I discovered Julia Pastrana's mummy at a forensic institute in Oslo, Norway. It was possible to secure hair samples from it and to have radiographs of the jaws made using up-to-date techniques. The results were not a little surprising. It turned out that Julia Pastrana had terminal hair, not lanugo hair. Since replacement of lanugo with terminal hair never occurs in a person with true hypertrichosis with lanugo hair, it could conclusively be stated that she did not have this disease. The radiographs showed that unlike the hairy toothless people such as Adrian and Lionel, she had a complete set of permanent teeth. When my colleague Professor A. E. W. Miles examined a set of plaster casts of her jaws, kept in the Odontological Museum of the Royal College of London, he found evidence that she had suffered from gingival hyperplasia, a form of overgrowth of the gums. With these findings in mind, it was possible to diagnose Julia Pastrana as an extreme case of congenital hypertrichosis (with terminal hair) and gingival hyperplasia, an established, autosomally dominant syndrome. From the good examinations of her by Julius Parreidt and Mme Royer, it seems very likely that Krao had the same disorder. The old classification into a "monkey-faced" and a "dog-faced" subgroup of congenital hypertrichosis lanuginosa is thus not only un-

36   couth, but also completely erroneous: the patients belong to two completely different genetic syndromes, with excessive hairiness as the only common denominator. Today this classification is accepted in the standard textbook on this subject, Professor McKusick's *Mendelian Inheritance in Man*.

In 1984, Dr. M. A. Macias-Flores and coworkers described a large Mexican family with congenital hypertrichosis running in five generations. Two young boys belonging to this family were active as circus acrobats, under the artist's name of The Werewolf Boys. Their pattern of hairiness was somewhat different from that in the classic European cases, with shorter and somewhat coarser hair. The pedigree and the mode of inheritance, coupled with the fact that males were much more severely affected than females, suggested an X-linked mode of inheritance. Some scientists doubted this, but in 1995, Dr. L. Figuera and coworkers actually mapped what they called "the congenital hypertrichosis locus" to a certain part of the X chromosome (Xq24–q27.1) using multiple blood samples from the Mexican family.

In an X-linked disease, an affected father marrying a normal mother has normal sons and affected daughters. Since the historical accounts agree that Schwe-Maong, the ancestor of the Hairy Burmese, had at least one normal daughter and at least one affected daughter, his variant of congenital hypertrichosis cannot have been X-linked. Nor is the pedigree of Petrus Gonzales, with an affected father siring affected children of both sexes, consistent with X-linked inheritance. The historical cases thus provide vital evidence that the mode of inheritance in congenital hypertrichosis lanuginosa is autosomally dominant, and that the "hypertrichosis locus" described by Figuera and coworkers is not the genetic defect responsible in these cases. In 1993, Dr. F. A. M. Baumeister and coworkers examined one of the rare modern cases of congenital hypertrichosis lanuginosa and found a slight chromosomal abnormality, what is known as a balanced pericentric inversion, in the eight chromosome. Very intriguingly, a group of Italian scientists recently made exactly the same finding in another child with congenital hypertrichosis lanuginosa, supporting that this balanced structural chromosomal aberration may well have been causative; such an aberration is of course perfectly compatible with an autosomally dominant mode of inheritance.

These recent advances imply that there are (at least) three major subgroups of inherited excessive hairiness. Firstly, there is the traditional congenital hypertrichosis lanuginosa, which affected many of the historical cases like Barbara Urslerin, the Gonzales family, the hairy Burmese, Adrian and Fedor, and Lionel. The inheritance is autosomally dominant, from a locus on the eighth chromosome. Although most cases are sporadic and the result of spontaneous mutations, there is one example of a three-generation pedigree (Gonzales family) and one example of a four-generation pedigree (hairy Burmese). Secondly, there is the syndrome of excessive hairiness with terminal hair and overgrowth of the gums, which affected Julia Pastrana and Krao. This syndrome is also autosomally dominant and clearly has variable expression. Some individuals have only mild gingival hyperplasia and others, more severe overgrowth of the gums and also excessive hairiness; the very extremes, like Julia Pastrana and Krao, are the only ones to have an extent of hairiness resembling the old historical cases of hypertrichosis. Thirdly, there is the X-linked hypertrichosis without gingival hyperplasia, recently described from Mexico; this syndrome cannot be implied in any of the historical cases.

The question regarding whether excessive hairiness is an atavism is still debated today. An atavism is defined as the reappearance of a lost character, either morphology or behavior, that is typical of remote ancestors and not seen in the parents or recent ancestors of the individual in question. Examples of such an ancestral phenotype are hind limbs in whales and three-toed (polydactylous) horses; in humans, supernumerary nipples, the presence of a tail, and excessive hairiness have been quoted as examples of atavisms. The model used to explain them is that the genetic and developmental information originally utilized in the production of these characteristics has not been lost during evolution, but lies dormant within the genome and can still be "turned on" by a mutation. Although the majority of earlier writers accepted the concept of congenital hypertrichosis as an atavism without question, it seems reasonable to raise a few objections to it. The fact that there are (at least) three separate genetic defects, some of them X-linked, others autosomal, causing congenital hypertrichosis would weaken the case for this condition being the result of the reactivation of an ancestral pattern of development. The associated defects—toothlessness or overgrowth of the gums—cannot be considered as ancestral qualities. Many of the historical cases, like Jo-Jo and Lionel, had an extremely hairy nose, something that is untypical of primates. Nor is there any evidence of any sinister primitive or "animal-like" characteristics in the individuals with congenital hypertrichosis. Most of them had normal intellect; some, like Petrus Gonzales and Lionel, were remarked upon as "learned" or particularly clever. The claims that Jo-Jo was "dog like" in his behavior was just a hoax to make him appear more interesting to the sideshow "rubes." It is more serious that the alleged "apelike" characteristics of Julia Pastrana and Krao are still widely believed by credulous and careless authors, even in recent books published

38   by university presses. For any person who has examined a chimpanzee, it is apparent that the shape of its face is due to the protuberance of the jaws, and not to any abnormality of the gums. The radiographs of the head of Julia Pastrana's mummy indicate that her jaws were of a normal shape, and the casts of her jaws indicate that her prognathic appearance was entirely due to overgrowth of the gums. It is impossible to directly disprove that congenital hypertrichosis is an atavism, since the concept of an atavism is in itself an arbitrary one, but there are several arguments against it. The sinister interpretation of the word atavism, implying that the affected individuals, like a hairy child or a baby with a tail, are generally "primitive" or "apelike," thus opening the door to racist and bigoted interpretation, is completely unfounded. This unsavory relict of nineteenth-century anthropology should be left to mold in the murky old tomes of old libraries.

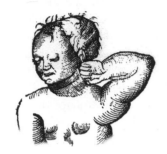

The Stone-child

THE ANCIENT FRENCH TOWN SENS, SITUATED ON the river of Yonne about 60 miles southeast of Paris, is famous for its gothic twelfth-century cathedral. In the sixteenth century, it was an influential archbishop's seat, as well as a prosperous market town. In early 1554, one of the townswomen of Sens, the forty-year-old Mme Colombe Chatri, became pregnant for the first time. She was the wife of M. Loys Carita, a tailor, described as being of small stature, but otherwise "well formed and corpulent, although of common stock." Mme Chatri's menstruations ceased, her breasts swelled, her stomach increased in size, and she could even feel the child move within her. Some time before her child was due, Colombe Chatri was seized with violent labor pains. A great quantity of amniotic fluid, tinged with blood, was passed. But, in spite of the predictions of the Sens midwives, there was no childbirth; instead, her labor pains ceased, the movements of the child could no longer be felt, and her breasts diminished in size. After this interrupted pregnancy, Mme Chatri felt quite unwell, and she had to remain in bed for three full years. She could feel a hard tumor of considerable size situated in the lower abdomen. Until the end of her life, she complained of tiredness, abdominal pains, and loss of appetite. Only by means of provoking her relish for food with herbs and vinegar sauces could she eat anything at all. There was much gossip among the Sens townswomen about Mme Chatri's strange obstetrical mishap: they whispered that she probably still had an unborn child within her, and that it would kill her one day. Mme Chatri and her husband consulted several physicians and surgeons, but none of them could suggest a cure.

In 1582, at the age of sixty-eight, Colombe Chatri was described as being broken down by disease and old age. She died later that year, and since there had been much gossip about her mysterious pregnancy many years ago, her husband requested that her body should be dissected by two skillful surgeons, Messrs. Claude le Noir and Iehan Couttas. At first, these two gentlemen thought that she had suffered from some kind of hard, scirrhous tumor. They cut through the stomach and peritoneum and viewed the prodigious growth, which was wrinkled and formed like a turkey's crest. It was hard and brittle like a shell, and covered with what seemed like scales. The surgeons "plunged their razors into it," but without being able to penetrate the hard shell. After wearing out the edge of their knives on the hard tumor, they fetched mauls and a drill and finally succeeded to break it. They felt something solid, rather like the head and right shoulder of some small statue, but it was not until they broke off a large portion of the covering shell, and saw the wonderful sight inside, that they understood what they were dealing with. They ran to fetch some physicians, M. Jean d'Ailleboust among them. He was astonished to see that inside the shell was a fully formed child, but petrified and hard like a marble statue. During this time, curious townsmen came running in to see this prodigy. The surgeons were busy telling the story, and to demonstrate the infant more clearly, they grasped the opening in the calcified shell with their iron hooks to tear it apart. After tearing with all their force, they broke it open and took out the stone-child. This was done with great haste, and Jean d'Ailleboust deplored that they had made it impossible to study closer the anatomy of the calcified shell and the nourishing vessels.

The shape of the stone-child was roughly that of its rounded, calcified shell. The knees were bent, and the legs drawn up toward the chest. The feet and lower legs were fused by the calcific deposits. All could clearly see that the fetus was of the female sex. The head was slightly tilted to the right and supported by the left arm. The right arm extended down toward the navel; its hand had been broken off through carelessness when the stone-child was extracted. The bones of the head were transparent and the fontanelles were not closed. In several places the skin of the head was covered with hair. The stone-child had one sole tooth, situated in the lower jaw.

&

The stone-child of Sens became one of the foremost curiosities of France. People traveled hundreds of miles to see and admire it. Jean d'Ailleboust needed no encouragement to write a Latin pamphlet about it, detailing the case history of Mme Chatri as well as the autopsy findings. It was published in 1582 by the Sens printer Jean Sauvine and soon became a medical best-seller. For the benefit of the curious populace, who did not read Latin, d'Ailleboust's colleague Simeon de Provancheres translated the entire work into French. The larger part of Jean d'Ailleboust's thesis was dedicated to a long-winded explanation, in the manner of the time, of the causes underlying the calcification of the fetus. Jean d'Ailleboust believed that the growing fetus had shriveled and calcified in the womb, through the excessive dryness of the mother's blood. Simeon de Provancheres, who wrote a supplement to the thesis, believed that Mme Chatri's womb had become too cold, from the pain and the efflux of amniotic fluids; this had caused all fluid in the fetus to evaporate, turning it into stone. A better-known contemporary, the obstetrician François de Rousset, who incorporated d'Ailleboust's thesis into a work on cesarean section, had another, more reasonable theory. For some reason, the tissues of the fetus had joined with those of the mother, which explained why it had not been born in a normal way. Later, it accumulated increasing amounts of a hard substance, which might be of the same nature as the hard swellings on the fingers of patients afflicted with the gout.

Jean d'Ailleboust also supplied a curious drawing of the stone-child and its "mother." It is believed to depict the corpse of Colombe Chatri lying on a richly padded bed, her abdomen dissected to show the stone-child in situ within its calcified shell. Beside the bed, the stone-child is laid out on a pillow. The woman seen in the drawing seems far younger than the sixty-eight-year-old Colombe Chatri. Considering her lifelike but languid pose, much unlike that of a half-dissected corpse, it is likely that the woman figure was copied from a contemporary erotic drawing, and that the stone-child and other anatomical details were superimposed later. This practice was not unknown at the time: for example, the obstetrical illustrations in Charles Esti-

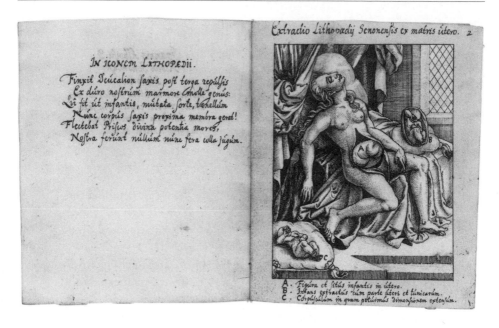

The original (?) drawing of the lithopedion, with the accompanying poem.
Reproduced with permission of the Royal Library of Copenhagen.

enne's famous *De dissectione partium corporis humanis,* which was published in
1545, owe much to the erotic drawings of Perino del Vaga, a pupil of
Raphael. Jean d'Ailleboust's illustration resembles those of Charles Estienne, with the woman luxuriously spread out on an ornamental bed with pillows, but the original has not been traced to the figures used by Estienne.
Jean d'Ailleboust himself cryptically added that the drawing was made in
imitation of the works of Phydias, the ancient Greek sculptor. In Germany,
the same illustration was used in a handbill entitled "Der Versteinerte Foet,"
described by Dr. Sonderegger in his *Missgeburten und Wundergestalten.*

❧

The famous surgeon Ambroise Paré, the founder of French surgery, was a
contemporary of Jean d'Ailleboust. He had occasion to see and examine the
stone-child, which was figured in his book *Des monstres et prodiges.* His drawing was probably made soon after Jean d'Ailleboust's pamphlet was published, and it remains the best sketch of what the stone-child of Sens really
looked like. Although Jean d'Ailleboust was unwilling to part from his great

treasure, it is recorded that in the 1590s, it was purchased by a wealthy merchant, M. Prestesiegle, who put it in his famous private museum of curiosities in Paris. It was examined there by Mme Louise Bourgeouis, the leading French midwife of her time, who wrote a brief account of it and reproduced Jean d'Ailleboust's original drawing. Later, the stone-child was purchased by M. Estienne Carteron, a wealthy Paris goldsmith. He sold it in 1628 to M. Gillebert Bodëy, a jewel merchant of Venice. Two formal documents of sale were drawn up. In one of these, six Paris burghers certified that the stone-child turned over to the brothers Claude and Henri Bossu, emissaries of M. Bodëy, by Marie Charpentier, wife of Estienne Carteron, was the same one described by Ambroise Paré and exhibited for many years in the museum of M. Prestesiegle. In the other document, signed in Venice on February 12, 1628, Carteron officially sold the stone-child to M. Bodëy. In the early 1640s, it was seen in Venice by Thomas Bartholin, the famous Danish anatomist. He was evidently much impressed by the stone-child, stressing that the price paid for it by its present owner had been a very great one.

Thomas Bartholin is likely to have told his royal master, King Frederick III of Denmark, about the marvelous stone-child he had seen in Venice. In the early 1650s, the king was building up a large cabinet of curiosities at his castle in Copenhagen. After the death of that great collector, Professor Olaus Wormius, the king purchased his entire museum, which was to form the core of the royal repository in Copenhagen, which thus acquired a solid stock of zoological, botanical, medical, and ethnological specimens. King Frederick III was eager to extend his collection further, and in 1653, he decided to purchase the stone-child from its owner in Venice. The document of sale and certificate signed in 1628 were also turned over to the king, as well as a handwritten copy of Jean d'Ailleboust's autopsy report, with the original illustration; all these documents are still kept in the Royal Library of Copenhagen. The sum paid was a well-kept secret, but it is unlikely that the shrewd Franco-Italian merchant let the king have it cheaply, particularly since he himself had paid a very high price for it. According to Bartholin's nephew Holger Jacobsen, writing in 1710, the price was one thousand Danish riksdalers; according to a later Danish writer, it was one thousand guilders. A few years later, Thomas Bartholin described the stone-child closer in one of his collections of anatomical anecdotes. By this time, it had become much the worse for wear, and it is likely that during its years in private hands, the stone-child of Sens had not always been treated with the reverence due to its age and fragility. Both arms were now broken off, the jaw was injured, and the skin lacerated. At some sites, the gypsum-like muscles were so badly worn (probably by the stone-child being examined by so many hands) that the skeleton had become partly visible. The sole tooth still remained in place. Unlike Jean d'Ailleboust, Thomas Bartholin gave some idea of the actual dimensions of the stone-child: it was the size of a fetus at full term.

The stone-child of Sens remained in the royal museum for many years. Thomas Bartholin's nephew, Holger Jacobsen, mentioned it in the extensive museum catalogues. In the 1696 edition of the catalogue, it was honored by the inclusion of a figure, and the king was praised "for bringing it to Denmark and putting it among the curiosities of his museum, where it was subjected to the examination of learned men." In the illustration, the miserable-looking specimen is depicted sitting lopsidedly on a box. Part of the missing arm had been refastened, but otherwise, the stone-child was unchanged since it was described by Thomas Bartholin. In Jacobsen's 1710 catalogue, it is more thoroughly described. The skin was now missing in large parts, and where it remained, it was quite black, giving the stone-child a strange appearance, as if it had been partly dressed. The orbits were

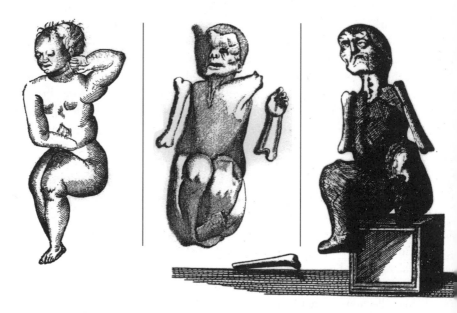

From left to right: Ambroise Paré's drawing of the lithopedion of Sens, from his *Des Monstres et Prodiges*; the drawing of the lithopedion reproduced by Thomas Bartholin in 1656; and the one published in the 1696 edition of Holger Jacobsen's *Musaeum Regium*.

empty, and the right side of the lower jaw was separated from the upper one.
The flesh of the right arm had been worn off, but the bone of the upper arm
still remained. The brief 1737 catalogue stated that whatever remained of the
stone-child was now kept in a glass box, probably to preserve it from further
rough handling. In 1770, it still remained at the royal museum, which was by
then a rather rundown establishment, the successors of Frederick III not
sharing his predilection for natural curiosities.

In the 1820s, the Danish government decided to dissolve the royal museum, and many preparations were scrapped or sold by public auction.
Many bizarre pieces changed hands under these circumstances, among them
the hand of a mermaid, solemnly described by Thomas Bartholin 170 years
earlier, a pair of slippers made from human skin, and an egg allegedly laid by
a Norwegian peasant woman. The stone-child was not among the preparations sold or thrown away, probably since it was still considered valuable. In
1826, it was transferred to the Danish Museum of Natural History, along
with several other human, animal, and vegetable specimens. In the late
1800s, the remaining exhibits from the Danish Museum of Natural History
were transferred to the Zoological Museum of Copenhagen University, and
a good many zoological specimens are still there. But the stone-child of Sens
disappeared somewhere along the way, as did many other medical curiosities
from King Frederick's museum, among them a two-headed child preserved
in spirits, and a minute fetus, alleged to be one of the 365 children of the prolific Dutch countess Margaret of Henneberg. The stone-child is not at the
Zoological Museum of Copenhagen, nor has it ever been there. Some antiquaries suspect that the director of the Danish Museum of Natural History
in the mid-1800s, Professor Reinhardt, disliked the old-fashioned specimens
from the museum, which he considered unfit for a modern scientific establishment. It may well be that the stone-child of Sens was scrapped at this
time, along with the other older medical specimens, of which no trace remains. Extensive searches for them in the existing Danish medical museums
have been fruitless.

❧

A stone-child, or *lithopedion*, is defined as the calcified remains of an extrauterine pregnancy, carried, usually in the abdominal cavity, beyond the
normal period of gestation. In the medical literature, more than 290 cases
have been described; except in developing countries, the condition seems to
be getting rarer as the resulting extrauterine pregnancy is usually discovered

at an earlier date. In a thorough review of older cases of lithopedion, written by Dr. Friedrich Küchenmeister in 1880, forty-seven cases were described, the lithopedion of Sens being the earliest among them. In the lithopedion material collected by Dr. T. S. P. Tien, the mean age of the mother, at the time the lithopedion was discovered, was fifty-five years, but several of them were octogenarians, and the oldest to date was exactly one hundred years old. An abdominal lithopedion did not prevent several of the women from subsequently bearing normal children. A good many of them carried their lithopedions for quite a long time: the mean was twenty-two years, and 9 of 128 women carried them for more than fifty years. Friedrich Küchenmeister had himself autopsied the corpse of an eighty-seven-year-old woman, who had carried her lithopedion for fifty-seven years.

Friedrich Küchenmeister defined three subgroups of lithopedion formation, and later writers adhered to his classification. In the lithokelyphos, or stone sheath, category, calcification occurs mainly in the membranes and does not involve the fetus itself. In the lithotecnon, or true lithopedion, group, the fetus itself is infiltrated with calcium salt deposits after it is deposited into the abdominal cavity after rupture of the membranes. Finally, in the lithokelyphopedion group, both fetus and sac are calcified. Of Dr. Tien's large lithopedion material, 26, 43, and 31 percent, respectively, belonged to these three categories. Of 114 lithopedion cases, 74 were the results of tubal pregnancies, while 13 originated in ovarian pregnancies; these lithopedions were located intra-abdominally after the rupture of these parts. Eight lithopedions were the results of primary abdominal pregnancies, and 5 lithopedions originated in the horn of a bicornuate uterus. The fetal age of the lithopedion is often difficult to estimate, owing to drying up and shrinking of the fetus; it should be noted, however, that 43 percent of the cases were described as being the size of a fetus at full term.

Not the least curious of the cases brought together by Dr. Küchenmeister was the stone-child of Leinzell. In 1674, a forty-eight-year-old German woman, Anna Mullern, living in the village of Leinzell in Schwaben, declared herself to be with child. She had all the usual signs of pregnancy, and at the expected time, her water broke and she was seized with labor pains. These labor pains lasted about seven weeks, however, and when they finally ceased, she still had a large, swollen belly. The tough countrywoman recovered her health, and worked in the fields as before, although troubled by pains in the lower part of her belly during prolonged exercise. Even more remarkably, she later became the mother of two healthy children, a son and a daughter. Notwithstanding this, she was, just like Colombe Chatri in Sens one hundred years before, firmly convinced that she was still carrying her first, unborn child. She requested that Dr. Wohnliche, the local physician, and Herr Knauffen, a barber surgeon active in Heubach, should open her body after death to resolve this matter. Both these gentlemen had to give their promise, in writing, to attend. Frau Mullern lived to a venerable age, however, and at the time of her death in 1720, at the age of ninety-four, the physician had predeceased her. When summoned by the local parson, the elderly surgeon showed up, assisted by his nephew. Herr Knauffen appears to have been a rather unskilled, coarse fellow; when he observed that her belly contained "a hard mass of the form and size of a large Ninepin-Bowl," he knocked it open with a blow from a hatchet. Whether he was seized with amazement when seeing the sinister-looking stone-child inside is not known. At any rate, a certain Dr. Steigerthal was summoned, and he described the lithopedion before the Royal Society of London, presenting an excellent illustration.

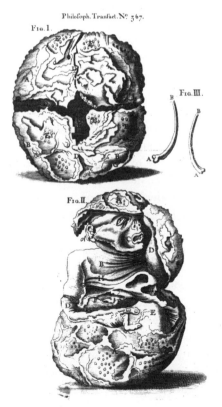

The stone-child of Leinzell. From Vol. 31 of the *Philosophical Transactions* of the Royal Society of London, 1720–23.

48   The stone-child itself was passed into the cabinet of rarities of the duke of
Württemberg. In 1854, Dr. Wilhelm Kieser, of the University of Tübingen,
published a doctoral thesis about this famous case. He managed to borrow
the preparation from the university museum and obtained permission to
study it closer by sawing it in two through the medial line. His detailed mi-
croscopical investigation identified the internal organs of the lithopedion and
provided valuable morphological evidence as to its structure.

Like the lithopedion of Leinzell, the famous stone-child of Sens was in
many respects a typical lithokelyphopedion. The mother was sixty-eight
years old and had carried it for twenty-eight years; furthermore, the symptoms caused by the lithopedion were typical, with the sense of a heavy, hard
abdominal tumor as the major complaint. What is odd is that Jean d'Ailleboust, without hesitation, declared that the lithopedion had been situated in
the intact uterus. The great majority of modern cases have been located
intra-abdominally, and only a few in one horn of a bicornuate uterus; no entirely intrauterine lithopedion has been described during the 1900s. It is evident from the original report that the dissection of Colombe Chatri was
performed rather hastily, and it remains a strong possibility that the two surgeons mistook the calcified shell around the lithopedion for the uterus. It is
well known that the uterus of a woman with an intra-abdominal lithopedion
is often much atrophied. It should be noted, however, that the efflux of amniotic fluid per vaginam would imply that the fetus, at that time, was in its
natural position. In his thesis on lithopedion formation, Dr. Kieser thoroughly discussed the problem of the intrauterine lithopedion. He accepted
the reality of this phenomenon, on the strength of two cases, described in the
eighteenth and nineteenth centuries. One of these was well substantiated,
with three excellent illustrations, the woman having carried the lithopedion
for 14½ years. In the absence of any modern cases, one would find it difficult
to accept the concept of a fetus at full term turning into a lithopedion while
still situated inside an intact uterus, however. The truth may well be that
Mme Chatri's fetus was situated inside the uterus until the onset of violent
labor pains. What then happened was that the distended uterus actually ruptured, which would explain the vaginal loss of blood. Instead of being born
by the natural route, the fetus was expulsed into the abdominal cavity and
gradually, over a long period of time, turned into a lithopedion. A rupture of
the uterus is a serious obstetrical complication and would have had a high
mortality rate in the sixteenth century. It is thus not surprising that unlike
Anna Mullern and the majority of other "mothers" of lithopedions, Colombe
Chatri was severely ill for a long time after the occurrence.

In many modern reviews on lithopedion formation, it is stated that the original case was described in 1557 by Israel Spach. In fact, the work in question appeared in 1597; it was the well-known anthology *Gyneciorum*, where Jean d'Ailleboust's thesis on the stone-child of Sens was reproduced. This mistake, which originated with Gould and Pyle's *Anomalies and Curiosities of Medicine*, has unfortunately been widely disseminated in both the medical and the popular literature. Although the lithopedion of Sens was without doubt the earliest recorded instance of this phenomenon, it is by no means the only one of its kind to be preserved and treasured in a pathology museum, or in a private cabinet of curiosities. The lithokelyphopedion of Leinzell, or rather what remains of it after Dr. Kieser's examination in 1854, may still be kept in the Stuttgart Museum of Natural History. Another German lithopedion was described by a certain Dr. Nebel in 1770, and later preserved in the pathology institute of Heidelberg. If the lithopedion of Sens had been preserved to this day, it would have been a treasure to any medical museum, and the circumstances concerning its disappearance in the mid-1800s, when it was already more than 250 years old, can only be described as gross vandalism.

If the ultimate fate of the lithopedion of Sens is unknown, what about the man who described it? According to a historian of the d'Ailleboust family, there were two brothers, both named Jean d'Ailleboust; both were successful medical practitioners. The elder brother was the one who described the lithopedion; he was the city physician of Sens as well as physician in ordinance to the duke of Alençon. The younger, more famous, brother was the physician of King Henri IV. It is odd that two brothers would have the same Christian name, and even odder that they would both be royal physicians; the duke of Alençon was a royal duke and the youngest son of Catherine de Medici. It would seem more reasonable that the two presumed brothers were one and the same person, and that the physician of the duke of Alençon would later hold the same appointment at the court of Henri IV. What seems to prove this argument is that in 1601, Caspar Bauhin described the Jean d'Ailleboust who had described the lithopedion as "protomedicus regis" (first medical attendant to the king). Furthermore, Mme Bourgeois, who knew the protagonists of the case, clearly identified the discoverer of the lithopedion as the same man who later became a royal physician, and Fortunio Liceti mentioned, in the 1634 edition of his *De Monstrorum Natura*, that the same Jean d'Ailleboust "later became the physician of Henri IV."

According to the court chronicles, Jean d'Ailleboust began his labors as King Henri's physician in 1593, when he was already quite an old man; it is unlikely that he was born later than 1518. In 1594, he was ordered to examine Gabrielle d'Estrées, the king's mistress, who was feeling unwell. When the king inquired what ailed her, Jean d'Ailleboust bluntly said that she was pregnant. The king was furious, to say nothing of Mlle d'Estrées, but the elderly physician did not budge; he even had the effrontery to predict, much to the king's displeasure, the exact day the royal bastard would be born. Very near the day he had predicted, on June 7, 1594, Gabrielle d'Estrées delivered a healthy boy, the future César de Vendôme. Jean d'Ailleboust did not have long to enjoy the victorious outcome of his dispute with his royal master; he himself died under highly mysterious circumstances on July 24 of the same year. According to the chronicles of Sully and d'Estoile, he was poisoned by the spiteful Gabrielle d'Estrées. The king grieved the death of his honest old physician and regretted that he had spoken harshly to him before.

I conclude with a beautiful Latin poem, written by Jean d'Ailleboust in 1582 to celebrate the lithopedion of Sens. He recalled the classical myth that after the Flood, the world was repopulated by the two survivors, Deucalion and Pyrrha, who walked the earth, throwing stones behind them, which, on striking the ground, became living people:

> *Pinxit Deucalion saxis post terga repulsis*
> *Ex duro nostrum marmore molle genus:*
> *Qui fit ut infantis, mutata sorte, tenellum*
> *Nunc corpus saxis proxima membra gerat!*

An English translation may be attempted:

> *From the rocks Deucalion had dropped behind,*
> *was fashioned the living flesh of humankind:*
> *How was it then done, that a tender babe well formed*
> *was, by reversal, into solid rock transformed?*

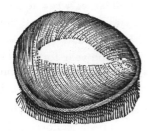

The Woman Who
Laid an Egg

THE READER OF *THE SCOTTISH GALLOVIDIAN Encyclopedia*, a curious work on Caledonian ethnography published in 1824, is likely to be surprised by the following entry, inserted somewhat haphazardly among the notes about various Scottish vernacular expressions:

> Jock Mulldroch—A fellow who lived at *Craigwaggie*, Galloway once, perhaps 150 years ago. Tradition has it that he *laid eggs*, ay eggs, larger than goose eggs, and strangely speckled black and yellow; he used to *cackle* too after he laid them.

Once a fortnight, Jock produced an egg. This was viewed with no little astonishment by the neighbors, who used to call Jock "Craigwaggie's meikle chuckie"! His mother, who had apparently received her fair share of Scottish financial astuteness, sold quite a few of the eggs as "bonny goose eggs." She set two others beneath a *chuckie* (hen) to hatch. When at last they chipped, out came two little lads clad in green. These "mongrell fairies" grew to adulthood and were well known in Galloway as Willie and Wattie Birly; despite the unique circumstances of their birth, they were accepted and well liked by everybody. They disappeared in a snowstorm "after the year forty," since their diminutive stature prevented them from keeping their heads above the drifts of snow.

If "the year forty" refers to 1740, and the assumption that he had lived about 150 years before the publication of the encyclopedia is correct, it is likely that the kilted Jock Mulldroch sat cackling on his nest some time in the late seventeenth century. To this day, Jock remains unique as the only egg-laying man in history. Even at his time, however, there had already been quite a few instances on record of *women* laying eggs. By far the most famous of them happened in the outback of Norway: in 1639, a peasant's wife, Anna Omundsdatter, laid two eggs after violent labor pains. Both eggs were accepted as her progeny by the Norwegian clergy, and one of them was sent to Denmark's leading authority on natural curiosities, Professor Olaus Wormius.

Olaus Wormius was born in Aarhus in the year 1588. The scion of a wealthy merchant family, he left Denmark at an early age for a lengthy *peregrinatio academica*, to study theology, philology, chemistry, and medicine at several leading European universities. In 1613, he returned to Copenhagen. It did not impede his academic career that Olaus Wormius married the daughter of the old professor of medicine, Thomas Fincke, and that he was the brother-in-law of the influential Caspar Bartholin. After the latter gentleman, suffering badly from the gout, retired in 1624, Olaus Wormius succeeded him as professor of medicine. For more than thirty years, Wormius remained one of Denmark's leading physicians. Every year, he wrote a dissertation on clinical or experimental medicine that was defended by one of his pupils; these medical theses demonstrated that he kept aware of the advances in contemporary anatomy and physiology. In spite of his considerable learning, he never performed any experimental research of his own; indeed, his stubborn defense of the teachings of Aristotle and Galenus and his opposition to Harvey's novel ideas about the circulation of the blood marked him as a reactionary. His only anatomical discovery of note was obtained through scrutinizing some human skulls kept at the Department of Anatomy: he found some sutural bones that may occur near the sutures of the skull and that are still called the *ossa Wormi*. Olaus Wormius was the founder of zoological and botanical lecturing in Copenhagen; during his time as professor, an anatomical theater was built, and a considerable botanical garden with medicinal herbs was planted. Five times, Wormius served as vice-chancellor of the university; he was one of the men who laid the foundation for the considerable Danish advance in natural science research during the second half of the seventeenth century.

In 1611, Olaus Wormius had been greatly impressed by the cabinet of curiosities collected by Prince Moritz of Kassel. He wanted to build up a similar repository in Copenhagen, and throughout the 1620s, he assiduously collected curious plants, minerals, and stuffed or preserved beasts and birds. In 1630, he finally built his museum in a large room in his professorial mansions. Through the years, it grew in size and importance, and many of the royal personages, noblemen, and scholars who visited Copenhagen considered it one of the sights of the town.

In an illustration to his museum catalogue, Wormius depicted the layout

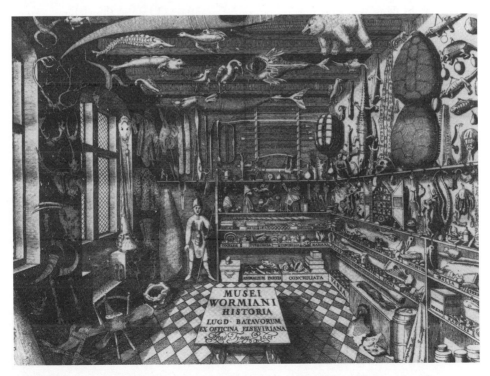

The frontispiece of the *Museum Wormianum*, which gives a fair idea of the interior of the museum.

of his museum. It was a jumble of objects from the animal, vegetable, and mineral kingdoms, arranged according to their geographical origin. Stuffed rodents, birds, and lizards crowded the shelves, and along the walls hung tortoiseshell, dried crocodiles, snakeskin, and deer's horns. Even the roof was used to suspend some prepared fish and fowl; the place of honor was taken by a stuffed polar bear's cub, which was given to Olaus Wormius by his Icelandic friend Gisle Magnusson. From other friends on the European continent, he obtained several other rare stuffed beasts, including an iguana and an armadillo. He also obtained a living coati and a penguin, both of which he kept as pets. For more than fifteen years, Wormius worked on a catalogue of the more than 1,600 objects in his museum. At the year of his death, in 1654, the manuscript was almost ready to be sent to the printers. His son, Willum Wormius, took care of the manuscript, and in 1655, the *Museum Wormianum, seu Historia Rerum Rariorum* was published. It was to become Olaus Wormius's most famous scholarly work and was widely disseminated throughout Europe.

Olaus Wormius was by no means unaffected by the flourishing superstition and fanaticism of his time. He took astrology quite seriously and considered the position of the moon to be of importance for the actions of various medicines. Several preparations in the Museum Wormianum, like a lemming presumed to have fallen from the skies, and a piece of the skin of the fabulous Vegetable Lamb of Tartary, illustrate his interest in the old monster lore. His friend Jan de Laët had given him a rib and several small bones from a mermaid caught by Portuguese sailors off the coast of Angola, where these creatures were said to be of common occurrence in the frothy waves. Learned men in Portugal used balls, or rather suppositories, made from the ribs of the poor sirens as a cure for hemorrhoids—indeed, a far from poetic use of the remains of the sweet-tongued daughters of the ocean!

Some historians of science have reproached Olaus Wormius for his credulity and superstition, but he was in fact the man who put an end to one of the hoariest zoological myths of all: that of the unicorn. This fabulous beast was well known among early seventeenth-century naturalists, and few doubted its existence, although no living or dead specimen had ever been shown in Europe. Wormius's predecessor Caspar Bartholin wrote a treatise on the unicorn in 1628 and stated that as long as some distant parts of the globe had not been searched by explorers, there was still hope that a unicorn would once be found in some desolate part. The unicorn was usually depicted as a wild and fiery horse, with a long, spirally turned horn in the middle of its brow. The unicorn's horn was a valuable museum exhibit, and no prince wanted his museum to be without one; it was also presumed to have miraculous medicinal properties. Olaus Wormius was one of the few who doubted the unicorn's existence. With some reason, he found it highly suspicious that just the horn, and no other parts of this fabulous beast, had ever been preserved. In 1636, he visited a friend, Chancellor Christian Fries, to discuss the unicorn. He particularly regretted that no complete cranium of a unicorn, with the horn in situ, existed. The chancellor replied that he had one in his private collection! Wormius examined it thoroughly and found evidence that it was certainly not the cranium of a four-footed beast, but of an animal of the whale kind, although smaller in size; even the blowholes for water were present. He concluded that the "unicorn's horn" was really the horn of a particular type of whale occurring in Scandinavian waters. His treatise on the unicorn, published in 1638, spread rapidly among European scholars and probably caused a rapid decline in the price of the valuable horns. Bishop Thorlak Skulason of Iceland provided Wormius with a complete drawing of the narwhal, including its long pointed horn; he later published it in his *Museum Wormianum*.

❧

Anna Omundsdatter, the modest and pious wife of the farmer Gudbrand Erlandsen, lived in the village of Sundby near Stavanger in Norway. They had been married for many years and had twelve children alive. Throughout their worthy and strenuous lives, they had achieved nothing to distinguish themselves compared to the other peasant families in the neighborhood. In early March 1638, Wife Anna was taken ill, with diffuse symptoms of weakness and vertigo; the local doctor, clergyman, and quack made their various diagnoses but were incapable of curing her. Her illness went on for more than a year. In the afternoon of April 17, 1639, she felt the early throes of childbirth and sent her husband to call the neighbor women to help her, in the belief that she was to give birth. In the evening, her labor pains increased, but instead of bearing a child, she laid an egg, to the horror and surprise of all those present. The egg looked rather like a hen's egg, and although Anna Omundsdatter wanted to preserve it, one of the neighbor women was bold enough to break the egg to see what was inside its shell; it proved to have a white and a yolk, just like an ordinary hen's egg. The following day, Wife Anna again fell into labor, and there was much speculation what prodigious birth would follow. Anna Omundsdatter did not disappoint these onlookers, as she laid another egg similar to the one laid the day before. She begged that the spectators should not break or destroy it, since she was certain that higher powers would punish both her and the villagers. Accordingly, the second egg was preserved with great care. A runner was sent to the rectory of Näs to tell the tale of these great wonders. Three clergymen, the curates Ericus Vestergaard, Rotalph Rakestad, and Thor Venes, were sent to Sundby, like the Three Kings, as witnesses of the miraculous birth. After they consulted Dr. Paul Tranius, the rector of Näs, the three curates wrote a detailed account of what had occurred; the wives Anna Grim, Elin Rudstad, Gyro Rustad, and Catharina Sundby testified that there was no evidence of fraud and that they had all witnessed the laying of the two miraculous eggs. All three clergymen signed this document and stamped it with their seals.

Dr. Tranius, into whose possession the egg had been passed, apparently considered that such a medical sensation was far beyond his field of expertise. He sent both the egg and the signed testimony of the witnesses to Olaus Wormius, whose interest in such wonders was well known in Scandinavia. Once the egg was in Copenhagen, Olaus Wormius examined it closely. He found that the egg was quite similar to an ordinary hen's egg with regard to size and shape, except that the whitish color common to fresh hen's eggs had been overtaken by a darker hue, like that of a putrefying egg. The rumor of the Norwegian miracle swiftly spread throughout Europe, and several doctors and collectors of curiosities wrote to Olaus Wormius, asking whether the woman's egg was for sale. Olaus Wormius answered in the negative, since he wanted to keep this wonder of wonders for his own museum. He never published any separate account of the egg-laying woman, but saved the story for his forthcoming museum catalogue. In a letter to his curious brother-in-law Henrik Motzfelt, written in January 1644, he discussed the egg-laying woman of Norway. Although the egg seemed very similar to that of a hen, Olaus Wormius did not suspect a fraud; the unanimous testimony of the witnesses and the certificate of the three curates did not fail to impress him. He also attached significance to the fact that Anna Omundsdatter had complained that the labor pains at the time of her laying the egg much exceeded those at her previous childbirths; indeed, she had been bedridden for several weeks after her abnormal confinement. Wormius did not think that the egg had developed naturally, but that the Devil had tormented the unhappy woman by exchanging her unborn child for an egg. In the twenty-first chapter of his *Museum Wormianum*, dedicated to his collection of eggs and birds' nests, Wormius put his famous *Ovum magicum*, the magical egg from Norway, in the place of honor. Once more, Wormius repeated his conviction that Anna Omundsdatter had been possessed by the Devil, and that the egg had been sired by the Prince of Darkness. He quoted a report by the old Cornelius Gemma concerning the presence of "needles, knives, razors, insects and other objects" within the bodies of individuals possessed by the Devil, either encapsulated in boils or hidden in the female genital system.

&

The old annals of monstrous births contain many idle tales of women giving birth to all kinds of unexpected objects. Had Olaus Wormius been better read in the anecdotal reports of medieval and ancient teratology, he might have found stories far stranger than the idle fantasies of Cornelius Gemma, which had little relevance to the Norwegian miracle. The elder Pliny mentioned the Roman lady Alcippa who gave birth to an elephant, and another lady who was delivered of a serpent. The medieval chronicler Julius Obsequens described two Italian women, one of whom had given birth to a dog and the other a cat. In 1278, a Swiss lady gave birth to a lion cub. In his *Monstrorum Historia*, the famous Italian savant Count Ulysses Aldrovandi had much to say about the strange births of the sixteenth and seventeenth centuries. In 1531, a woman accursed by the Devil gave birth to an unprepossessing set of triplets: a human head, a four-legged serpent, and a piglet. A lady from Thüringen gave birth to a toad; other women gave birth to piglets and chickens. Queen Bertha, who had been excommunicated for marrying her cousin Robert the Pious, gave birth to a child with the head and neck of a goose. According to the monks of Corbie, a French lady had given birth to a black cat, which was burned alive at the orders of the Church, since only the Devil could be the father of such a monstrous birth.

Perhaps the most ridiculous of these idle tales, which were all seriously

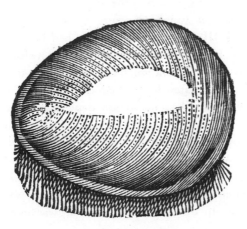

The magical egg of Norway, as depicted in the 1655 edition of the *Museum Wormianum*.

58   debated in the obstetrical literature of the time, was reported in the collected medical observations of the old Salmuth. A noble countess had given birth to an infant whose skin was discolored red on one side. The reason for this, stated the learned observer, was that within the womb there also lived a little bird without feathers, which had bitten and wounded the wretched child. The featherless bird was pulled out from its lair by the midwife, but it gave a shrill squeak, freed itself by pecking her hand with its sharp beak, leapt off the table, and ran swiftly along the floor of the room. Nowadays, the doctors and midwives would have succumbed to a series of severe nervous attacks when faced with such a perilous situation, resembling a scene from one of the most exaggerated horror movies of the present time; their sixteenth-century counterparts dashed after the bird, caught it with a rugby tackle, and smothered it with the countess's bed pillows.

There were also quite a few old tales of women laying eggs. The earliest one was that of Leda, who laid two eggs after having consorted with Zeus in the form of a swan; both of these eggs produced twins: Castor and Pollux in one and Helen and Clytaemnestra in the other. In the *Monstrorum Historia*, Ulysses Aldrovandi repeated a fanciful tale, which originated with the chronicler Conradus Lycosthenes, about the moon being populated by gigantic, humanoid, oviparous creatures. In a remarkable illustration, a woman is depicted sitting on her eggs in a huge basin. Ambroise Paré never encountered any egg-laying women, but he did see a very peculiar egg, which seemed to contain a human head. It was discovered in 1569 and later passed into the collection of King Charles of France.

In the seventeenth and eighteenth centuries, the foremost museum in Denmark was the *Kunst-kammer*, or Royal Museum, at Copenhagen Castle, founded by King Frederick III. This king previously had been a learned cleric, becoming archbishop of Bremen. A patron of the arts, he founded the Royal Library of Copenhagen and spent much time and money to establish his great museum. To an even greater degree than that of Olaus Wormius, the Royal Museum was planned to be a microcosm depicting the world that surrounded it. It contained a wealth of stuffed animals, birds, and fish; prepared insects, plants, and fungi; antiquities, ethnographical objects, coins, medals, and objets d'art. When the king received word that the heirs of Olaus Wormius were willing to sell their father's collection, he purchased the entire Museum Wormianum, including the magical egg, which was a treasured part of the collection. In July 1655, the museum was moved from

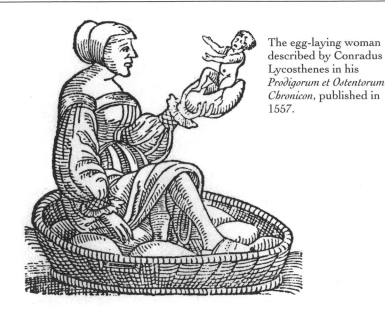

The egg-laying woman
described by Conradus
Lycosthenes in his
*Prodigorum et Ostentorum
Chronicon*, published in
1557.

Wormius's house to the royal castle. The earliest inventory of the Kunst-
kammer, made in 1674, stated that the magical egg from Norway was kept in
a box on top of a high chest of drawers.

Thomas Bartholin, Olaus Wormius's foremost pupil, was even more interested in human abnormalities. He had a real scientific genius and was one
of the founders of modern anatomy, through his discovery of the lymphatic
system. Like Wormius, he was influenced by the superstitious old monster
medicine, and some of the most ridiculous tales can be found interspersed
among his valuable anatomical and pathological discoveries in his collection
of case reports, *Historiarum Anatomicarum Rariorum*. Thomas Bartholin described spontaneous human combustion, a cow giving birth to puppies, and
a woman who was frightened by a cat while pregnant and who later had a
daughter with a cat's head. One of his case reports concerned a noblewoman
of Elsinore who gave birth to a large rat, which darted out of its lair and
eluded the pursuing obstetricians and midwives by creeping down a crack in
the floor of the bedchamber, never to be seen again. Another told of a cat in
Frederiksborg, which surprised its owner by giving birth to kittens by its
mouth. He was also interested in the magical egg of Norway. Unlike
Wormius, Thomas Bartholin considered it unlikely that the egg had been
born by the natural route, or indeed that Anna Omundsdatter had been possessed by the Devil. He questioned whether the magical egg had developed

in the uterus or in the rectum, and quoted an observation by the old Salmuth, who claimed to have seen an egg laid by a woman. When opened, the egg proved to contain a two-headed, evil-looking worm. If Anna Omundsdatter's egg really came from the womb, the case was even more interesting. Thomas Bartholin knew well that William Harvey had published his famous *Exercitationes de Generatione Animalium*, in which it was first postulated that the human being, and all other mammals, had once originated in an egg. Many other anatomists had difficulties accepting this novel concept, but not the visionary and far-sighted Thomas Bartholin, who earlier had been one of Harvey's henchmen in the question of the circulation of blood. He entered the realm of high speculation, however, when he attempted to relate Wife Anna's egg to Harvey's great theory.

In 1696, the earliest proper catalogue of the Royal Museum of Copenhagen was written by Thomas Bartholin's brother-in-law, Holger Jacobsen, the same individual who had traveled to London to examine the Hairy Maid. Jacobsen's impressive *Musaeum Regium* became one of the finest museum catalogues in this time of many great collectors. Already on the second page was a thorough description of Olaus Wormius's magical egg; in a later edition of the catalogue, published in 1710, the egg was also included in one of the plates, using the image previously reproduced in the *Museaum Wormianum*. Holger Jacobsen agreed with Thomas Bartholin that the egg was unlikely to have been created through magic, but that it probably had been engendered by natural means. By this time, Regnier de Graaf had discovered the anatomy of the ovaries, and that the fertilized ova passed to the uterus via the fallopian tubes. Jacobsen had observed that hens and other domestic birds sometimes laid eggs without shells; was it then any more anomalous that a woman would lay an extraordinary large egg with a shell, through any defect in its natural development?

Holger Jacobsen had also searched the contemporary medical literature for similar instances of women laying eggs. The astonishing outcome of his search was that after Thomas Bartholin's description of the Norwegian miracle, several European scholars and medical men published similar case reports of women laying eggs; indeed, a veritable epidemic of abnormal egg-laying had occurred throughout Europe during the past fifty years. In 1671, the Dane Johan Rhode saw a woman, living near Vincentium, lay an egg after usual labor pains. A similar occurrence was described by the Dutchman Antonius de Heyde. In his account of this miraculous birth, he insulted Anna Omundsdatter by querying whether there was a large rooster on the farm in Sundby, and if the egg may have been the hideous result of an illicit affair with this amorous bird. Thomas Bartholin provided another Danish case in the book *De insolitis Partus Viis*. A lady in Copenhagen, pregnant since twelve weeks, awoke in the middle of the night with a colicky pain; she believed she would pass wind, but instead, to her great astonishment and terror, she laid an egg.

In 1669, a German woman laid an egg under circumstances much resembling those of the Norwegian miracle. She was six months pregnant, and after violent labor pains, she laid an egg, which was larger than that of a pigeon but smaller than that of a hen. The egg was broken and examined by Dr. Hieronymus Conrad Virdung. It seemed to contain a minute human fetus inside its usual membranes, but with a hard, calcified eggshell surrounding it. Like Thomas Bartholin, Dr. Virdung was well aware of Harvey's work on generation, and he offered the egg-laying woman as another argument that human beings really originated in an egg.

Another German scholar, Dr. Georg Sebastian Jungius, described an even greater curiosity, the famous Egg-laying Dog of Vienna. This animal, a large mongrel cur, laid many large eggs through the anus. After each of these strange births, it seemed weak and exhausted, but it soon recovered from its confinements and was jumping about its owner, who showed it as a curiosity in a popular show. To impress his spectators and to show that the eggs were genuine, the enterprising Austrian broke one of the dog's eggs, fried it in a pan, and ate it. In spite of his scientific curiosity, Dr. Jungius did not want to taste the egg; nevertheless, he felt convinced that the eggs were really produced inside the dog. In his *Cynographia Curiosa*, published in 1685, the zoologist Christian Paullin declared himself quite unconvinced, however: the notion that a dog could lay eggs was contrary to both sense and reason, and the bizarre dog show in Vienna had been a disgusting fraud.

❧

The only reasonable explanation of the tale of the magical egg of Norway is that it must have been a deliberate fraud: Anna Omundsdatter must have pretended to give birth to the eggs, with enough skill to deceive her helpers. It is impossible to figure out any exact motive for this or to determine if some other person might have put her up to it. It is unlikely that an illiterate Norwegian peasant's wife knew the tale of Leda and the swan, but the village gossips may have told some garbled version of this or any other old tale of egg-laying women. Although the old Æsir cult contained no element of egg-laying women, there definitely was, at this time, a Scandinavian tradition of mighty heroes and Vikings born from eggs. An important element in the legend of the hero Holger Danske, who lived in France during the time of Charlemagne, is that he would once be reborn from an egg laid by a magpie, and return to save Denmark from destruction. There is no Norwegian national hero of this kind, but several tales of Vikings or "strong boys" born from eggs were current at the time. It should be noted, in this context, that Anna Omundsdatter said that she was sure the egg had supernatural properties and that it was inadvisable to break it. It is likely that not only the three curates, but also throngs of curious people from all over Europe, came to view the magical egg and the woman who laid it; Anna Omundsdatter must have been revered among her neighbors as the only egg-laying woman in history. If her purpose was to obtain long-lasting herostratic fame before posterity, she has succeeded: her short biography has been repeated in quite a few books on Scandinavian medical history.

The best known of all the women who gave birth to animals or other unexpected objects was Mary Toft, of Godalming in Surrey. In 1726, she managed to trick King George I, the Prince of Wales, and the court medical experts that she had given birth to seventeen rabbits. The court anatomist, Dr. Nathaniel St. André, wrote a scholarly treatise about this miracle. It was later exposed, however, that Mary had bought the rabbits in the marketplace, before pretending to give birth to them with enough skill to trick the dull-witted "experts" who examined her. It is recorded, in M. Witkowski's curious *Histoire des accouchements chez tous les peuples*, that just a few years after the Mary Toft scandal, a Frenchwoman laid two eggs, which were taken to the Academy of Sciences in Paris. The eggs were incubated by the academicians, and two pigeon chicks hatched in due course. The birds were exhibited before a commission of scientists, who concluded that they had been imposed upon. The ultimate fate of this egg-laying Frenchwoman is not known.

What finally happened to the magical egg of Copenhagen? As late as 1726, it was mentioned in a novel catalogue of the foremost preparations in the royal collections, but in later inventories, the egg appeared to have lost its former fame and glory. It remained at the Royal Museum until 1824. That year, the old museum building was emptied at the orders of the court marshal, Adam Wilhelm Hauch, and the museum curator, Johan Conrad Spengler; the former royal collection was to be split up to form parts of the state museums of antiquities, art, and natural history. About one-third of the old Royal Museum is still kept in this way, but more than 90 percent of the specimens relating to medicine and natural history have been lost, discarded, sold, or destroyed. Only thirty-one objects remain from the old Museum Wormianum, few of them from its section for natural sciences. Although the magical egg had been treasured by Wormius, Bartholin, and King Frederick III, the museum officials decided that this bizarre remnant of seventeenth-century superstition was not worth preserving. In 1824, many of the discarded specimens from the Royal Museum were sold in a series of public auctions. Listed as lot no. 241 in the catalogue is "a box of different natural history specimens," containing Olaus Wormius's siren's hands and the magical egg. An unnamed Dane bought this box for the not-unreasonable sum of one mark in silver, which he paid in cash. It is unknown how he planned to use these objects, and where they are today; if it was his intention to use the 186-year-old egg in an omelet, he was to face a grave disappointment.

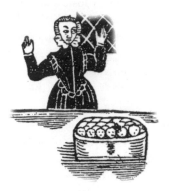

The Strangest Miracle
in the World

I N MAY 1660, THE FAMOUS DIARIST SAMUEL
Pepys visited the Netherlands. He traveled to the village of Loosduinen,
which at first did not impress him greatly: it was "a little small village"
and at the tavern were "a great many Dutch boors eating of fish in a boorish
manner." Although the villagers were "very merry in their way," Samuel
Pepys did not remain long in their company; he had come to Loosduinen to
see a memorial of "the strangest miracle in the world," a monument so justly
famous that many thousands of people had already made the same pilgrim-
age to the sleepy little Dutch village. He went to the church of Loosduinen,
where he saw a wooden tablet with an inscription relating the story of
Countess Margaret of Henneberg, who had given birth to 365 children at
one time, on Good Friday in the year 1276. Samuel Pepys also saw the two
basins in which the children had been baptized.

Although the church of Loosduinen has changed its appearance since
the time of Samuel Pepys, the wooden plates commemorating Countess
Margaret and her strange birth of 365 children can still be seen, hanging on

the church wall. The Dutch text is on the left and the Latin on the right. An English translation is as follows:

> Margaret, the wife of Herman Count of Henneberg, daughter of Floris IV, Count of Holland and Zeeland, and sister of Willem, King of Rome and later Emperor of the Realm . . . . This noble Countess, who was then about 42 years old, was on Good Friday 1276, at about 9 o'clock, brought to bed of 365 children, who were all baptized in two basins by Guido, Suffragan of Utrecht; The boys were all christened Jan and the girls Elizabeth; the children all died, together with their mother, and were buried here in the church of Loosduinen; This happened because the Countess had met a poor woman who was carrying a pair of twins in her arms, and the Countess, being amazed, had insulted her by declaring these twins must have two different fathers. The poor woman, being annoyed, had cursed the Countess by wishing that she herself would at one gestation have as many children as there are days in a year, and this miraculously happened, as related here on this tablet, from handwritten as well as printed old chronicles. God may therefore be feared, honored and praised to all eternity. Amen.

Two basins, representing the ones in which the 365 children were baptized, are still hanging over the wooden tablets. In the present day, just like in Samuel Pepys's time, the church of Loosduinen is visited yearly by several thousand people interested in the legend of Countess Margaret and her 365 children, henceforth referred to as "the Legend." There is much speculation about the tradition's origins and whether the whole thing is fabulous or the Legend might contain a grain of truth; despite the work of many scholars, these problems have never been solved satisfactorily.

The Countess in History

There is no doubt at all that Margaret of Henneberg was a historical person. She was born in 1234, the daughter of Floris IV, count of Holland and Zeeland, and his wife Machteld of Brabant. Her eldest brother Willem was a distinguished warrior and nobleman. At Pentecost 1249, Countess Margaret was married to Count Herman von Henneberg, a distinguished German nobleman who belonged to the ruling family of Henneberg-Coburg. An ambi-

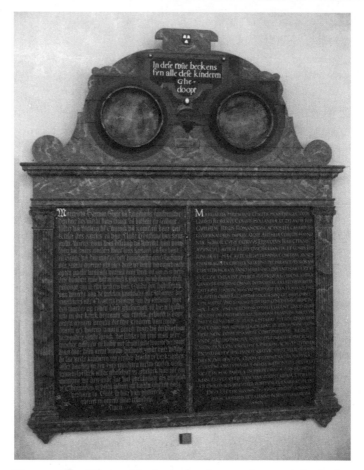

The wooden tablets and the basins, as they can be seen today in the church of Loosduinen Abbey. Reproduced by permission of the Stichting oud Loosduinen.

tious warrior in the civil wars that ravaged Germany at this time, he aspired to become king of the Holy Roman Empire and ruler of the German states. In the election arranged in 1246, he failed to gain the crown, and Countess Margaret's brother Willem was elected king of the Holy Roman Empire in his place. To gain further influence in Germany, Willem wanted the friendship of Count Herman, and at length he managed to win over the influential count to his own side. King Willem arranged the marriage between Margaret and Count Herman to strengthen this alliance further.

The count and countess of Henneberg had their permanent residence at Coburg, but they also had a castle near Loosduinen, at Hooghe Werf. The first child of the Hennebergs, a son named Herman, who died very young, was buried in the church of Loosduinen Abbey in 1250. Countess Margaret was deeply religious, and after the death of her son, she spent much time with the nuns in the Loosduinen convent. Her seal, a drawing of which has been kept for posterity, has on one side a seated woman with a book in her lap, apparently the countess herself, and on the reverse the crest of the Hennebergs, a hen standing on the top of a hill. Countess Margaret's mother, Machteld van Holland, died in 1267. A letter from Countess Margaret, written on May 12, 1273, concerning the distribution of the inheritance between Margaret and her sister Aleide van Henegouwen, is reproduced in the *Oorkondenboek* of Holland. Another letter, from the Roman king Rudolph, written on January 13, 1276, mentioned that the Hennebergs had at this time a son and heir named Poppo (or Boppo). Probably, Poppo was about twenty years old at this time. The Hennebergs also had a daughter named Jutta, who was married to Margrave Otto of Brandenburg in 1268. Nowhere is it stated that Poppo and Jutta were twins.

On Good Friday 1276, tragedy struck the Henneberg family. Countess Margaret, who was then staying at Loosduinen, either at the convent or at the castle at Hooghe Werf, was taken ill and died. There is no record implying that she had any lingering illness, but the sources are incomplete, since the event took place more than seven hundred years ago. Count Floris V, Margaret's nephew, visited her when she was very ill and wrote a letter at her request, distributing various gifts and bequests to two ladies-in-waiting. Jutta, the daughter and heiress of the countess, objected strongly to this last-minute will. The original documents quoted in these accounts do not mention any miraculous birth. Nor do other contemporary records mention any extraordinary circumstances about the deathbed of Margaret of Henneberg. The countess was buried in the church of Loosduinen Abbey. Although some other tombs, probably those of Countess Margaret's mother Machteld of Brabant and her nephew Floris V, were discovered in the Loosduinen church during restoration work, the exact location of Countess Margaret's tomb and that of her son Herman is unknown. The inscription on the sarcophagus of Countess Margaret does not mention any extraordinary circumstances attached to her death. Nor do two documents written by Count Herman of Henneberg, in 1281 and 1282, concerning the hereditary rights of his children after the death of his wife. They explicitly state that both

68   Poppo and Jutta were still living, and that the Hennebergs had no other children alive.

The Earliest Mentions of the Legend

As we have seen, the scarce contemporary sources admit nothing remarkable about the deathbed of Countess Margaret. The earliest document mentioning her strange birth of 365 children at one time is the late-fourteenth-century Tabula of Egmond, which is kept in the Utrecht University Library. It is an annotated chronicle of notable events from 863 until the 1300s. For the year 1276, it reads:

Jacob Stellingwerf's early eighteenth-century drawing of the Henneberg castle. Reproduced by permission of the Stichting oud Loosduinen.

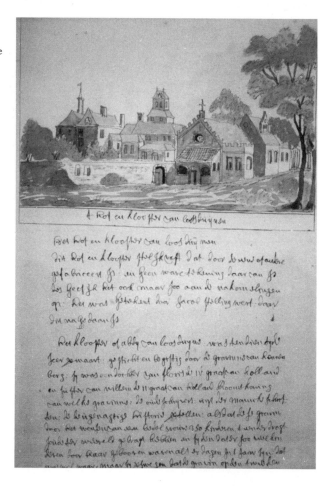

> During Easter, Countess Margaret of Henneberg gave birth to 364 sons and daughters and died quietly, together with them. Her tomb is in Loosduinen, with a stone sarcophagus adorned with an epitaph in metal letters . . .

This cryptic note leaves several matters unexplained. Like the contemporary sources, it places the death of the countess in 1276, during Easter. Then follows the brief and stark statement about the 364 sons and daughters, and that she died with them. Why the epitaph on the countess's sarcophagus does not mention her numerous children is left unexplained; such a birth was surely the most remarkable circumstance in the life of this pious and venerable lady.

Another important fourteenth-century source on the Legend is the *Kronyk van Holland*, by "de Clerc uit de laage landen bij der see," which was written between 1349 and 1356. It is not known whether the writer of this chronicle was named de Clerc or whether he was a clerk (secretary) of some other writer. He wrote that the countess did not believe that a woman could have more than one child at one birth by the same father. She said that a woman who gave birth to twins must have had several men, and refused to believe any other opinion. Through the power of God, she was punished for her stubborn refusal to believe that twins could not have the same father, and gave birth to 365 minute children, who were all baptized in a great basin. They were as large as mice, and all died together.

A third version of the Loosduinen miracle can be found in the *Chronica Novella* of Hermann Korner, a German historiographer; this work was prepared between 1416 and 1435. Under the year 1300, Korner tells the following strange story:

> In the city of The Hague lived a noble lady named Katherine. She was married to a knight named Simon, who was greatly valued by all, including King Willem II. Since she was merry in her ways, and took pleasure in meeting people, she was generally much liked, and a popular guest at feasts and gatherings. Only the Countess Margaret, the wife of Count Johan of Holland, was her enemy, and the more the others revered the honorable Katherine, the more she hated her. It then happened that Katherine became pregnant by her lawful husband, and bore him twin boys. When the Countess heard of this, she said "This is the result of the immoral life of this woman, since I believe

that it is as impossible for a woman to bring forth twins by one and the same father, as it is for me to give birth to as many children as there are days in the year." Due to these words from the Countess, Simon divorced his wife, and she was imprisoned in a convent. Here, she fervently prayed to God, that he would reveal her innocence, and her prayers were heard. Shortly after, the Countess gave birth to 364 children at once; they were all small like crabs, although completely human in structure, and with all members intact; when the midwives had put them in a large basin, they were baptized in holy water. After that, they all died, every one of them. . . . When Simon had been convinced of his wife's innocence, he took her back as his wife with much ceremony. He again loved her, and they lived happily together.

Korner's version of the Legend follows that of de Clerc in several respects. In both, the protagonist is a countess of Holland, and she is punished by God for her erroneous belief that twins must have different fathers. The children are likened to small animals, they are baptized in a basin, and then they die. While de Clerc has the countess survive the strange birth, Korner does not mention that she dies. These similarities may indicate either that Korner knew of the de Clerc version, or more likely, that they share a common source, which is not known. There are also several discrepancies between de Clerc's and Korner's versions, some of which are of importance. Firstly, Korner makes the story more dramatic by naming all the main protagonists. Another important development is that the countess now insults one specific woman by her erroneous belief, rather than merely stating her opinion that a woman bearing twins must be an adulteress. This version may actually be the original one.

The *Croonijcke van Hollandt* of Jan van Naaldwijck provides some further information. It is beautifully written, with some curious illustrations, but was badly damaged by fire in 1731, when Sir Robert Cotton's manuscript collection was still in private ownership. Had it not been tossed from the window of Ashburnham House by one of the Cottonian trustees, it would have been consumed by the flames. The remaining text in the section on Countess Margaret contains several new details. Firstly, that her husband had been present in Loosduinen on that fateful Good Friday. Apparently, Jan van Naaldwijck thinks it amusing that Count Herman invited several princes to his Loosduinen castle, for them to become godfathers of his child; he would have had to invite half the German nobility for them to suffice for his numerous offspring! An important new development in the versions of Aurelius and van Naaldwijck is that a poor beggar woman with twins was insulted by the haughty countess, and that her prayers to God called down his wrath on Countess Margaret. This version might be an adaptation from de Clerc, but it is much more powerful; it would recur in almost every later retelling of the Legend. The noble witnesses and the naming of the children Jan and Elisabeth by Bishop Guido are new details added by Jan van Naaldwijck, and their source is unknown; he might have had access to earlier chronicles, or else, since he lived near Loosduinen, he was in a very good position to absorb elements of local tradition.

Some Sixteenth-Century Sources on the Legend

In the sixteenth century, the Legend was mentioned in many historical books, cosmographies, and books on notable events. A very full account was published by the historian Ludovico Guicciardini in 1567. He had obviously been to Loosduinen, since he quoted the epitaph and the text on the tablets quite correctly. Already during this time, several perverted versions of the Legend were current. One of them, supported by the *De Monstris* of Irenaeus, said that Margaret, countess of Cleve, had given birth to 365 children in 1555; another, on the authority of Jobus Fincelius, that she had been a princess of Ireland, who had given birth to 364 children in the year 1313. The *Hennebergische Chronica*, written by Cyriacus Spangenberg and published in 1599, hints that a Latin epitaph of Countess Margaret, giving the number of children as 364, half of them boys named Johannes and the other half girls named Elisabeth, was really inscribed somewhere in the Loosduinen church. Some handwritten notes in the copy of the *Hennebergische Chronica* that is kept in the Dresden National Library affirm that this was really the case, and that in the late 1500s, some kind of tombstone or monument could be seen inside the church. These annotations were made by the German historian Nathaniel Carolus. He had received a letter from the countess of Stolberg, who was related to the Henneberg family. The sister of this noble lady had been in the Loosduinen church more than once and seen the basin in which the children were baptized, as well as "the monument of the tombstone and the picture." On the wall was written:

Here were baptized 365 children
born on one and the same day
through one woman:
Recognize oh people the power of God Almighty.

A castle at the Dutch village Pouderoyen was called Arx Puerorum, since it had 365 windows, one for each of the children of the countess.

Already in the early sixteenth century, Loosduinen and its abbey had become famous as a result of the Legend of Countess Margaret. The monk Wilhelmus of Heda, who was canon of Utrecht, and who died in 1525, related that a painting or sculpture was kept in the church to illustrate the Legend. Furthermore, a wooden tablet was hanging on the wall, and with it a basin, in which Countess Margaret's children had been baptized. It was the habit of childless women to come to Loosduinen Abbey and wash their hands in the basin, hoping that the potent magic of the Legend would make them fertile again. It is recorded that in 1549, Crown Prince Philip of Spain visited Loosduinen; he went to the abbey and heard the story of the Legend. In 1572, there was a civil war in Holland, between Philip II and the insurgent troops of William of Orange. The abbey of Loosduinen was demolished by the Spanish troops, in order to prevent the insurgents from using it as a fortress. When the adherents of William of Orange occupied Loosduinen, the old abbey was completely ruined, and the old wooden tablet, as well as the original basin, were among the items destroyed by the iconoclasts. Some years later, when the Loosduinen Abbey became a Protestant church, one of its first rectors, Reverend Jacobus Meursius, wanted to revive the Legend. He had a new wooden tablet made, with another text (the one quoted initially) in both Dutch and Latin. Two copper basins, which the rector bought in a shop in Delft, were hung on each side of this inscription. The basins revered in the church today are thus nothing more than counterfeits. The superstitious people did not care about this: it is recorded that even after the Reformation, many sterile women came to Loosduinen to wash their hands in the basins the rector had hung up for them.

Another commemorative plate was made in these years; it was not hung in the church, but in the Loosduinen tavern "Het wapen van de Prins van Oranje"; an inscription dates it to be "from the time of Prince Mauritz," that is, before 1625. It is decorated with a drawing by Pieter Kaerius, dating from the early 1600s. Today, it hangs on the northern side of the Loosduinen Abbey church. On the top of the plate are the images of the two basins, and the text "Door Duynen Bevrijdt," implying that Loosduinen was protected from the sea by the dunes. The drawing of Pieter Kaerius was issued as a print in France during the seventeenth century. On the far left can be seen "Les enfants dans le bassin" and on the right the poor countess with her midwives, who are busy boiling water and preparing fresh linen. The Kaerius drawing is not the only illustration of the Legend. In the chapel of the Castle Thierberg in Kufstein is a painting by Michael Waginger, depicting both its main events. On the left, the countess insults the poor beggar woman (who, incidentally, is carrying triplets), and on the right, the minute children are baptized by the bishop, in the presence of noblemen and church dignitaries.

Early Pilgrims to Loosduinen

The accounts of the Legend in many sixteenth-century popular and scholarly works made it well known throughout Europe. Many travelers visited the church of Loosduinen to see and admire the basins and inscription, some of them crossing half the continent to see it with their own eyes. The English nation seems to have been particularly interested in the countess and her nu-

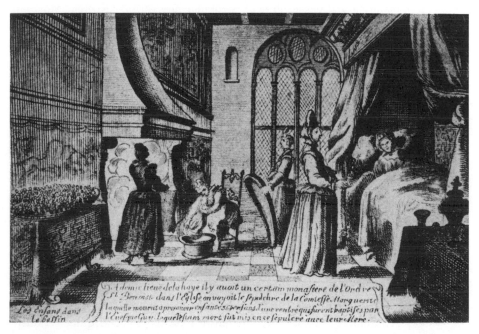

A seventeenth-century French engraving of the Pieter Kaerius drawing. From the author's collection.

merous brood. Already in 1593, Mr. Fynes Moryson visited "the village Lausdune" and its church during a stay in The Hague. He copied the text on the monument, which he was apparently already acquainted with, since the earl of Leicester had taken another copy of it to England. The two brass basins were hanging on the church wall. In 1622, James Howell went to The Hague and Loosduinen to see:

> a Church-Monument, where an Earl and a Lady are Engraven
> with Three Hundred Sixty Five Children about them, which
> were all Delivered at one Birth; they were half Male, half Fe-
> male; the Bason hangs in the Church which carried them to be
> Christened, and the Bishops name who did it.

On September 1, 1641, the diarist John Evelyn rode out from The Hague to visit "the church of *Lysdun*, a desolate place," where he saw "the monument of the woman, pretended to have been a countess of Holland, re-ported to have had as many children at one birth as there are days in the year." He also saw the basins and "a large description of the matter-of-fact in a frame of carved work." It is of particular interest that Evelyn, Moryson, and Howell all mentioned a monument in the church; according to Howell, this monument had the figure of the count and countess, with their 365 chil-dren about them. This strongly hints that in the early 1600s, there was some kind of wood carving in the church, to commemorate the Legend and its ori-gin. There is no later mention of this monument; it was certainly not to be found in the church in the late 1600s. The wooden tablets with the Dutch and Latin versions of the Legend, which can be seen today in the Loos-duinen Abbey church, are the same ones seen by these writers at the turn of the seventeenth century.

In 1693, Loosduinen was visited by the Danish Judge Mathias Poulsen, who went to the church to see "a tablet on the right side of the Alter, on which is written the story of the 365 children born at one time by the Countess of Henneberg." In September 1719, the English traveler John Rawlinson went to Loosduinen to see the memorials there. The two basins were hanging on the north side of the church, near the pulpit, and Mr. Rawl-inson also saw the wooden tablet with its inscription in Dutch and Latin. Another early eighteenth-century visitor to Loosduinen was the French trav-eler Maximilien Misson. He apparently took the Legend quite seriously, since he was taken to task by M. de Blainville, the erstwhile ambassador to

London who had visited Loosduinen in the 1730s and seen the church, basins, and wooden tablets. It was de Blainville's decided opinion that the old story had not the least air of probability, and that the histories of these times were full of similar untruthful accounts of wonderful happenings.

The Legend in Poetry

The earliest appearance of the Legend in poetry occurs in a late sixteenth-century Spanish song. A poor woman, followed by her numerous children, went begging. She encountered "madama Margarita," who was a princess of Ireland. When the noble lady saw the many children, she taunted the beggar woman by presuming that they all had different fathers. The poor woman fell on her knees and called on God to punish "madama Margarita," wishing that she would herself have more children than she could count and tell apart. Soon after, the princess gave birth to 360 children, all as small as young mice, but alive and healthy. A bishop baptized them all in a silver basin, which was later exhibited in a church. It was once seen there by Emperor Charles of Spain.

In the early 1600s, the Legend was described in several well-known English books. In 1608, Edward Grimeston's *General Historie of the Netherlands* appeared, and in 1611 Coryat's *Crudities*; both had long and dramatic accounts of the Legend. Coryat added that the story of Countess Margaret "is so absolutely true, as nothing in the world more." Another contemporary work, John Stow's *Annales; or, A General Chronicle of England*, gives the insults of the haughty countess toward the poor woman with quadruplets as "Goe gette thou hence thou harlotte, thou shalt neuer make me beleeue, but those thy brattes had foure Fathers, thou insatiate strumpet!" Either of these works may have inspired an illustrated black-letter ballad entitled *The Lamenting Lady*, printed in London in 1620. This anonymous, twenty-one-stanza poem was directly inspired by the Legend. As a Divine punishment for her insults toward a poor woman with twins, an unnamed noble lady gives birth to as many infants as there are days in a year, "in rememberance whereof, there is now a monument builded in the Citty of *Lowdon*, as many English men now liuing in *Lowdon*, can truely testifie the same and hath seene it." The writer himself probably had not seen the church and the monument, and he changed the story as it suited him. The childless noblewoman envies the poor beggar woman who has twin children, and taunts her with the words:

Thou art some Strumpet sure I know,
and spend'st thy dayes in shame,
And stained sure thy marriage bed
with spots of black defame:
Else vnto these two louely babes
thou can no mother be,
When I liue in greatest grace
no such content can see.

The twins' mother answers her with a terrible curse, and the lady grows increasingly nervous during her pregnancy. When she sees the ghost of the beggar woman appear at night, she receives a terrible shock:

A coarse drawing
from the English
black-letter ballad of
1620 of the countess
insulting the poor
beggar woman.

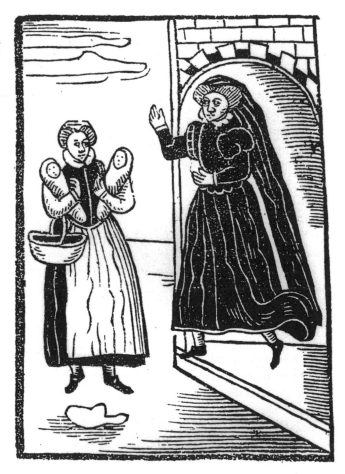

At which affright my bigg sweld wombe
  deliuered forth in feare
As many children at one time
  as daies were in the yeare:
In bignesss all like newbred mice,
  yet each one shap'd aright,
And euery male from female knowne,
  by Gods great power and might.

The children were then taken from her, and "in Countries farre and neare a wonder thus be showne." When the lamenting lady repents her sins, God has mercy on her. The minute children all die, to be buried in a grave with a monument over it, which becomes a well-known curiosity all over Europe.

Several other English poets were inspired by the story of the Legend, and it frequently occurs in seventeenth-century literature. In Act III of William Strode's *The Floating Island* from 1639, *Concupiscence* says,

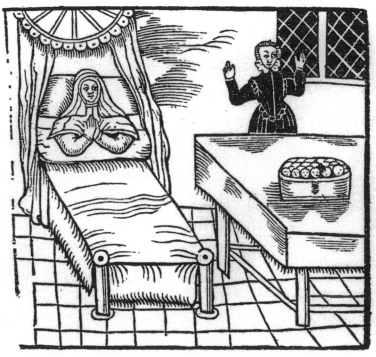

Another drawing from the English black-letter ballad of 1620 of the countess and her children.

> "the Femal passions
> As soon as they are born, turn all to sins;
> And they are all my children.
>   Memor. Then have you
> More daughters far than Danaus, or Margaret
> Countesse of Henneberg; whereof one did equal
> The weekes, and th'other the dayes of the year
> With numerous issue."

The poet Robert Waring also mentioned the Legend, in a memorial poem to his friend William Cartwright, printed in the 1651 edition of Cartwright's *Comedies*:

> As the Dutch Lady, who at once did bear
> Numbers, not Births, to date each day i' th' year,
> Grew barren by Encrease; and after all,
> None could Her, Mother, or them Children, call.
> So whilst All write, None judge, we multiply
> So many Poems, and no Poetry.

Another poet, Abraham Cowley, used the Legend in his introductory poem "Upon Mrs K. Philips Her Poems," praising the diligence of a contemporary lady poet, Mrs. Katherine Philips, who was publishing a new book of poetry:

> So easily they from thee come,
>   And there is so much room
> In the unexhausted and unfathom'd womb;
> That, like the Holland Countess, thou might'st bear
> A Child for ev'ry day of all the fertile year.

Another poetical celebration of the Loosduinen miracle is in the book *Ockenburgh* by the physician Jacob Westerbaan, which was published in 1654. In his remarkable 202-page poem in Dutch, Dr. Westerbaan described the parts around Ockenburgh and Loosduinen in great detail, with a sizable section devoted to Loosduinen Abbey and the legend of Margaret of Henneberg. On the way to the church can be seen a green hill, which had been the site of the castle of Henneberg. Its high towers had once soared toward the sky. One day, some time after the miraculous birth, the ground swallowed up the castle, towers and all, as a punishment for the dissolute lives of the Hennebergs. Nothing was ever built again on this accursed ground, but in the evenings, people could hear sounds as if a great feast was going on there: the ovens were roaring, the kettles boiling, and the roasting spits turning. Loosduinen itself was just a small village with low houses, and all foreign visitors had to go to the church, where they would find a plate, two basins, and a tombstone to commemorate the Legend. According to Jacob Westerbaan, who was a firm Protestant, Loosduinen Abbey had been quite a gay place in olden times. Young noblemen frequently visited the abbey to "entertain" the nuns. These immoral goings-on were said to have occurred until the Reformation. Westerbaan then described the Legend in great detail. He added the important information that the tombstone of the countess had the effigy of a grave with mother and children, thereby adding further evidence to the version of the English visitors of the early 1600s that there was really such a "monument" in the church. Westerbaan also affirmed that in the 1650s, the Loosduinen fertility cult was still extant. It was the habit of childless women to come to the abbey to touch the basins exhibited in the church, hoping that the magic of the Legend would make them have children later. In spite of Westerbaan's dramatic story of the Henneberg castle being swallowed up by the ground, several old drawings of the Hoogh Werf castle are in existence, indicating that it was still in reasonably good condition in the sixteenth and early seventeenth centuries.

In the seventeenth century, the Legend achieved its widest distribution. Records of it survive from well-nigh all European countries, including Denmark, Spain, Wales, and Ireland. It was considered a *Historia valde memorabilis*: a very memorable happening. The Legend was reported, often in detail, not only in historical and topographical works, but also in books on theology, philosophy, and medicine, and even in schoolbooks and books of popular anecdotes. It is particularly surprising that one of the few writers of this time who tried to dispose of various vulgar errors, Sir Thomas Browne, also accepted the Legend in his *Pseudodoxia Epidemica*: "Though wondrous strange, it may not be impossible what is confirmed at *Lausdun* concerning the Countess of Holland." The two versions of the original Legend, that the countess gave birth to 364, or 365, children, were freely intermixed. A problem for the adherents of the latter variation was whether the 365th child was male or female; they solved it by inventing a tale that it was declared to be a hermaphrodite after much theological debate! This addition to the Legend is thus of seventeenth-century origin and occurs nowhere in the original sources.

In the late 1700s, most people disbelieved the Legend, and it was less often mentioned in encyclopedias and historical works than before. The visitors to Loosduinen gradually became fewer during this time. One of them was the English traveler Samuel Ireland, who went from The Hague to Loosduinen in 1789. He considered the Legend very silly and trifling, and although he was shown the copper basins, he remained incredulous. Interestingly, he was told that once, there had been a picture or monument in the church, to illustrate the Legend; this was probably the one seen by the early pilgrims to Loosduinen. In 1836, another visitor to Loosduinen, the Danish aesthete Niels Laurits Høyen, was even more scornful. He had been on a guided tour through the church, and the sight of the two basins inspired the following tirade: "How whimsical Fate is! Two thin, wretched brass basins are kept for hundreds of years through a ridiculous tradition, while in the same time, so many works of art and things of permanent value were destroyed through sloth and fanaticism."

The Missing Infant in Copenhagen

Although most accounts of the Legend agree that the countess and her children were buried in the church of Loosduinen Abbey, some sixteenth-century writers claimed that the small fetuses were preserved as a curiosity. It is stated that they were taken to the city hall in Amsterdam to be preserved in a bottle. According to Battista Fregoso, writing in 1565, Emperor Charles V once took them out, held some of them in his hand, and admired them.

In 1681, the French dramatist Jean François Regnard visited Scandinavia, traveling from Denmark to Sweden and Lapland. He liked the city of Copenhagen very much, being particularly pleased with the beauty and vivacity of the ladies. He found time to see some of the sights of the town, among them the famous Kunst-kammer of King Frederick III. Here he saw a large horse tail, a female mandrake, and a monstrous nail from a beggar called "the Grandson of Neducadnezar." The most famous curiosity of all was one of Countess Margaret's 365 children, which was kept in a small glass case. It had probably been kept in the Kunst-kammer for several years; the earliest catalogue from 1674, mentioned a "small fetus not longer than two fingers' bredth." The 1696 catalogues stated it to be as long as a thumb and kept in an oblong, translucent glass case. It had been taken to Copenhagen by Count Hannibal Sehested, who had "bought it in Belgium as one of the 365 children of Countess Maria of Holland." Another description was given by the servant Mathies Skaanlund, who saw it hanging from a small golden chain in a little bottle. It was as long as one joint of a finger and almost entirely black; only the minute nails were of a white color. In a later museum catalogue, Dr. Holger Jacobsen reported that the missing infant of the countess had been brought to Copenhagen by Count Hannibal Sehested, a famous political adventurer who had purchased it during his travels in Holland. He gave it as a present to King Frederick III, whose favor he was seeking.

For many years, the child of Countess Margaret remained in the Kunst-kammer. The missing infant in Copenhagen was mentioned in an anonymous work entitled *A Description of Holland*, published in 1741, with the words: "One of them (the 365 children), or at least an Abortion given out to be one of them, is to be seen in the Musarum Regium at Copenhagen." The writer of this may actually have seen the specimen, although he misspelled the name of the museum, and it is interesting that he likened it to an abortion; from the existing descriptions, it can be deduced that this was probably its real origin. In the 1820s, the Kunst-kammer was dissolved by the government. Many specimens were sold at public auctions, and others were distributed among the other state museums. Countess Margaret's fetus was taken over to the Royal Museum of Natural History, along with several other zoological and medical specimens. The document of reception, dated December 26, 1826, is still extant. This is, however, also the last trace of the specimen. Probably, the chairman of the Royal Museum of Natural History, Professor Reinhart, had it scrapped along with the stone-child of Sens and several other medical specimens, which he did not consider worthy to be contained in a museum with mainly zoological exhibits.

The Legend in Medicine

Many medical writers of the sixteenth and seventeenth centuries were interested in the abnormal and macabre; in their commentaries and collections of case reports, anything out of the ordinary was certain to be included. They naturally took particular interest in the Legend, which was reproduced in most scholarly works on obstetrics and in many books on general medicine, as well as in popular books on the workings of the body. Some medical men found the Legend hard to swallow already at this time, but the majority accepted it uncritically. Ambroise Paré reported Cromer's version that a Polish countess had given birth to thirty-six infants, while Pierre Boaisteau preferred the traditional version, which is retold at length in his *Histoires prodigieuses*. The French obstetrician François Mauriceau was much more skeptical regarding the Legend, which he nevertheless reported in detail, "pour miracle ou pour fable." The Dutch anatomist Theodor Kerckring was another disbeliever. Some other writers used the Legend to prove the concept that a woman could have an indefinite number of children. The Dutch anatomist Ludolph Smid described the Loosduinen miracle at length in his *Schatkamer der Nederlandsche Oudheden*. He regarded it as a reality, since he had once dissected an ovary with a very large number of ova. This would, according to him, make it feasible for a woman to have even as many as 365 children, provided that the ova were impregnated simultaneously.

One of the last medical men to take the Legend seriously was the English obstetrician Dr. John Maubray, who had probably visited Loosduinen. In his book *The Female Physician*, published in 1724, he wrote, "The basons are still to be seen in the village church of Losdun, where all strangers go on purpose from The Hague, being reckoned among the great curiosities of Holland." Maubray was an extremely credulous character, and he became notorious among his contemporaries for endorsing, in the same book, the odd notion that the Dutch women, if they spent too much time before their hot stoves, might give birth to an ill-looking, ratlike little animal called *de Suyger* or *Sooterkin*. He was also involved in the scandal surrounding the notorious Mary Toft, an illiterate English peasant woman from Godalming who managed to trick King George I, the Prince of Wales, and several distinguished obstetricians and men of science that she had given birth to seventeen rabbits. Maubray was severely ridiculed in a pamphlet titled *A Letter from a Male Physician in the Country, to the Author of the Female Physician in London*, which was published in 1726. According to the pamphlet writer, if the Godalming rabbit breeder had not been exposed, her place of birth would have "been as famous in History to After-Ages, as ever *Losdun* in *Holland* was; and drawn in as many People to pay for seeing the Rabbet there, as ever were in *Losdun* to see the basins, wherein the 365 Children, born at one time, were baptized."

Today, as in the time of Paré and Mauriceau, it is well known that humans, like other larger mammals such as the cow, the horse, and the orangutan, are usually uniparous. It is true that the ovaries of a three-year-old girl have been estimated to contain 800,000 ova, and that she would thus be able to populate a large city, but only if she is given enough time (more than half a million years) to do so. Several writers have suggested that there is a mathematical relationship between the occurrence of twins, triplets, and higher multiple gestations. According to this model, one of 87 pregnancies results in twins, one of 87^2 is a triplet pregnancy, and one in 87^3 results in quadruplets. In 26 million births in England and Wales during the years 1952–1988, there were 112 sets of quadruplets, 16 sets of quintuplets, 6 sets of sextuplets, and 1 set of septuplets.

An early, probably apocryphal example of septuplets are the tenth-century "Seven Lords of Lara." The noble family of Lara played an important part in Spanish medieval history, and according to tradition, all seven children, all of them boys, survived to become famous warriors. A perhaps more credible historical case of septuplets were born in January 1600 in the German town Hameln, of Pied Piper fame. Frau Anna Römer gave birth to two boys and five girls, all of whom died within a few weeks. A memorial plate was erected in Hameln to celebrate this event.

Today, it is obvious that it is physiologically impossible for a woman to give birth to as many as 365, or even 36, children in one birth. The highest plural birth recorded in modern times is a set of nine children born in Sydney, Australia, in 1971. There is no evidence that the human being is capable of giving birth to more than nine children at once, although the annals of strange events mention several old stories of varying reliability, dealing with

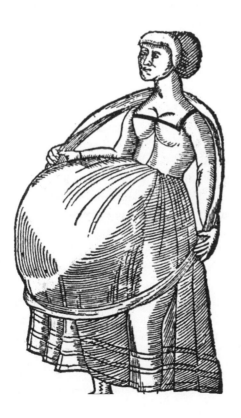

An old print of the pregnant Dorothea Losel. From the author's collection.

even higher multiparous births. One of the most remarkable of these tales concerns the German woman Dorothea, the wife of a gentleman named Kristel Losel, living in Salzach in the Tirol. In her first pregnancy, she had twins; in her second, she had nine children; and in her third, occurring in the year 1501, she gave birth to not less than eleven children at one time. A Nuremberg chronicle mentioned that her belly was of prodigious bigness, and in several medical works of the time, she was portrayed with a sling around her neck to hold it up.

In the late nineteenth century, the Legend of Countess Margaret and her 365 children has become almost totally forgotten in medical circles, but in the 1930s, it reappeared in quite another context. Two gynecologists, Dr. Schumann and Dr. Brews, independently suggested that the 365 children had really been a hydatidiform mole. Several later writers on this subject have agreed, and Countess Margaret has even regained some of her lost fame by being quoted as the first known patient to lose her life after the expulsion of a hydatidiform mole. This kind of mole is really a diseased condition in the chorion part of the placenta, with hydropic degeneration of its villi; these changes occur very early in pregnancy. It has a strange appearance, resembling a bunch of grapes held together by thin strands of fibrous tissue; its volume might be close to 3 liters. The "grapes," or rather hydropic cysts of chorion tissue, are 3–10 millimeters in diameter and filled with a clear or opalescent fluid. Frequently, there is bleeding associated with a hydatidiform mole, and after a spontaneous expulsion of the mole, the patient might bleed to death. A hydatidiform mole may well contain a hundred cysts or more, all of different sizes and shapes. The proponents of this theory, several distinguished obstetricians among them, suggest that the cysts were likened to children by people who had never before seen a hydatidiform mole, and that the countess died from a hemorrhage after its expulsion. It should be noted, though, that it would take an extremely vivid imagination to see any likeness between these cysts and human fetuses; this observation is an obvious one to any person who has once held a hydatidiform mole in his or her hand. To accept this theory, it must also be presumed that the obstetrical attendants of the countess, at the Loosduinen Abbey church, were quite unfamiliar with hydatidiform moles. Nowadays, these moles occur once in about two thousand pregnancies, and they are nearly ten times more common in developing countries owing to nutritional factors; this speaks in favor of this disease being by no means unknown in Holland of the thirteenth century.

An interesting section in Albertus Magnus's *Historia Animalium* deals

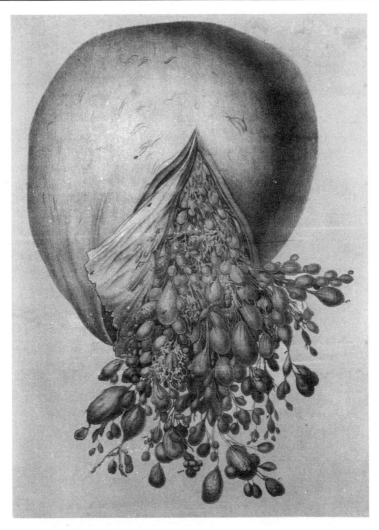

A hydatidiform mole. From the obstetrical works of the French midwife Madame Boivin.

with human multiple births. The famous Dominican had once met a German physician who encountered a noblewoman in Germany, who had given birth to not less than sixty infants, five at a time. The same physician also claimed that he had once been called to treat a noblewoman who believed that worms were issuing from her private parts. He found that they were instead small children, about 150 of them, each as long as a human finger. Their eyes were incomplete, and the toes and fingers thin like hairs. They had a movement of contraction and dilatation, and other signs of life; they were all put in a basin, where they were lying before his eyes. Dr. Claudius Mayer suggested that the noble lady was in fact Countess Margaret, and that it was her Loosduinen physician who had informed Albert the Great of the miraculous birth. This would presume that Albertus Magnus, who was eighty-three years old in 1276, was still busy making additions to his manuscripts. According to Albertus Magnus's biographers, the *Historia Animalium* had already been written and laid aside in the 1260s, making Mayer's presumption even more unlikely. Nevertheless, there are some puzzling similarities between Albert the Great's story and the Loosduinen Legend. Are they mere coincidences, or had the Dutch medieval chroniclers read Albertus Magnus's account? Another alternative is that both were fanciful early descriptions of hydatidiform moles.

Did the Countess Only Have Twins?

In 1758, the French antiquary M. Struik published a new theory about the Legend in *Journal des scavans*. He repeated the old story without any new details and erroneously presumed that the Legend was only mentioned by various modern writers, and not in the older annals of Holland. He had seen the inscriptions in the church, which led him to formulate a novel theory. If the countess had given birth to her children on Good Friday, that is on March 26, she would have conceived on the second day of the new year, since in those times, the year started on March 25, just before Easter. Thus, if she had given birth to as many children as there had been days in the year, she would have had two children, the twins Jan and Elizabeth.

This theory has been repeated by many writers; in fact, the twin theory has been accepted by the majority of later historians of the Legend. They presumed that there had been some very early chronicles, which had been lost later, and that in these presumed chronicles, the Legend had been reported merely with the words that the countess had given birth to as many children as there were (or had been) days in the year. Some writers presumed that this had been intended as a joke. A remarkable discovery, regarded by some as another strong argument that the countess had had twins, was reported by the Dutch historian van Heusden in 1719. A certain Mr. Rosemale, the son of the mayor of Rotterdam, claimed to have discovered, in a church in that city, a piece of a tombstone with the inscription that Countess Margaret of Henneberg had died on Good Friday after giving birth to the twins Johan and Elizabeth. It was not stated that Johan and Elizabeth also died, but instead hinted that Johan might have reached adulthood, since his seal was in the possession of the antiquary van Alkemade.

Several later writers on the Legend have re-invoked the Rotterdam tombstone as evidence for the twin theory. The story of the tombstone is rather mysterious, however, and it cannot be accepted at its face value. No writer earlier than van Heusden mentioned it, and only the elusive Mr. Rose-male ever saw it. Its present whereabouts, if it ever existed, is unknown. Already in the eighteenth century, there was some doubt about its authenticity, and the Dutch antiquary Christian Vermey termed the whole thing "a fairy story." The numerous sixteenth- and seventeenth-century descriptions of the Loosduinen Abbey give no indications that a tombstone of these character-istics was kept there; indeed, the "tomb-stone or monument" mentioned by several early writers had quite a different inscription, one that was fully con-sistent with the traditional version of the Legend. It is particularly unlikely that any of the twins survived. Such an event would surely have been recorded in the annals of the House of Holland and those of the counts of Henneberg, but these sources are unanimous that the Hennebergs only had three children: Herman (who died young), Jutta, and Poppo. The seal dis-cussed by van Heusden may have been that of the countess herself, which is known to have been drawn by van Alkemade.

The Lady with Nine Little Pigs for Her Children

A closer study of the medieval mythology about multiple births makes it ob-vious that the Legend is only one in a group of similar myths, which we may term "The Beggar with Twins and the Wicked Noblewoman," although it differs from the other folktales in this group through its extremely prominent position in European culture. The medieval tale of the origin of the noble house of Guelph has many similarities to the Legend. Irmentrude, countess of Altdorf, one day scolded a poor mother of triplets for her immoral life, since she firmly believed that the triplets must have different fathers. She herself gave birth to not less than twelve boys, and this shocked her very much, since she believed that people would think that they had twelve dif-ferent fathers! She ordered the midwife to drown eleven of the boys, but at the river, the midwife chanced upon the count, who asked her what she was doing. She said that she was drowning some newborn puppies (or *Welfs*), but this lie was its own undoing, since the dog-loving count wanted to keep some of them to be trained as hounds. He then discovered the truth and ordered the midwife to feed and rear all twelve infants. When they were six years old, the count pardoned his erring wife and ordered that his twelve sons henceforth were to be called not counts of Altdorff but Guelphs.

A similar legend concerned the French family de Trazegnies. In 1276, a noble chatelaine encountered a poor mendicant woman with twins and insulted her for her immoral life. The beggar cursed her, hoping that she would give birth to as many offspring as a sow, an animal that was just then passing them by in the street. Nine months later, the noble lady gave birth to thirteen children, and she tried to hide her shame by ordering them all to be drowned. They were saved by her husband, who was just returning from the wars; these children took the family name de Trazegnies (Treize-nés in thirteenth-century French). An almost indistinguishable tale, but with twelve children instead of thirteen, was current about the French noble family d'Urfé. Several new elements are encountered in the legend of the Porcelets. The pregnant wife of the lord of Arles met the inevitable mendicant woman, this time carrying triplets in her arms, and dismissed her with the usual taunts. The beggar woman answered her with the words, "You are wicked as a sow, and like that unclean animal, you will disgust all those present at your childbed." Then, according to one version, the lady herself gave birth to nine little pigs! After doing penance, she was pardoned by her husband, and her later pregnancies were normal. Another version tells that she gave birth to nine children, whom she planned to drown, but her husband saved the children and had his wife executed. The legend of the chatelaine of Montigny-le-Ganelon is even more dramatic. After the customary cursing that the lady was to have as many children as a pig, she gave birth to nine infants. She kept one of them and sent a maid to drown the rest. Her husband was just returning from the crusades, and he saved the children in the nick of time, sending them to be brought up secretly. When the children were seven years old, he had them brought to the castle, all dressed alike. When they burst into their mother's room, the distraught lady was unable to distinguish one from the other. Then, the cruel knight had his wife tortured and executed, so "that she almost died nine deaths."

It is probable, but by no means certain, that the Loosduinen Legend is the earliest version of the "Beggar with Twins and the Wicked Noblewoman" type of tale. It can be found in a rudimentary form already in fourteenth-century sources and appears fully fledged in the augmented version of the Annals of Jan van Naaldwijck. The garbled accounts of de Clerc and Korner were each a forme fruste of the tale, perhaps representing stages in its development. It should also be pointed out that the year of the Trazegnies' multiple birth is exactly the same as Countess Margaret's year of death, which speaks in favor of the French tradition being dependent on the Loosduinen Legend. The earliest versions of the Trazegnies and Porcelets legends are from the sixteenth century, but it cannot be ruled out that they, in their turn, were based on even earlier popular traditions. It is certain that the concept of multiple births as a shameful thing goes far back in medieval times.

The Countess and the Mouse-tower

It is both instructive and illuminating to compare the "Beggar with Twins and the Wicked Noblewoman" legend type with another curious medieval myth, which also occurs in many variations: the legend of the mouse-tower.

In the year 913, southern Germany suffered from a severe famine. Only the wealthy miser Archbishop Hatto of Mainz had his granaries full of corn. Every day, the starving poor crowded around the bishop's palace, begging for food and corn. Bishop Hatto was annoyed by the cries of the people, and one day, he bade them all come to his great barn, where bread was to be offered for sale. When the barn was crammed full of people, the bishop executed a nefarious scheme, as expressed in a quaint old English poem:

> *Then, when he saw it could hold no more,*
> *Bishop Hatto he made fast the door,*
> *And while for mercy on Christ they call,*
> *he set fire to the barn, and burnt them all.*
>
> *'T'faith, 'tis an excellent bonfire!' quoth he,*
> *'And the country is greatly obliged to me*
> *For ridding it, in these times forlorn,*
> *Of rats that only consume the corn.'*

Bishop Hatto slept easily after his black deed, but the next day, a servant came to tell him that rats had eaten all the corn in his granaries, and another terrified valet shouted that an army of rats was marching toward the palace. When Hatto saw the gray hordes approaching through the fields and hedges, he dashed out of doors, jumped in a boat, and was rowed to a stone tower built on a steep rock in the Rhine, which had apparently been pur-

90 posely built to serve as a refuge for him in such an emergency. Here, the bishop believed himself secure, but the rats swum the Rhine, scaled the rock, and poured in through the windows:

> *From within and without, from above and below,*
> *And all at once at the Bishop they go.*
> *They have whetted their teeth against the stones,*
> *And now they pick the Bishop's bones;*

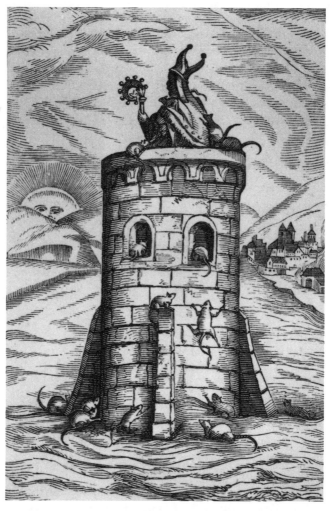

An old engraving of the grisly fate of Bishop Hatto. From the author's collection.

They gnaw'd the flesh from every limb,
For they were sent to do judgment on him.

The Mäuseturm, or mouse-tower, which was pointed out as the bishop's place of death, can still be seen standing in the Rhine, at Bingen. Nor is there any doubt that Archbishop Hatto I of Mainz was really a historical person. An ambitious prelate and politician, he ruled Mainz and its surroundings with an iron hand. He even raised a private army and personally led it into battle on several occasions. Nor was he incapable of using dirty tricks to further his political intrigues, and a certain Count Adalbert was basely betrayed by him. Hatto had offered him support against the emperor, but turned his back on him when it became clear that their forces were insufficient. The wicked prelate even informed the emperor of his whereabouts, and when Adalbert was captured, Hatto was present to gloat. Before the count was beheaded, he solemnly cursed Hatto for his treachery. In the year 913, another old enemy of Archbishop Hatto's, Duke Heinrich of Saxony, was killed by an assassin, and many people believed that Hatto had paid a ruffian in his employ to murder him. Later in 913, Hatto himself breathed his last breath, probably from "an Italian fever," as expressed in the archives of Mainz. Some enemies of Hatto made up lurid stories about his death. One of them wrote that as a Divine punishment for killing Duke Heinrich, he had been struck by lightning. According to another German chronicler, the archbishop had fallen down Mount Etna into the volcano!

There is no contemporary evidence for the tale of Bishop Hatto being devoured by rats and mice. The earliest mentioning of this tale seems to occur in the writings of Siffridus the Presbyterian, who died in 1307. Furthermore, German antiquaries have demonstrated that the mouse-tower at Bingen was built in the thirteenth century, long after the bishop was dead, to be used as a toll station.

The story of the wicked bishop and the mouse-tower also occurs in several variations. Another medieval legend states that Bishop Widerolf of Strasbourg was devoured by rats and mice in 997, as a Divine punishment for having suppressed a convent; Bishop Adolph of Cologne suffered a similar fate in 1112. The curse of the rats was not merely for wicked prelates. The Freiherr von Güttingen was a wealthy landowner in Switzerland. During a famine, he lured the starving people into a large barn and burned them, mocking their cries with the words "Hark! how the rats and mice are squeaking!" Shortly after, the rats attacked, and the Freiherr took refuge to a castle on a rock in the Lake of Constance, but to no avail. Similar tales were told about the Austrian mouse-tower at Holzölster, and the so-called Mouse-lake near Inning in Bavaria, once the place of a tower where the wicked Count of Seefeld was devoured by mice, even though he had suspended his bed with iron chains from the roof. Second to Hatto in the hall of fame of mouse-tower victims is King Popiel of Poland. He poisoned his uncles when they complained about his bad government, but the bodies of the poisoned victims metamorphosed into mice, which attacked the king when he was holding a banquet to celebrate his murderous deed. King Popiel took refuge to a ring of fire, but the mice broke through it. He then repaired to a mouse-tower, which he had had built in advance, but to no avail: the animals followed him and he was devoured there, along with his wife and two sons.

The "Mouse-tower" and the "Beggar with Twins and the Wicked Noblewoman" tales share several important characteristics, which can explain their strong effects of fascination on the medieval mind, and their wide dispersion through oral tradition. In both types of tale, there is a polarity between the refined and powerful, but wicked and immoral, bishop or noblewoman on one side, and the brutally killed starving people, or the innocent and injured beggar woman, on the other. God takes the side of the poor and injured party and punishes the wealthy sinner. These two types of legend create an illusion of a just society, with God as the ultimate guardian of individual justice. The macabre and gruesome punishments meted out to the cruel and unjust rulers were another part of the legends' fascination.

Concluding Remarks

According to Dutch antiquary van der Aa, writing in 1867, the Legend of Countess Margaret and her 365 children was still revered in Loosduinen in the mid-1800s. The simple villagers used to point out a hill on a meadow named Bergweij as the situation of the former Henneberg castle. Here, the count and countess lived extravagantly and immorally, wining and dining while the poor people starved. After the death of the countess, this second Sodom was laid waste by God, as a punishment for the dissolute lives of the Hennebergs. It was rumored that the hill was haunted, and many Loosduinen villagers ruined their night's sleep by listening in vain for the sounds of a ghostly party, with the rumbling of kitchen utensils, coming from the former site of the Henneberg castle.

In the late 1800s, there were fewer visitors to Loosduinen, and they used to dismiss the Legend as a mere vulgar tradition. In 1922, the church was visited by Professor A. E. H. Swaen, who found the basins and wooden tablet hanging in the entrance of the church, under the organ loft. The basins had become very much oxidized with time, and although they were made of copper, the material appeared more like zinc. The inscriptions had suffered less and could be traced without difficulty. Many visitors had cut their initials in the frames or even into the tablets themselves, sometimes with the date added; the earliest date was 1620.

Today, knowledge of Countess Margaret and her extraordinary birth in 1276 is restricted to the people of Loosduinen and The Hague, as well as the occasional ethnologist. The age of the tradition is revered, and it has few parallels in Europe. The tale of Bishop Hatto comes to mind, as well as the English medieval conjoined twins, the Biddenden Maids, who were said to have been born in the year 1100. It is truly amazing to contemplate the widespread, pan-European acceptance of the Legend in the seventeenth century, among historians, antiquaries, and medical men. It was indeed a *Historia valde memorabilis* that fascinated all and sundry. Many people found the moral of the story edifying: the haughty noblewoman was punished for her high-handed treatment of the beggar with twins, creating the illusion that God was on the side of the poor, and he was ready to avenge the ills brought on by the evil rich people.

By far the best-known theory of explaining the Legend is that it was originally the result of a chronological intricacy. The proponents of this theory remain undecided about the exact nature of this intricacy, but the main points are that in the 1270s, the new year started during Easter, and the countess had as many children as there had been days in the new year (or, according to some, as many children as there were days left in the year). In any case, the countess had only two (or three) children, and this was noted in the chronicles as "as many children as there were (or had been) days in the year." These presumed "chronicles" are not in existence today. In both the Tabula of Egmond and the de Clerc chronicle, the number of children is specifically given as 365. Acceptance of the twin theory would also imply that this odd habit of chronology was current in the 1270s and not only defunct but virtually *forgotten* in the 1350s.

Another hypothesis worth considering is that the countess died after the expulsion of a hydatidiform mole. This would explain both the death of the countess, through hemorrhage or infection, and the extraordinary illusion of a great many children. One objection to this theory may be that these moles were not of uncommon occurrence, and that a trained obstetrical attendant would not be unfamiliar with them, but it is by no means certain that the

Loosduinen nuns had much experience in midwifery. In this age of superstition, the most startling misconceptions about disease were current.

From the arguments presented here, it is likely that the Loosduinen Legend was the foremost version of a widespread medieval myth, which can be called "The Beggar with Twins and the Wicked Noblewoman." Probably, it was also the origin of all the other versions of this myth. Whether the Legend had any foundation in reality cannot be resolved. One possibility is that the mythical paraphernalia—the beggar woman, the insult, and the curse—may have been added to a preexisting popular tradition that something odd had happened at the deathbed of the countess on Good Friday 1276. This just possibly may have been due to a calendaric intricacy, as suggested by many writers, but strong arguments speak against this theory; the suggestion of a hydatidiform mole seems rather more credible. Another possibility is that the whole thing belongs to the realm of fantasy, like the mouse-tower tale of Bishop Hatto, and that Countess Margaret of Henneberg was wholly undeserving of her great fame before posterity.

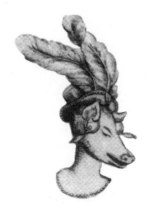

Some Words
about Hog-faced
Gentlewomen

This lady was neither pig nor maid,
And so she was not of human mould;
Not of the living nor the dead.
Her left hand and foot were warm to touch;
Her right as cold as a corpse's flesh!

THUS BEGINS A "QUAINT BRETAGNE BALLAD"
intoned by the ghastly Madame de la Rougierre in Joseph Sheridan
Le Fanu's famous novel *Uncle Silas*. Nominally the governess of the
young Victorian girl Maud Ruthyn, this sinister hag is secretly in the employ
of Maud's wicked uncle, who tries to lure her into marrying his own boorish
son. The ballad continues:

And she would sing like a funeral bell, with a ding-dong tune.
The pigs were afraid, and viewed her aloof,
And women feared her and stood afar.

95

She could do without sleep for a year and a day;
She could sleep like a corpse, for a month and more.
No one knows how this lady fed —
On acorns or on flesh.

One of the first to acknowledge Sheridan Le Fanu as one of the nineteenth-century masters of horror was the distinguished antiquary Montague Rhodes James, who was also a ghost story writer par excellence. M. R. James recognized, as have some perceptive modern literary critics, that Le Fanu was no mere horror-monger, but a writer of considerable depth and hidden meaning. In his introduction to a new edition of *Uncle Silas*, M. R. James wrote that he had been greatly intrigued by the "Breton ballad of the lady with the pig's head, which is introduced with such sinister effect." He had valiantly tried to trace its original source, but without success. Later researchers also were unable to locate a source for this poem. To do so, one must disregard, at least for the moment, its immediate literary context in Le Fanu's writings and investigate the hoary myth that lies beyond it: the tale of the Hog-faced Gentlewoman and her avaricious suitors.

Some say she's one of the swine possessed,
That swam over the sea of Genesaret.
A mongrel body and demon soul.
Some say she is the wife of the Wandering Jew,
And broke the law for the sake of pork;
And a swinish face for a token doth bear,
That her shame is now and her punishment coming.

In the Grenville Library of the British Museum is a slender, calf-bound volume, formerly the possession of the Right Honorable Thomas Grenville, like so many others, and carrying his seal. It is unique only in its astounding title emblazoned on the spine: "Hog-Faced Gentlewomen." Its no less remarkable contents are a lengthy pamphlet, published in London in 1640, giving "A Certaine Relation of the Hog-faced Gentlewoman called Mistris Tannakin Skinker"; in Grenville's collection, it was bound along with Mr. Fairburn's portrait of the Pig-faced Lady of Manchester-Square and a pamphlet entitled "A True Description of the Young Lady born with a Pig's Face, now living in London."

It is the first mentioned of these pamphlets that provides some valuable

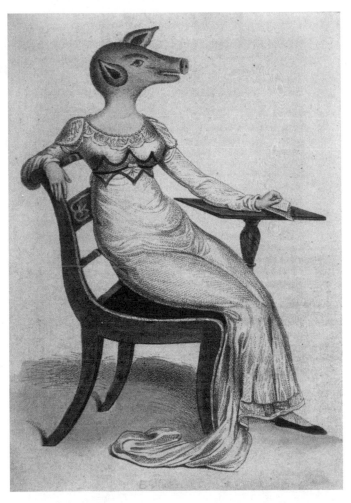

A hand-colored engraving of a Hog-faced Gentlewoman, by
Fairburn Senior. From the author's collection.

information about the origin of the legend of the Hog-faced Gentlewoman.
She had come from Holland, all accounts agree, and was in London looking
for a husband. When the Hog-faced Gentlewoman first made her curtsy to
the London public in December 1639, her fame spread rapidly. In one
week's time, not less than five ballads about her were registered; they were
respectively entitled: "The Woman Monster," "A Maiden Monster," "A

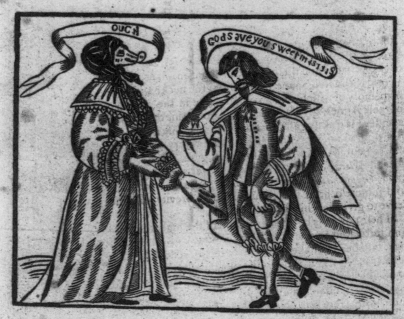

A certaine Relation of the Hog-
faced Gentlewoman called Miſtris *Tannakin*
Skinker, who was borne at *Wirkham*
a Neuter Towne betweene the Emperour and the
Hollander, ſcituate on the river *Rhyne*.
Who was bewitched in her mothers wombe in the yeare 1618.
and hath lived ever ſince unknowne in this kind to any,
but her Parents and a few other neighbours. And
can never recover her true ſhape, tell ſhe
be married, &c.

Alſo relating the cauſe, as it is ſince conceived, how her mother
came ſo bewitched.

London Printed by *J.O.* and are to be ſold by *F. Grove*, at his ſhop
on *Snow-hil* neare *St. Sepulchers Church.* 1640.

The title page to the original London pamphlet about Tannakin Skinker, published
in 1640. Reproduced by permission from the British Library.

Strange Relation of a Female Monster," "A New Ballad of the Swines-faced Gentlewoman," and "A Wonder of These Times." Neither of these ballads is in existence today, but Samuel Pepys preserved, in his collection of black-letter broadside ballads, a copy of the astonishingly titled:

> *A Monstrous Shape.*
> *Or*
> *A shapelesse Monster.*
> *A Description of a female creature borne in Holland,*
> *compleat in every part, save only a head like a swine,*
> *who hath travailed into many parts, and is now to be seene in LONDON,*
> *Shees loving, courteous, and effeminate,*
> *And nere as yet could find a loving mate.*

According to the Grenville pamphlet, the hog-faced Miss Skinker was born in 1618, the only child of a wealthy Dutch couple residing in Wirkham, a town on the border between Holland and the German Empire. Her parents were much ashamed of their daughter's monstrous appearance and brought her up in a private chamber. She was always wearing a veil and was fed and taught only by her parents. They pondered over the cause of her deformity and strongly suspected that she had been bewitched within her mother's womb. When Mme Skinker was pregnant with Tannakin, a witch-like old woman approached her, begging for alms. Unfortunately, Mme Skinker did not appreciate the moral of the legend of her famous countrywoman Countess Margaret of Henneberg: that one should be kind to beggars, particularly when pregnant. She turned the crone away with petulance, and the sinister old witch was seen to skulk away, "muttering to her selfe the Divells pater noster, and was heard to say; As the Mother is Hoggish, so Swinish shall be the Child shee goeth withall." It was considered very likely that the "malitious Spells, and divelish murmurations of this wicked woman" caused poor Tannakin's deformity. The witch was tried and convicted, but even when at the stake, she refused to reverse the spell, because of either perverse obstinacy or simple lack of power.

When Tannakin Skinker was seventeen years old, the strange deformity of her face had become well known in Wirkham and its surroundings. People who saw her eat were astonished that she fed from a silver trough "to which she stooped and ate, just like a Swine doth in his swilling Tub." They were no less amazed to hear her speak: her only language was the Dutch hoggish "Hough" and the French piggish "Owee! Owee!" The anti-Dutch author of the ballad *A Monstrous Shape* wrote:

And to speak further for her grace,
She hath a dainty white swines face,
Which shews that she came of a race
that loued fat porke and bacon.

The more Tannakin was mocked and laughed at by these heartless visitors, the more diligently her parents sought a cure for their poor daughter. Finally, her father consulted an astrologer and mathematician named Vandermast, who was well known to dabble in the black arts. He pondered her case at length and finally recommended that the only way to cure her was to marry her off, the sooner the better. As long as she remained "in the estate of a Virgin," there was no hope at all of her recovery, but if she was married, not to a "Clowne, Bore, or Pesant; but to a gentleman at least," there might be some chance that she could escape her semiporcine guise; the learned gentleman did not digress on exactly how this strange transformation would take place. The parents, seizing on their only hope, purchased a very rich and costly dress for their daughter, who was then about seventeen years old. Her face, or rather snout, was still kept veiled and covered. They then announced that any gentleman marrying her would receive a dowry of forty thousand pounds. The front page of the Grenville pamphlet is decorated with a curious woodcut, in which a gallant in gentlemanly dress greets Tannakin with the words "God save you sweet mistress": her only reply is "Ouch!"

As expected, there was no shortage of suitors: "His Gates were thronged as at an Outcry, or rather as a Lottery, every one in hope to carry away the great Prize of forty thousand pound; for it was not the person, but the prize at which they aimed." The suitors' comments were probably as amusing to the rowdy Londoners at the alehouses as they will be abhorrent to the feminists of the present age. "Put her head but in a blacke bagge, and what difference betwixt her and any other woman," queried one of them. Another gallant comforted himself that he would at least never have a scold for his wife, since "if shee cannot speake, shee cannot chide." A parsimonious individual congratulated himself that since the monstrous girl only ate gruel and pig food, she would not "be very chargeable to him for her Dyet." The suitors to the pig-faced lady came to Holland from all over Europe: from Italy, France, England, and Scotland. First came a Scottish captain, who had spent the greatest part of one month's pay on a fine suit of clothes. Tannakin's parents were much impressed and thought that he was some great laird from the Highlands. They introduced him to their daughter, and the captain paid her many compliments for her elegant dress and handsome proportions. But as soon as she lifted her veil, the captain ran out of the room saying that they must pardon him, since he could "indure no Porke"! Next came a Sowce-man (cook) from England, who comforted himself that his familiarity with the members of the porcine race and their habits would make him an excellent husband to the monstrous girl. But as soon as he saw her face, he exclaimed, "So long I've known Rumford, I never saw such a Hogsnout!" He did not know whether his stomach was strong enough for such a Dish, since he preferred his pork "well boyled or rosted" and never took it raw. A tailor and several other suitors came to see her, but retired in disarray the moment she unveiled her face. The author of the ballad *A Monstrous Shape* wrote:

> *Great store of suters euery day,*
> *Resort vnto her as they say,*
> *But who shall take this girl away,*
>   *as yet I doe not know:*
> *But thus much dare I undertake,*
> *If any doe a wife her make,*
> *It is onely for her moneys sake*
>   *he loues her.*

Tannakin Skinker's parents, having failed dismally in their attempts to get their daughter married on the continent, decided to set out for London, the capital of folly, where they took up residence in either Black-Friars or Covent Garden (the pamphlet writer was not sure which). The parents did not wish to announce their address, since the house might be stormed by the multitude of the curious and pulled down about their ears. Some people had already seen Tannakin in London, and were much impressed by her courteous manners and elegant dress, and even more by her fortune of forty thousand pounds. The sneering, anti-Dutch author of the ballad *A Monstrous Shape* solemnly warned those young gallants who wanted to seek her out, with the words:

> *If any young man long to see*
> *This creature wheresoere she be*
> *I would haue him be rul'd by me,*
>   *and not to be too forward,*
> *Lest he at last should fare the worse,*
> *Although she haue a golden purse,*
> *She is not fit to be a nurse*
>   *in England.*

The legend of the pig-faced lady became part of seventeenth-century culture, and is alluded to several times in the contemporary literature, much more often in England than in Holland or France. The "Swines-fac't Lady" is the subject of an epigram in Robert Chamberlain's *Jocabella*, and she is again alluded to in *Ad Populum, or a Low-Country Lecture*, published in 1653. The *Mercurius Democritus* newspaper of the same year spoke of a monstrous giant exhibited by an English merchant in America, and joked that "The Hogges-fac't Gentle-Woman is sent for out of Holland to be his godmother." Another newspaper, the *Mercurius Fumigosus*, mentioned that in 1654, one of the signs at Bartholomew Fair was "the Signe of the Hoggs-fac'd Gentlewoman." "The Long-Nos'd Lass," a popular song of the 1670s, began with the lines:

> *O did you not hear of a Rumor of late,*
> *Concerning a person whose Fortune was great;*
> *Her portion was seventeen thousand good pound,*
> *But yet a good Husband was not to be found:*
> *The reason for this I will tell to you now,*
> *Her visage was perfectly just like a Sow,*
> *And many to Court her came flocking each day,*
> *But seeing her, straight they run frightened away.*

The song was a coarse satire on various London tradesmen—tailors, millers, tinkers, tanners, and glovers—who went out in force to see the pig-faced lady, but were so frightened by her beastly countenance that they swiftly withdrew. Another popular song, commonly sung in the music halls by a character in the dress of a country yokel, began with the words:

> *Your zarvant all round and you zee I be here*
> *And what I left plough for will soon make appear,*
> *For I's come to Lunnon an outlandish place,*
> *To marry the lady that's got the Pig's face!*

In the eighteenth century, there were many pig-faced ladies, all shapely and elegant except for their deformed faces, and all eagerly seeking a husband. The prolific pseudo-gothic novelist Thomas Peskett Prest described one of them in his *Magazine of Curiosity and Wonder*. His account was stated to have its origin in a German book published in 1704, but Prest was unreliable with regard to his source material, and I have not been able trace any original source. The tale of the hog-faced gentlewoman is embellished by a woodcut, stated to have been taken from this same German book; it has a suspicious similarity in style to Prest's other woodcuts in his magazine, however. At any rate, the lady was thirty-four years old and lived in Amsterdam. Her figure was perfection itself, and she had beautiful long dark hair, but her face exactly resembled that of a pig. She could not venture outdoors, due to "the curiosity of the spectators, who followed her in vast crowds, and excessively annoyed her with their rude remarks." Confined to her own townhouse, she was waited upon by a devoted, elderly servant. She talked fluently and could converse elegantly upon the most difficult subjects, but she laughed just like a grunting pig. Unlike Tannakin Skinker, she ate normally and did not use a silver trough. The German writer concluded his account with the words: "I called upon her several times, during my stay in Amsterdam, and by her own permission took her likeness, and had her consent to publish this account, which the reader may depend upon it is strictly true." Another hog-faced gentlewoman was described in a German broadsheet published in 1717. She was of Dutch origin, and her parents were extremely wealthy. She sat in her castle, awaiting her suitors, but when they saw her deformed face, they ran away.

Mr. James Paris du Plessis, a writer on monstrosities active in the early eighteenth century, described yet another hog-faced gentlewoman who was not a native of Holland, but resided at St. Andrew's Parish, Holborn, in the heart of London. She belonged to a wealthy, noble family, and was well built, with beautiful black hair, although her face resembled that of a sow or cow. When traveling, her face was covered with a large black velvet mask. She spoke distinctly, but in a grunting voice. James Paris du Plessis is usually a reliable observer, but unlike the majority of his teratological case studies in his manuscript *History of Prodigies*, he did not claim to have seen the woman himself.

A contributor to *Chambers's Edinburgh Journal* was informed by a venerable and clear-headed old lady of ninety that her mother had been well acquainted with a noble lady of Scottish ancestry who was called the Pig-faced Lady due to some "peculiar conformation of her features." This lady had been at large in the 1750s, and the elderly informant asserted that her mother had frequently visited this lady at her home in Sloane Square.

⤐

In the winter of 1814–1815, there was a widespread rumor in London that a pig-faced lady was actually living in the metropolis. She was reported to be young, immensely rich, and the daughter of a noblewoman residing in London; there were hints that she lived in a closely guarded, fashionable town-

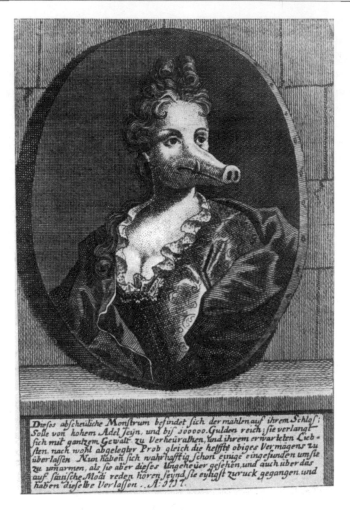

A print issued in 1717 of a fierce-looking German pig-faced lady. From the author's collection.

house in Manchester Square, and sometimes took exercise in a carriage, protected by a heavy veil. Several letters in the more fanciful newspapers of the day were submitted by excited or horrified Londoners who claimed to have observed the veiled silhouette of a pig's head in a passing, elegant carriage, or seen a snout emerge from its window.

In early 1815, an elegant colored portrait of the Pig-faced Lady of Manchester Square, by Fairburn (Senior), was published and went into several editions. On this engraving, some additional information about this phenomenon was provided, allegedly from the source of "a female who attended on her." She was about twenty years old, a native of Ireland, of high family and fortune, "and on her life and issue by marriage a very large property depends." Like the earlier pig-faced ladies, she was flawless in body and limb, but her head and face were those of a pig. She spoke only in grunts and ate her victuals from a silver trough. In spite of being paid the princely salary of one thousand guineas per annum, her female attendant was too frightened by the less lady-like habits of her monstrous mistress. She resigned from her position and apparently felt free to tell the press all about her strange employer afterward.

The Pig-faced Lady was stated to have been the general topic of conversation in the metropolis at this period of time. Thousands, particularly those living in the West End of town, believed in her existence. An article in

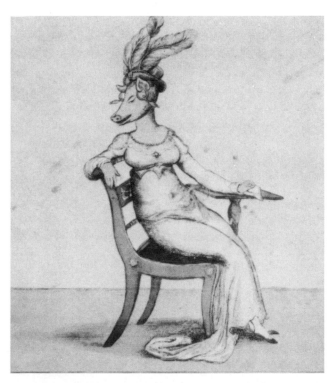

An 1815 engraving of the Pig-faced Lady of Manchester
Square. From the author's collection.

the *Times* of February 16, 1815, deplored the credulity of Londoners in general, and the Pig-faced Lady craze in particular. A few days earlier, an earnest young woman had put an advertisement into the *Times*, offering herself as the Lady's paid companion. She made it perfectly clear that a handsome yearly income and a premium for residing with her for seven years were required; this scheming swineherdess in spe may well have read the statement that the earlier attendant of "her Sowship" had received one thousand guineas per annum, and hoped for a similar salary.

An even more ridiculous advertisement was submitted to the *Times*, along with a one-pound note, by a young London gallant hoping to become the husband of the Pig-faced Lady. Enraged already by the previous idiotic addition to the Pig-faced Lady section of the *Times'* Lonely Hearts column, the editor decided to burn the advertisement and give the money to some charity. The *Morning Chronicle* had no such censorial aspirations with regard to its contents and published the following bizarre advertisement:

> SECRECY. A single Gentleman, aged thirty-one, of a respectable Family, and in whom the utmost Confidence may be reposed, is desirous of explaining his Mind to the Friends of a Person who has a Misfortune in her Face, but is prevented for want of an Introduction. Being perfectly aware of the Principal Particulars, and understanding that a final Settlement would be preferred to a temporary one, presumes he would be found to answer the full extent of their wishes. His intentions are sincere, honourable, and firmly resolved. References of great Respectability can be given. Address to M.D. at Mr Spencer's, 22 Great Ormond Street, Queen's Square.

It is unknown whether this earnest young suitor to the Pig-faced Lady had any success, and whether any scented letter with the noble crest of a boar's head was dropped by a trembling hand into the letter box of 22 Great Ormond Street.

The editor of the *Times* wrote a further article to point out that the story of a pig-faced lady was an old one. Some elderly people of good memory could well recall that in 1764, exactly the same tale had been current in London. A note in a 1764 newspaper told that a man had offered to make the Pig-faced Lady an ivory trough to feed from. The editor deplored the credulity of the Londoners, remarking that if there had been just one actor in this first folly, there were now twenty, and a man had just written to the

Times offering to make the Pig-faced Lady a silver trough. A letter writer seconded the editor's article the day after and ridiculed the Pig-faced Lady craze further by comparing it to the scandalous activities of the prophetess Joanna Southcott. The pig-faced woman was probably the daughter of Joanna, he wrote, and the "Swinish Lothario" who had sent a letter to the *Times* was advised to "woo her in grunts." When faced by this onslaught, the editor of the *Morning Chronicle* saw it proper to defend the Pig-faced Lady. He stated that for several months, there had been a story that a young lady of family and fortune, on whose issue by marriage a very large estate depended, had a head of such deformity as to resemble that of a pig. Although the doctors he had consulted declared such a deformity to be unknown to them, the editor boldly declared that it might well be true that such a female existed, but that her deformity had been exaggerated by the credulous people. As to the letter from the "desperate fortune-hunter," the editor had not found it immoral or indecent enough to decline it for publication. It was his decided opinion that when any respectable newspaper deemed an advertisement improper for publication, it should also return the money.

⁓❧

Despite the efforts of the editor of the *Times* and other skeptics, the Pig-faced Lady craze continued. During the illuminations that took place to celebrate the peace between Britain and France, a great crowd assembled in Piccadilly and St. James's Street, and the carriages moving by could only travel very slowly, like in the present-day traffic jams in these parts. From one of them, an enormous pig's snout was seen to emerge, protruding from beneath a fashionable-looking bonnet! The startled crowd called out "The Pig-faced Lady! The Pig-faced Lady! Stop the carriage! Stop the carriage!" but to no avail. The coachman whipped up his horses and drove through the crowd at a dangerous pace. It was later stated that the coach had put down its monstrous load in Grosvenor Square, the home of a well-known lady of fashion; it was presumed that the Pig-faced Lady was her daughter or ward.

Several satirical caricature prints were inspired by the Pig-faced Lady craze of 1815. One of these, Waltzing in Courtship, suggested that the short and hunchbacked Lord Kirkcudbright was one of the Pig-faced Lady's suitors. He is depicted waltzing with the tall, elegant lady with a pig's head. In another caricature, also published in March 1815, the Pig-faced Lady stepped into foreign politics. In an amusing drawing by George Cruikshank, the Pig-faced Lady of Manchester Square sits playing the piano. She is elegantly dressed and her snout is covered by a transparent veil. The back of

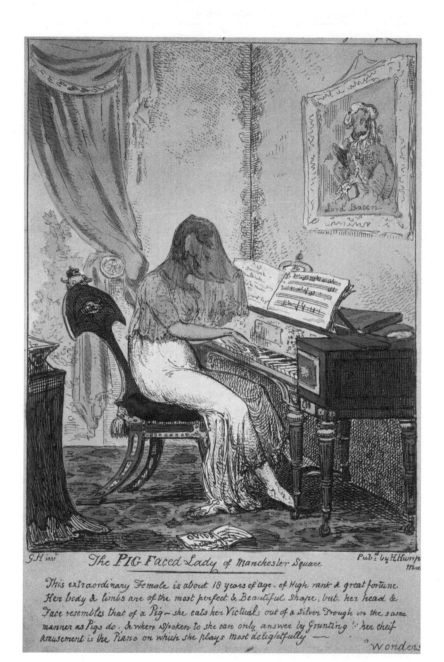

The Pig-faced Lady of Manchester Square plays the piano in this amusing caricature, facing that of the "Spanish Mule of Madrid." Note that the sheet music is "A Swinish Interlude set to Music by-Grunt esqr." and that the portrait on the wall depicts Lord Bacon with a pig's face. From the author's collection.

her chair is topped by a coroneted pig; the title of her music is "Air-Swinish Multitude set to Music by-Grunt esqr"; on the wall is a portrait of Lord Bacon, a man with a pig's head. Below the title are the words:

> This extraordinary Female is about 18 years of age — of High rank & great fortune. Her body & limbs are of the most perfect & Beautiful Shape, but, her head & Face resembles that of a Pig — she eats her Victuals out of a Silver Trough in the same manner as Pigs do, & when spoken to she can only answer by Grunting! her chief Amusement is the Piano which she plays most delightfully.

In another image, next to her, is a caricature of King Ferdinand VII of Spain as "The Spanish Mule of Madrid," complete with a mule's head. An insert, designed as a picture on the wall entitled "Amusement at Madrid," depicts a friar pointing toward two men on a gibbet full of hanging corpses, saying, "Here's some more Patriots"; the King with a mule's head replies "O! that's right Kill'em Kill'em." The text underneath this image parallels that of the Lady, parodying the monster handbills of the time and doing an excellent job of it:

> This wonderful monster (to the great grief of his subjects) is a King!!! He was caught 7 years ago by Buonaparte, & during his confinement in France, amused himself by singing Anthems & Working a Robe in Tambour for the Holy Virgin! but since his liberation, he has amused himself, by Hanging his best Friends!!!!!

Another amusing Cruikshank caricature, published on March 22, 1815, was entitled "Suitors to the Pig-faced Lady." Various tradesmen and upstarts court the Lady, who rejects them all eloquently: "If you think to gammon me, you'll find you've got the wrong sow by the ear — I'm meat for your masters, so go along, I'll not be plagued by any of you." Another drawing was published by Palmer in 1815. It was entitled "The Wonderful Miss Atkinson" and based on a drawing by the artist George Morland. Since Morland died in 1804, the drawing could not have been directly inspired by the craze in 1815. The original 1815 drawing merely stated that this prodigy was "Born in Ireland, has £20.000 fortune, and is fed out of a silver trough." This information was on the back of the original drawing, which was, at the time of publication, in the possession of Morland's nephew; one rather suspects that this individual had dug the old drawing out of Morland's portfolio just in time to cash in on the Pig-faced Lady craze. It is curious that a later, undated version of the same colored print, in my collection, tells quite another story. Again, the information is said to derive from Morland's original inscription on the back of the drawing, but now, "The Wonderful Mrs. Atkinson" is "Born and Married to a Gentleman in Ireland of that Name, having 20,000 fortune. She is fed out of a Silver Hog-Trough, and is called to her Meals by Pig-Pig-Pig." According to a note on the print, the original source of this information, and the description of the Lady's appearance, was Morland's servant George Simpson, "who will swear to the truth of it, having heard it on board the *Vesuvius* Gun Boat, from some Irish Sailors who he says cannot tell lies."

Another story told that Sir William Elliot, a young baronet, was once visiting a lady of fashion in Grosvenor Square. He was ushered into the drawing room, where he saw a elegantly dressed lady standing with her back turned to him. Intrigued, he walked up to her, but recoiled when she turned round sharply and revealed a hideous pig's face. Sir William gave a shout of horror and rushed for the door. The Pig-faced Lady obviously thought him quite impolite, since she gave a furious grunt, ran after him, and bit him on the back of the neck. This very credible story ends by stating that Sir William's wound had proved a severe one, and that he was under the care of Mr. Cesar Hawkins, surgeon, in South Audley Street. A caricature, in the same manner of those mentioned previously, was made to celebrate Sir William's misadventure; it was entitled "Beware of the Pig-stye!"

An unexpected postscript to this strange Pig-faced Lady craze of 1814–1815 is provided by some correspondence in the *Notes and Queries* magazine of 1861. A gentleman signing himself "M. A." inserted a query regarding whether there was any further information about the Pig-faced Lady who had lived in London about forty years earlier. He knew of two authentic observations of her, one by a gentleman still living. He earnestly inquired whether there had been any more recent cases of pig-faced ladies, since "in spite of the natural horror of the phenomenon, its interest, both physiological and psychological, is so considerable that I am surprised to find so little information afloat on the subject." He was answered by a certain George Lloyd, who had seen a pig-faced lady exhibited in Wakefield in 1828 or 1829; he had been too young to take any note of this phenomenon "further than a mental one, which has haunted me ever since." Another correspon-

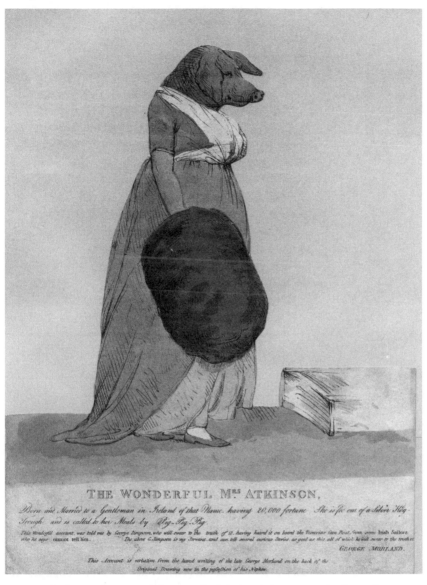

THE WONDERFUL MRS ATKINSON,

Born and Married to a Gentleman in Ireland of that Name, having 20,000 fortune. She is fee out of a Silver Hog Trough. and is called to her Meals by Pig-Pig-Pig.

This Wonderfull account, was told me by George Simpson, who will swear to the truth of it, having heard it on board the Vanguard Man Boat, from some Irish Sailors who he says cannot tell lies. The above G. Simpson is my Servant and can tell several curious Stories, as good as this, all of which he will swear to the truth of.

GEORGE MORLAND.

This Account is verbatim from the hand writing of the late George Morland on the back of the Original Drawing now in the possession of his Nephew.

George Morland's drawing of the Wonderful Mrs. Atkinson. From the author's collection.

112   dent to the *Notes and Queries*, Mr. F. FitzHenry, provided a more sinister
reply. He knew a certain lady, whom he termed Lady H. W., who was much
admired as a beauty in the 1820s. When at a dinner party forty years earlier,
all the party goers were solemnly cautioned not to say a word about pigs, out
of delicacy to Lady H. W., since it was widely believed that her sister, Lady
C. B., was the original pig-faced lady.

⤷

In eighteenth- and nineteenth-century Ireland, speculation was rife about
"Madam Grisly Steevens, the Pig-faced Lady of Dublin." She was said to be
fabulously rich and had financed the building of a large hospital, where she
spent the remainder of her days, hiding from the rough and insensitive populace who wanted to gawk at her. The cause of her malformation was that
her pregnant mother had refused a beggar woman carrying several children
alms with the words "Take away your litter of pigs!" Many Irishmen had
seen the large silver trough from which she used to feed every day. For many
years, there were also people who claimed to have seen Madam Steevens in
person, during fairs and markets; they willingly asserted that she really had
the head and face of a pig.

Sources agree that, unlike Tannakin Skinker and the Wonderful Miss
Atkinson, Miss Grizel Steevens was undoubtedly a real person. She was the
daughter of the Reverend John Steevens, a wealthy clergyman. In 1710, her
twin brother, Dr. Richard Steevens, died, and she was left a considerable
fortune; she was to have 650 pounds a year, and the remainder was to be
used for the erection of a hospital in their hometown Dublin. Miss Steevens,
who was well known for her zeal in working for various charities, decided to
go one better: the hospital was to be built in her own lifetime. The philanthropic lady succeeded in this enterprise, and Steevens' Hospital still remains as a memorial of her benevolence.

In her youth, Grizel Steevens suffered from some disorder of the eyes,
which forced her always to wear a veil. She was a lady of retiring disposi-
tion, and during her charitable rounds to the poor districts of Dublin, she
preferred to remain seated in her carriage while her servants doled out the
various alms to the needy. It has been supposed that her veiled countenance,
seen through the carriage window, gave rise to the rumor about her monstrous appearance, which soon spread like wildfire through Dublin. Grizel
Steevens was of course much dismayed by this ludicrous rumor, particularly
since she had not the slightest deformity of the face. Although there is no
record of her receiving any impudent offers of marriage from impecunious

Dubliners, it must have been quite an ordeal for a shy, nervous lady to have rude boys grunting at her in the streets, and drunken Paddys jumping up on the footstep of her carriage to try to catch a glimpse of her snout through the window. To scotch the rumor of her pig-faced countenance, she used to sit in an open balcony near the hospital, allowing all and sundry to see her. When she tired of this, she had her portrait painted, and ordered it to be hung in the hospital main hall for inspection by curious visitors.

The visitors preferred to visit a neighboring public house, however, which had a silver trough and a portrait of her with a fine pig's head on show to impress the customers. Poor Miss Steevens must have despaired of human vulgar credulity, and the representation of her with a pig's head may well have added to her determination to become a hermit inside her own hospital, where she died in 1746 at the ripe old age of ninety-three. Her memory and that of her many charitable acts were revered by the hospital governors and doctors, but the ludicrous legend of her having a pig's face was equally revered by a large proportion of the Irish nation; even today, it remains the major claim to fame of this pious, charitable lady.

When William Wilde, the father of Oscar, arrived at Steevens' Hospital as a medical student in 1832, one of the memorabilia he was shown was a silver trough, which many curious visitors presumed to be the one from which Grizel Steevens had eaten her gruel. He had already seen an engraving of her feeding from it in a penny peep show, one of many that upheld this unfortunate lady's undeserved notoriety. To visit the hospital and see this silver trough seems to have been quite a fashionable pastime in early nineteenth-century Dublin. Dr. T. P. C. Kirkpatrick, author of the *History of Doctor Steevens' Hospital*, wrote that several hospital officers were in the habit to tell the story of the pig-faced Madam Steevens to credulous visitors, and to show them a silver trough. It even appears, according to the same work, as if a plaster cast of a human face with a large pig snout was on show at that time. Later, the hospital governors seem to have doubted that this spectacle had the *gravitas* suitable for an establishment dedicated to the healing arts, and forbid this ludicrous practice, on pains of dismissal for the individuals involved.

In 1864, the *Dublin Medical Press* mentioned that it was still a popular legend among the poor in Dublin that Madam Steevens had a pig's face. This belief was by no means confined to the Irish people living in Dublin. An American sailor of Irish descent wrote a letter, dated "Jan. 30th, 1864, On board U.S. Ship of War Portsmouth, off New Orleans," directed to Madam Steevens senior, whom he believed still to be alive. The letter contained a proposal to marry her pig-faced daughter, since the sailor had heard that she would "give any Man A fortune to any one who will Marry her." The *Dublin Medical Press* published this letter to ridicule the poor sailor, who had probably not intended his earnest, badly written missive for publication in a medical journal.

In the 1880s, an Irish lady correspondent of Mr. Richard Chambers, editor of the *Every-Day Book*, wrote that when she was a girl, everybody believed that Madam Steevens had the face of a pig, and the idea was still prevalent. Many people went to the hospital to see the silver trough and a painting of her with a pig's head that were said to be on show there; the matron of the hospital received them graciously, but said that she was currently not allowed to show these treasures. She never denied that they existed and never refused the tips that were offered to her. According to another account, a Dublin gentleman used to show a large silver punch bowl, displaying the noble crest of a boar's head, as Madam Steevens's silver trough. Dr. T. G. Wilson, the biographer of Sir William Wilde, writing in the early 1940s, commented that even in his own time, the Dubliners still commonly supposed Madam Steevens to have had a pig's face.

෴

In the eighteenth and nineteenth centuries, pig-faced ladies were hot property in British show business. There had been exhibitions of pig-faced ladies molded in wax or papier-mâché, and such was the perpetual fascination of this subject among the Irish that even a print of the Wonderful Miss Atkinson was one of the prime exhibits at an early nineteenth-century fair, visited by, among others, the aforementioned William Wilde. At the Hyde Park Fair, in the year of Queen Victoria's accession, Madam Steevens, the Wonderful Pig-faced Lady, was advertised to be *living*! This Irish celebrity, who was eager to get married and grunted to give replies to questions from the audience, had many visitors and was mentioned several times in the newspapers. There is evidence that a live pig-faced lady appeared at Bartholomew Fair in 1828, and probably also in previous years. The living pig-faced lady seen by the impressionable Mr. Lloyd in Wakefield in 1828 or 1829 may well have been the same one.

The modus operandi was that the showmen procured a fine black bear and shaved the hair off its snout, neck, and front paws. The beast, which had been drugged with a tub of warm, strong ale, or with some concoction of Mickey Finn, was then lugged into a comfortable armchair and dressed in an elaborate lady's costume with a padded bosom, frills, and ribbons. Elegant shoes were fastened to the bear's rear paws, and stuffed satin gloves to the shaven front paws, to hide the claws and give the resemblance of human fingers and toes. Finally, a large wig with elaborate blond ringlets was stuck on its head, and a large fashionable hat on top of the wig.

As soon as these brutal stylists made "Madam Steevens" ready to make her bow to the audience, the yokels were admitted into the tent to admire Her Sowship, who was reclining benignly in her easy chair. It was explained to them that "Madam Steevens" could not speak to her court of visitors, but only grunt, once for yes and twice for no. Then the interrogation went on: Are you the heiress to a great fortune? One grunt. Do you feed from a silver trough? One grunt. Are you yet betrothed to any man? Two grunts. If one of the visitors was still unsatisfied, the pig-faced lady was treated to a meal of ale, gruel, and apples, all served in a silver trough. Toward the end of the fair, the situation must have become precarious indeed: the alcohol had worn off, and the bear was becoming restive; it had taken exception to being surreptitiously prodded by a stick to provoke the answers to the questions, and was generally not amused by its situation. When its bonds were eventually released, it is not unlikely that some of the knaves got a resounding box on the ear for their trouble — I rather hope so.

There were rumors that gangs of rowdy Dublin medical students were adept at this game, and that they delighted to exhibiting "Madam Steevens" before the crowds of wide-eyed Irishmen who had come to visit the manifold curiosities of the Irish capital. It is recorded that the many Irish exhibitions of pig-faced ladies were all uniformly successful; and no charge of fraud was made against the 1828 Bartholomew Fair exhibition, or that held in Hyde Park in 1843. During a fair in Plymouth some time in the 1880s, a quarrel broke out, and a mob broke into the pig-faced lady's tent and tore her wig and cap off. The showmen were not treated gently; nothing is known about how the bear fared in this encounter.

❧

In two papers published in the journal *Volkskunde*, the Dutch antiquary G. J. Boekenoogen attempted to trace the earliest sources of the legend of the pig-faced lady. After searching various Dutch and British archives, it was clear to him that the legend had first appeared in 1638 or 1639, and that no earlier versions could be traced. Neither Mr. Ricky Jay nor I have been able to find any earlier source. In ballads, handbills, and pamphlets, the pig-faced lady was celebrated in Holland, France, and Britain, and it is clear that something of the legend's universal popularity was due to its novelty. It is of particular interest that one early illustrated Dutch print reproduced by Dr. Boekenoogen contains a version that may well be the original one. A wealthy Dutch lady named Jacamijntjen Jacobs, living in Amsterdam, was one day approached by a filthy beggar woman who asked her for alms. The lady did not want to give her any, however. The mendicant was carrying three unprepossessing children and pleaded that her poor children were starving, but the hard-hearted Jacamijntjen Jacobs just said, "Take away your filthy pigs, I will not give you any thing!" The beggar woman wept bitterly and said, "Are these my children pigs? May the Lord God then give you such pigs as I have here!" Jacamijntjen Jacobs was pregnant at the time, and she later gave birth to a daughter with the head and face of a pig. This took part in 1621, and at the time of writing, this daughter was twenty years old. She ate from a trough and spoke in a grunting voice like a pig.

It is not fanciful to link this very early version of the pig-faced lady legend to that of her countrywoman Margaret of Henneberg. Indeed, one version of the latter legend says that the gentlewoman insulted the female beggar with the taunt that her children were like a litter of pigs. In the French version of the Porcelets, the noblewoman likening the beggar woman's children to a litter of squeaking piglets herself gave birth to nine little pigs. In this transitory version, the mother is punished both by the great number of "children" and by their deformity. The added horror of the child's pig face had great power and considerable popular appeal; in the mid-seventeenth century, it actually eclipsed the original version. It is thus very likely that with regard to the origin of the legend, the pig-faced lady is Countess Margaret's 366th godchild.

There have been several other theories as to the origin of the pig-faced lady legend. One of them assumed that the birth of some severely malformed child at the time, with a piglike visage and incapable of speech, might have given rise to a rumor that gradually got wilder and wilder, with colorful details like the silver trough and the immense dowry added to make the tale more interesting. The old annals of human monstrosities list an ape-woman, an elephant-man, a turtle-boy, a fish-boy, a bear-boy, a cat-woman, and several porcupine men, but no instance in which the unfortunate individual in the monster show was likened to a pig. In late-nineteenth- and early-twentieth-century Britain, there were several newspaper rumors that a pig-faced child had been born at some (named) hospital, but no further particulars of this unfortunate child were ever published, and the whole thing has many characteristics of the contemporary newspaper canard. A teratological case report, published in the *American Journal of Obstetrics and Gynecology* of 1952, described a stillborn fetus with a snoutlike face and many other malformations. But although the authors of this report were audacious enough to draw parallels with the nineteenth-century prints of the pig-faced lady, they wholly failed to convince the reader of any link between the malformations in question. In particular, while the "pig-face fetus" was incapable of extrauterine life, the traditional legend of the pig-faced lady presents her as being in the prime of health, her malformation notwithstanding.

There have also been, in otherwise-healthy individuals, instances of facial deformity, making the individual's face resemble that of a member of the porcine tribe. My early military service was in a small Swedish town. In certain isolated areas nearby, the deleterious effects of inbreeding were only too evident when one surveyed the intellectual ability and exterior appearance of the recruits that were natives of these parts. An extreme example of this was one of the enlisted sergeants, generally known (but never in his presence!) as the Pig-man. He was a remarkable sight with his large, snoutlike facial configuration, which was further adorned with an unkempt handle-bar mustache. The collar of his untidy, spotted uniform nearly choked him as he strode out to inspect his platoon through bulging, bloodshot eyes. His loud grunting voice, uneven tusklike teeth set in narrow jaws, and large floppy ears all added to the overall impression. For a short while, he had been a cabdriver, but few people had wanted a ride with such a sinister-looking creature. Perhaps the military authorities had hoped that the Pig-man would have a similar deterrent effect on invading Soviet storm troopers, or at least that he would be capable of scaring some discipline into the young National Service recruits. As second in command of his platoon, I witnessed the latter objective being achieved to perfection.

✺

In her earliest, mid-seventeenth-century incarnation, the pig-faced lady was treated as an object rather than a person; in spite of her costly dress and various lady-like accomplishments, she was just a malformed wooden dummy. No one ever felt sorry for the pig-faced lady, whose fate it was to be ridiculed, insulted, and surreptitiously rejected by her horrified suitors. The real objects of the satire in the ballads and pamphlets were the vainglorious upstarts, the tailors, captains, and sowce-men, people with whom the readers could identify: their ludicrous attempts to secure her hand in marriage, and their ignominious retreat. In the eighteenth and nineteenth centuries, the origin of the tale as a garbled version of the legend of Margaret of Henneberg gradually became forgotten. The persona of the pig-faced lady was still treated with the same jocularity and cheerful unconcern, however, even during the 1815 craze in London and the nineteenth-century exhibition of "Madam Steevens." A switch of gender would have been as unthinkable in 1815 as it was in 1639, and the story would have lost its entire fascination if it had dealt with a hog-faced *gentleman*. Today, the legend of the Pig-faced Lady is almost completely forgotten, although it may not be entirely fanciful to draw a parallel to Miss Piggy in the Muppets and her desire to marry her reluctant suitor, Kermit the Frog.

Joseph Sheridan Le Fanu was by no means a typical nineteenth-century horror novelist. He was a writer of considerable hidden depth who delighted in subtle hints and devious subplots. He used the standard Victorian sensation novel as his medium and accepted the obvious limitations this put on the artistic side of his work. Furthermore, his novels were of a very variable quality, and some of them were dashed off quickly due to pecuniary adversities. In contrast, he left the plot of *Uncle Silas* to mature for twenty-six years. As "Chapters in the History of an Irish Countess," a short version of the novel was published in the *Dublin University Magazine* of 1838, and later, as "The Murdered Cousin," in his 1851 collection *Ghost Stories and Tales of Mystery*. M. R. James was quite right that *Uncle Silas* was Le Fanu's best work by far, and it is still acknowledged as such by literary historians, including Le Fanu's biographer, Dr. W. J. McCormack. *Uncle Silas* is very carefully plotted, and it is clear that Le Fanu must have had some particular reason for including the poem about the lady with the pig's head. Neither M. R. James nor any other literary historian has ever found the original of this "Bretagne ballad"; the reason is probably that Le Fanu, a published poet in his youth, had written it himself with the purpose to add yet another of his clever puzzles to the complex narrative of *Uncle Silas*. All sources agree that the legend of the pig-faced lady was well known in mid-nineteenth-century Dublin, and Le Fanu must have heard of it, particularly as his house at Merrion Square in Dublin was not far from Steevens' Hospital. He may well have read one of the earlier pamphlets or poems about the hog-faced gentlewoman and her suitors and must certainly have been aware of the metaphorical meaning of the avaricious suitors to the pig-faced lady. Its meaning is likely to be that, in the eyes of Madame de la Rougierre, Maud Ruthyn is the Hog-faced Gentlewoman. Although she is described as a beautiful young girl rather than a deformed monster, her situation in life resembles that of the Pig-faced Lady. Her family is very rich, and she leads an isolated life in a large country house, along with her father, a retiring misanthrope who barely speaks to her. She is the sole heiress to his vast fortune. A certain

Captain Oakley, a foppish young military man, shows her attention and wishes to marry her for money. Her wicked Uncle Silas is also after her money, and as the scheming Madame de la Rougierre sings the ballad about the pig-faced lady, she is actually leading her naive charge to a concealed rendezvous with another avaricious suitor, her cousin Dudley, Silas's son. Can it be doubted that these two individuals, one a fortune seeker and the other the boorish, ill-mannered son of a murderer, are to symbolize the suitors to the Pig-faced Lady?

The inclusion of the wife of the Wandering Jew in Le Fanu's poem again testifies to his knowledge of Pig-faced Lady lore. Just as in the case of the marvelous birth of Margaret of Henneberg, there were several garbled versions of the legend of the Hog-faced Gentlewoman. One, allegedly immortalized in a sculpture in a Belgian cathedral, tells that a Christian man had converted to Judaism, but that shortly after, his wife gave birth to a girl with the face of a pig. The distraught man consulted a priest, who advised him to return to the faith of his fathers. He did so, and at the same moment, his daughter's porcine face changed into a divinely beautiful human face. Just like this version of the legend of the Pig-faced Lady, Le Fanu's *Uncle Silas* has a happy ending, although it is somewhat contrived. In the original concept of the story, outlined in *The Murdered Cousin*, the ending is that Dudley Ruthyn murders his own sister, using a pickax, since he mistakes her for Maud in the dark. Maud herself later becomes a gloomy old maid, who sits pondering her joyless and miserable life, saying that she would have preferred her cousin's fate for herself. Le Fanu thought this ending a bit too dismal for a popular novel and changed it when parts of the novel probably had already been written: it is not Maud's cousin, but Madame de la Rougierre herself, who is killed by mistake by the brutal Dudley. The novel leaves it unexplained how even a blood-crazed murderer could have made such a mistake: while Maud is described as shapely and slender in build, her former governess is a tall, strongly built woman with feet almost the size of a *pain riche*. At any rate, Maud is saved from the clutches of the villainous Uncle Silas, who later takes poison and dies. She marries a distinguished nobleman and thus also avoids the fate of the Pig-faced Lady: to live surrounded by wealth, but unmarried, unloved, and alone.

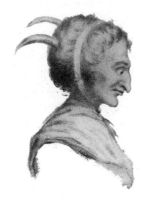

Horned Humans

IN HERMAN MELVILLE'S NOVEL *WHITEJACKET*, the reader encounters the somewhat sinister Surgeon of the Fleet Cadwallader Cuticle and his private museum of pathological specimens. The prize of his collection is a plaster cast of a human face, expressly stated to have been taken from life. Melville described this cast in such an eloquent way as to indicate that he had seen its original himself:

> It was the head of an elderly woman, with an aspect singularly gentle and meek, but at the same time wonderfully expressive of a gnawing sorrow, never to be relieved. You would almost have thought it the face of some abbess, for some unspeakable crime voluntarily sequestered from human society, and leading a life of agonized penitence without hope, so marvelously sad and tearfully pitiable was this head. But when you first beheld it, no such emotions ever crossed your mind. All your eyes and

all your horrified soul were first fascinated and frozen by the sight of a hideous, crumpled horn, like that of a ram, downward growing from the forehead, and partly shadowing the face; but as you gazed, the freezing fascination of its horribleness gradually waned, and then your whole heart burst with sorrow, as you contemplated those aged features, ashly pale and wan.

A rather less well-known writer, W. H. Davies, an eccentric Welshman who was a friend of George Bernard Shaw and who wrote the popular *Autobiography of a Super-tramp*, described a no less sinister encounter with a *homo cornutus* (horned human). In his youth, long before he set out touring the world as a tramp, he knew an old woman who always, indoor and out, was in the habit of wearing a cap that fitted her head very closely. One day, as she was sleeping in a chair before the fire, the mischievous young Davies crept up behind her and pulled her cap off. He was horrified to see that she had a pair of horns growing out of her head.

The literary imagination of the author of *Moby Dick* is undeniable, as is that of the globe-trotting Super-tramp, and many readers have probably considered their tales of these strange horned women as mere dramatic excesses. But it is a well-established fact in medical science that horned people have always existed, and neither Herman Melville nor W. H. Davies need to have exaggerated. In fact, both their accounts are likely to have been inspired by famous real-life cases of *homo cornutus*.

❧

In early times, horns symbolized wisdom and supernatural power. Both Moses and Alexander the Great were sometimes depicted with horns, to symbolize their omnipotence. Even Michelangelo's famous sculpture of Moses sports a pair of horns. Sorcerers and shamans wore headdresses with antlers, and the worship of a horned god, known as Pan or by other names, was widespread at the time when Christianity emerged. In England, worship of a horned god was particularly long-lasting, and at one time, in the seventh and eighth centuries, formed such a serious threat to early Christianity that bishops and archbishops anathematized the old rites severely. It was not until the attributes of Pan, including his horns, were attributed to the Christian Satan that the idea of a humanoid figure with horns acquired a wholly negative image.

The medieval chronicles have a good deal to say about horned human beings, but unfortunately little that belongs in the realm of reality. Conradus

122   Lycosthenes tells us that in the year 1225 in Raustadt in Germany, a child was heard to cry loudly in the womb before birth, to the terror of the mother and all around her. When the child was finally born, it had a pair of horns on its head. The learned Lanfrancus, writing toward the end of the thirteenth century, had once seen a man with seven horns on his head. He wanted the largest of them cut off, but Lanfrancus refused to perform such a hazardous operation and told the man that he should not waste time and money consulting other physicians, since he was completely incurable. Gilbert Nozerenus once saw a child with the face backward, a horn on the head, and the paws of a bear. Fincelius, in his aptly titled *De Miraculis*, told of a farmer's wife near Wistock who gave birth to a monstrous horned child, purple in color, with huge eyes, a wide mouth reaching from one ear to the other, and a cloven tongue.

Ambroise Paré, the founder of French surgery, several times mentioned horned humans. In his *Des Monstres et Prodiges*, he recorded that a woman near Turin had given birth to a five-horned child. He probably never saw this child himself (if it ever existed) and does not seem to have come across any other instance of *homo cornutus*. His collected case reports contain a not less startling observation, however: having *imaginary* horns was quite a common disease in sixteenth-century France, and Paré had seen several patients "who stubbornly persuaded themselves of having horns." This delusion could not be eradicated by any means from "the melancholy and bizarre brains" of the patients with this singular ailment. To effect a cure, Ambroise Paré blindfolded the patient and scratched him on each side of the forehead with a sharp cow's horn; the resulting effusion of blood often succeeded in persuading the patient that the horns had been torn out with force.

❧

Mrs. Margaret Gryffith, an elderly Welshwoman who appeared in London in 1588, has the dubious honor of being the earliest horned human being to be more thoroughly described. This was not due to the exertions of any member of the medical profession, however, but to a cunning showman successfully advertising his most recent "artist." In a pamphlet laboriously entitled *A Miraculous, and Monstrous, but yet most true, and certayne discourse, of a Woman (now to be seene in London) of the age of threescore years, or there abouts, in the midst of whose fore-head (by the wonderfull worke of God) there groweth out a crooked Horne, of foure ynches long*, her attractions were fully described. Margaret Gryffith was the widow of a husbandman named David Owyn, living in Llhan Gaduain in the county of Montgomery; they had three children alive. The cause for the horn was supposed to be that in her youth, her husband had suspected her of "some light behaviour" and chided her severely. She had denied this with much vehemence, and rejoined that if she had given her husband the horn through adultery, she wished that a horn would grow from her own forehead. To her great mortification, a small hard knob soon appeared in the middle of her forehead, and although she tried to cut it off or to file it, it grew steadily, and no surgeon could cure her.

In her widowhood, Margaret Gryffith lived quietly, and she maintained herself on a small parcel of land. The pamphlet does not state whether it was her own idea to go to London or whether some itinerant showman had "discovered" her in Wales; one would presume the latter. She appears to have been quite a success when put on show before the curious in London; it is recorded that even the Queen's Privy Council took time off from their preparations to receive the Spanish Armada, to see the horned old Welshwoman being exhibited. Her horn was probably kept for posterity. In 1599, when Thomas Plater of Basel visited the repertory of a London magnate, Sir Walter Cope, he saw "a round horn which had grown out of an Englishwoman's forehead."

Interestingly, several Elizabethan poets and playwrights alluded to Margaret Gryffith and her horn. Thomas Nashe, in *Have with You to Saffron Walden*, wrote that a certain gentleman, at an entertainment for Queen Elizabeth at Audley End, danced with a woman "thrice more deformed than the woman with a horne in her head." In John Marston's *The Malcontent*, published in 1604, the fool Passarello says that "the horn of a cuckold is as tender as his eye, or as that growing in the woman's forehead twelve years ago, that could not endure to be toucht." Thomas Dekker made even more direct use of the horned Welshwoman in his *Olde Fortunatus*, published in 1599. The plot is that the English princess Agripyne is tricked to eat the fruit of the Tree of Vice by her rival Andelocia. She then grows two horns from her forehead! When she complains to Andelocia that she has lost a magic purse, the wicked sorceress replies, "Sigh not for your purse, money may be got by you, as well as by the little Welshwoman . . . that had but one horne in her head, you have two." It is curious that both Marston and Dekker seem to have accepted the showman's tale that the horn had grown as the result of unchastity and vice, and used this imagery in their own plays.

∾

In 1598, ten years after Margaret Gryffith was exhibited in London, a party of French gentlemen were hunting in the forest near Mezières. They saw a group of rustic-looking mountain men standing nearby and engaged them in conversation. All the mountain men respectfully doffed their caps, except one surly-looking fellow. A certain M. de Laverdin reproached him for his insolence, but the man, a coarse character dressed in a jacket and trousers made from fox's furs, obstinately refused to remove his headgear. Enraged, M. de Laverdin then rode forth and tore the hat from his head. The gentlemen gave a great outcry of horror and surprise when they saw that the man had a large horn growing from the upper part of his bald forehead. It was curved like a ram's horn, and of considerable length and thickness.

After M. de Laverdin and his companions recovered their *sangfroid*, they spoke to the horned mountain man and examined him further. His name was François Trouvillou, he said, and he was thirty-five years old. He was a native of the village of Firmi. Since the age of seven, he had been aware of the horny growth on his forehead and had tried his best to hide it. But the horn grew at an alarming rate and had reached the length of a human finger when he was seventeen years old. One day, someone caught sight of it, and there was a great uproar in the village. Sorcery and witchcraft was of course suspected, and poor François was expelled from his village. Since then, he had earned a meager living as a huntsman and coaler up in the mountains. He kept his own company and always wore a hat. The horn appeared to have been fixed to the skull, but had some degree of movement. It grew in a curve and bent backward as far as the coronal suture. The sharp tip of the horn would have embedded itself in the scalp had François not filed it regularly.

Although François Trouvillou was a morose, unprepossessing character, and his behavior altogether rustic, his discoverers knew at once that they had come on to a good thing. Although many human and animal curiosities had previously been exhibited before the Parisians, a horned man would become quite a sensation. M. de Laverdin went to Paris and succeeded in obtaining an audience before King Henri IV. He gave such an eloquent description of his horned charge that the king immediately expressed a desire to see him. In a house near Saint-Eustache, François Trouvillou was introduced to the king. The reaction of either party unfortunately was not preserved for posterity, but it is known that certain irreverent courtiers remarked that with his reddish beard, bald head, and grotesque, curved horn, the mountain man was certainly the image of one of the satyrs of ancient legend. As a reward for this singular audience, Henri IV gave M. de Laverdin a signed permission to put François Trouvillou on show before the Paris townspeople. With this valuable help from the king, the enterprising showmen soon earned quite a fortune off their horned charge. The upkeep of this coarse country bumpkin cost them little, since he turned away the Parisian delicacies in favor of a rustic meal of gruel, cabbages, and lard. He stubbornly refused to use modern clothes and wore his strange costume made from fox's furs at all times, even in bed. A profound misogynist, he wanted nothing whatsoever to do with women. An excellent engraving of François Trouvillou, by Garnière, was sold at the exhibition, together with a brief account of his life.

During the two months he was on exhibition in Paris, François Trouvillou was seen by several scholarly observers, some of whom traveled to Paris

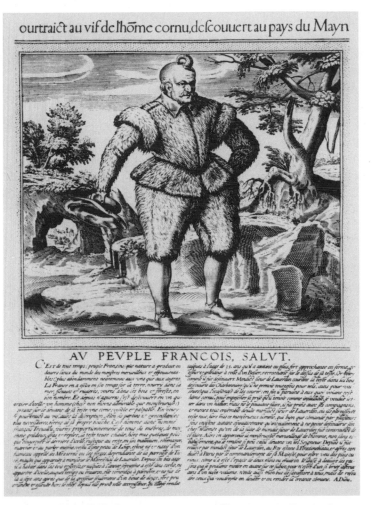

The original handbill about François Trouvillou. From a plate in the author's collection.

on purpose to see him. In the company of Dr. Jacob Fesch and his pupil Johannes Echenstein, Professor Emmanuel Ursitius had occasion to examine Trouvillou in 1598. Ursitius had read a tall story about a horned Benedictine monk who ruminated, and he wanted to examine Trouvillou's teeth, but the horned mountain man refused, in no uncertain terms. Another notable visitor was the philologist Isaac Casuabon, who left a thorough description of him. François Trouvillou told him about his sad childhood and how he had been banished from his village. He always kept his head covered during his stay in the mountains, since he was certain that if any person saw his horn, he would have been killed or imprisoned as a monster. His forehead, where the horn was situated, was completely bald. The horn was hard as a ram's horn and yellowish brown. Isaac Casuabon was apparently much impressed by this strange horned man and wrote that after seeing him, he no longer doubted the old legends of horned satyrs and aegipans.

After his successful stay in Paris, François Trouvillou was taken to Orléans, where he suddenly died in 1599, after previously appearing to be in good health. According to one account, he died from a broken heart after being exhibited like a wild beast before the coarse, unfeeling crowd, but this is probably an invention by some sentimental French writer. He was buried in the Saint-Côme cemetery in Paris, where his gravestone could still be seen in 1820, according to Dr. A. P. Dauxais, the author of a doctoral thesis on horned people. It had the suitable epitaph:

> *Dans ce petit endroit à part*
> *Gît un très-singulier cornard;*
> *Car il le fut sans avoir femme,*
> *Passans, priez Dieu pour son âme.*

This can be translated as:

> *A strange horned man departed this life,*
> *And lies buried under this gravestone.*
> *Since he got his horn without a wife,*
> *Pray for his soul, passer-by, ere you're gone!*

The engravings of François Trouvillou were widely disseminated all over Europe, and several medical men described the horned Frenchman in their scholarly tomes. Since it was now definitely proved that horned people really existed, many savants searched for other instances and tried to figure out what natural and supernatural causes could explain this anomaly. No one

was more eager to do so than Thomas Bartholin, the Danish anatomist
whom we have encountered several times in the pages of this book. He saw
Lazarus Colloredo and examined the Hairy Maid twice; he pondered the
mystery of the Stone-child, handled the Countess Margaret's missing infant,
and described the Magical Egg. Throughout his long career, Bartholin kept
a sharp lookout for horned human beings. In 1642, he was reading Judge du
Thou's historical anecdotes and encountered, in the 123rd book of this extensive collection, an account of François Trouvillou. He suspected that the
other descriptions of Trouvillou were taken from du Thou's work, but his old
friend and tutor Olaus Wormius wrote to tell him that Johannes Ursitius
himself had seen Trouvillou in Paris and touched the horn. An elderly Dane,
Dr. Christian Fabritius, had also been in Paris at the time and could well remember seeing François Trouvillou being exhibited.

The year after, Thomas Bartholin sent Wormius a picture of Trouvillou's
horned son, who was also shown in the marketplace as a curiosity. Olaus
Wormius scented knavery, however. He knew that it was possible to cut the
comb and spurs off a cock and transplant the spurs into the remnant of the

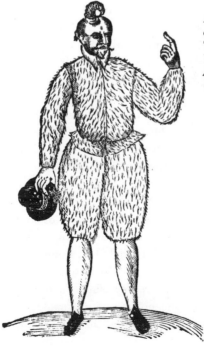

Another contemporary
drawing of François
Trouvillou. From
Ulysses Aldrovandi's
Monstrorum Historia
(1642).

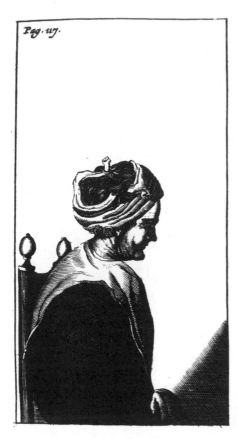

Pag. 117.

Thomas Bartholin's engraving of the horned Dutchwoman Margaretha Mainers. From the 1654 edition of Bartholin's *Historiarum Anatomicarum Rariorum, Centuria I–II*.

comb to make them appear like horns, and suspected that both François Trouvillou and his "son" had been subjected to some strange operation to make them into horned "curiosities" for the lucrative freak-show industry. Thomas Bartholin had heard from his friend Johannes Rhodius about the horned Benedictine monk who ruminated, and was amazed to find out that Trouvillou's alleged son was also reported to ruminate: had his father transmitted this character to the son, by virtue of the ruminant character both carried so conspicuously on their heads?

In 1646, Thomas Bartholin finally fulfilled his ambition to see a horned human being with his own eyes. In the northern parts of Holland, he saw the seventy-year-old woman Margaretha Mainers, who had a long, curved horn growing from the right temple. By some strange reasoning from the old woman herself, the appearance of the horn was attributed to the bitter quarrels she had had at the time with her prodigal son. The horn appeared like a goat's horn and grew curved almost in a bow. Interestingly, Bartholin noted that it grew from a reddish skin tumor, which the woman said was itching abominably; when she scratched it, it bled freely.

Thomas Bartholin later collected several other cases of horned humans. His friend, the famous anatomist Johann Caspar Bauhin, had seen a tailor who had a painful fleshy tumor behind the right ear. From this tumor grew a horn resembling a ram's horn, although smaller. It was possible to move it somewhat, but this caused the man much pain. Since the tumor from which the horn grew was a considerable one, no attempt was made to remove it. A sixty-year-old nun who consulted the anatomist Johann Vesling for a small horn growing from an encysted tumor on her forehead was more fortunate. The surgeon cut it off in the presence of Thomas Bartholin and tried to prevent its recurrence by etching her forehead with blue vitriol. The horn regrew, however. Although the poor nun objected to such a brutal method of treatment, Vesling then burned away the skin tumor with a red-hot branding iron. The eloquent Thomas Bartholin wrote that this operation was a complete success, thus verifying the words of Hippocrates: "What is not cured by fire, is incurable."

Thomas Bartholin's work inspired the German savant Georg Franck to write the earliest treatise entirely devoted to human horns. His thirty-one-page *Tractatus Philologico-Medicus de Cornutis*, published in Heidelberg in 1676, promised to cover all possible theological, legal, philosophical, historical, mathematical, ethical, philological, political, medical, and pathological aspects of horned human beings. It was a worthy review, although much devoted, in the manner of the time, to repeat the statements on the subject from all possible sources, the older the better. The reverence he felt for the old chroniclers prevented him from offering much in the way of a critical discussion, however, and some of his arguments belong in the age of superstition. Nevertheless, Georg Franck managed to draw up a list of twenty-five cases, several of them from the old monster chronicles, but others from Bartholin, Ulysses Aldrovandi, and other medical luminaries of the time.

In 1680, just a few years after Georg Franck's thesis was published, another horned Englishwoman made her curtsy from the London stage. Her name was Mary Davies and she was quite old at the time: one source says that she was born in Great Saughall near Chester in 1594, another that she was born in Shotwick in 1604. According to a letter from the Squire Owen Salus Evett of Brereton, to Sir Joseph Banks, she was born in 1591 and lived on the squire's family estate in Cheshire. Mary Davies was exhibited by the sign of the Swan, in the Strand, and a pamphlet entitled *A Brief Narrative of a Strange and Wonderful Old Woman that hath a Pair of Horns growing upon her head* was published to promote her career in show business. It contained the poem:

> *Ye who love wonders to behold,*
> > *Here you may of a wonder read:*
> *The strangest that was ever seen or told;*
> > *A Woman bearing Horns upon her head.*

130   Mary Davies was stated to be a wonder greater than any in Mr. Trades-
cant's famous cabinet of curiosities, and exceeding all the marvels the greatest travelers could, with truth, affirm to have seen. Mary Davies was the
widow of Henry Davies, who died twenty-five years previously; she was a
midwife by profession. In her youth, she was much troubled by a soreness in
her head, occasioned, the old gossips thought, by wearing a straight hat. This
soreness continued for twenty years and then ripened into a wen the size of
a hen's egg. Five years later, solid and wrinkled horns of a texture like a
ram's horn began to grow from this "wen, and sadly grieved the old woman,
especially upon changes in the weather." She shed her first pair of horns
after four years, and they were preserved by the vicar of Shotwick. The second pair, shed four years later, was purchased by Sir Willoughby Aston. The
third set of horns grew together to reach a length of not less than 9 inches,
but were broken off one day when Mary Davies slipped and fell backward.
This horn was purchased by a wealthy nobleman, who later presented it to
King Louis XIV of France.

     Mary Davies was still going strong in London late in 1680, and the ad-
vertisement promised that her fourth pair of horns would outgrow all the
others. What finally happened to the wonderful horned old woman is not
known, but one of her horns, and a portrait of her, were preserved in the
British Museum in the mid-eighteenth century. In the van Rymsdyk brothers' *Museum Britannicum*, published in 1778, the portrait of Mary Davies is
mentioned, but not her horn; this volume instead described an 11-inch horn
taken from a woman named Mrs. French, living near Tenterden. In 1685,
another of Mary Davies's horns was demonstrated by Dr. Robert Plot before
the Philosophical Society of Oxford. Mr. Elias Ashmole, the famous collector and antiquary, ordered that it be put in his repository. It was seen there
in 1710 by the German Zacharias Conrad von Uffenbach, who wrote that it
had been shed by the then seventy-one-year-old Mary in 1668. It was of a
blackish color, not very thick, but well proportioned. The same museum also
had two horns taken from the forehead of a man, and Uffenbach rather imprudently deduced, from this slender patient material of two, that the men
generally had their horns on the forehead and the females had theirs on the
back of the head. He illustrated Mary Davies's horn, which had a long and
graceful curve, just like her others, and postulated that England must have a
climate specifically predisposing for the formation of horns. He had never
seen goats and rams with such huge horns before he came to England, and
was not amazed that even the human beings sprouted horns in this *terra
maxime cornifera*. According to the Reverend John Pointer's *Oxoniensis*

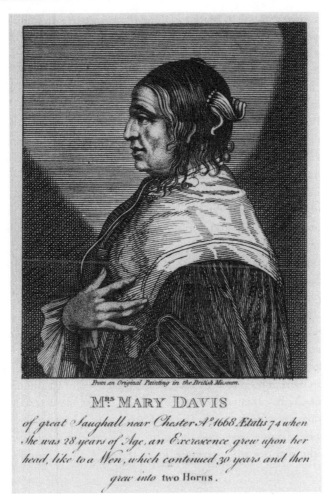

From an Original Painting in the British Museum.

M.ʳˢ MARY DAVIS

*of great Saughall near Chester A.º 1668 Ætatis 74 when
She was 28 years of Age, an Excrescence grew upon her
head, like to a Wen, which continued 30 years and then
grew into* two Horns.

A print of Mary Davies, the Horned Woman, aged 74. This
1792 print is allegedly based on an original painting of her in
the British Museum. Reproduced by permission of the
Wellcome Institute Library, London.

Academia, published in 1749, Mary Davies's horn could be seen in a room adjacent to St. John's College Library. The 1836 printed catalogue of the contents of the Ashmolean Museum mentions the horn. Dr. Erasmus Wilson, writing in 1844, confirmed that both Mary Davies's horns were still in their respective repositories. Neither of these horns is in existence today, however. They could have been lost through carelessness, or scrapped by some rationalist Victorian museum keeper lacking in reverence toward these early curiosities, just like the overzealous Danish museum curators who threw out the stone-child of Sens.

Mary Davies was described in several antiquarian works of the time, particularly in Charles Leigh's *Natural History of Lancashire*. A plate depicted her in 1668, aged 72, and another plate showed Alice Green, the Horned Woman of Whalley Abbey, who had two long horns growing out from the back part of her head. Leigh's portrait of Mary Davies was probably engraved from the British Museum portrait of her; another curious engraving of her, in Ormerod's *History of the County Palatinate and City of Chester*, was probably made from another portrait, also now lost, that had been in the Ashmolean Museum. Scotland has its own horned celebrity: Elizabeth Lowe, who was a contemporary of Mary Davies. In May 1671, when she was fifty years old, the surgeon Arthur Temple cut off a 4-inch horn growing from her skull, 3 inches above her right ear. It had been growing for seven years. An added note stated that Elizabeth Lowe was still living in 1682 and had another horn growing from the same site. The amputated horn was 4½ inches long, hard, and dark brown, in the shape of a stretched-out letter "S." It was kept in the anatomical museum of Edinburgh University for many years and was thoroughly described in Bennett's *Clinical Lectures* in 1858. The Scottish anatomists have been more reverent toward their horned celebrity than their colleagues in London and Oxford, and Elizabeth Lowe's horn is still in the Anatomical Collections of the Department of Biomedical Science, University of Edinburgh Medical School. It is kept in a cylindrical glass jar and held in place by a silver chain; an inscription on an oval silver plaque tells the story of the operation in 1671 by "Arthur Temple Chirurgion."

❧

It took a long time before the first systematic study of horned human beings was published, and well into the eighteenth century, the odd treatise of Franck von Franckenau remained the standard work on this subject. It was not until 1791, when the surgeon Everard Home read a paper on horny growths before the Royal Society of London, that the question was reviewed by a trained observer with up-to-date medical knowledge. Everard Home was the brother-in-law of the great John Hunter and served as his assistant surgeon at St. George's Hospital. Hunter was at this time the leading surgeon in London and a scientist of great talent and versatility. Hunter and Home were interested to note that the exhibition of horned "human curiosities" was still going strong in London two hundred years after the demise of Margaret Gryffith; at the time Everard Home was writing, two horned women were on show in the metropolis. One of them, the fifty-six-year-old Mrs. Lonsdale from Horncastle in Lincolnshire, had four horns growing from encysted scalp tumors. A certain Mrs. Elizabeth Allen from Leicestershire had a considerable horn growing from a burst encysted tumor. She was younger and more attractive than the horned old women described earlier, and became known as "the Female Satyr." Mrs. Allen achieved a brief noto-

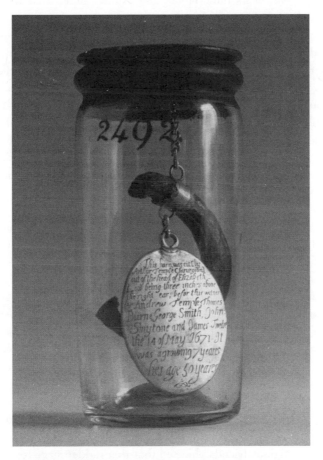

The horn of Elizabeth Lowe. Reproduced by permission of the Anatomical Museum Collection, Department of Biomedical Sciences (Anatomy), University of Edinburgh Medical School.

riety before the Londoners, but her neighbors back in Leicestershire were appalled by her brashness in putting herself on show, and her husband came to London and took her back home.

It is well known that John Hunter and Everard Home collaborated closely, and it is interesting to note that a newspaper article in the *British Mercury* stated that Elizabeth Allen had been presented to John Hunter, without even mentioning Home. It may well be that as in some other instances, Home had been provided with his busy master's notes on a certain subject, with instructions to write them up for publication. The article is certainly well ahead of its time. Home and Hunter noted that in both Mrs. Lonsdale and Mrs. Allen, the horns grew from encysted tumors on the head. This was apparently the case in many of the older instances of horned people, including the celebrated Mary Davies and the "wens" on her head, and had in fact been noted already by Thomas Bartholin 150 years earlier. Horny growths could occur all over the body, although those on the head and face had of course been particularly noticed. They had a perfectly natural explanation: a skin tumor, or repeated local trauma, changed the normal growth of the skin and caused it to produce a horny substance. Human horns were thus just another skin disease, like a birthmark or a wart. Although unsightly, most of them were not cancerous in nature, and the individual could live for a prolonged period of time, as demonstrated by Mary Davies and her horns, which grew for more than ten years.

This clear demonstration of the natural cause of human horns was published in the *Philosophical Transactions* of the Royal Society of London, a prestigious journal that was disseminated all over the world. The great German pathologists of the early nineteenth century agreed with Hunter and Home that human horns had a perfectly normal explanation, that they could arise not only on the head but also on any part of the body, and that they arose as a result of a diseased state of the skin. The acceptance of this theory among the medical scientists did not extend to the common people, however, and for many years to come, a horned human being was regarded with superstitious awe. A worthy example is the sad story of Mrs. Burnby, originally presented in the *Hampshire Telegraph* newspaper of April 13, 1812. This pious and worthy lady had remained single and worked as a schoolmistress until she was fifty years old. She then rather imprudently decided to marry, and although some of her religious friends objected that this sudden urge for matrimony might have arisen from impure motives, her decision was firm. But just as she was walking back from church after the wedding ceremony, "a mental derangement took place," and for the rest of her long life, poor Mrs. Burnby never recovered. As a final frisson of horror, it was added that during her prolonged residence in the local madhouse, a 6-inch, crooked horn grew from her forehead.

Another strange story is that of Anna Schimper, the horned nun of Filzen. She was born in 1747 and entered the Filzen nunnery at an early age. In 1795, French revolutionary troops occupied the area. One day, they suddenly charged the nunnery and chased the German nuns out of their cells and chapel, shouting, breaking windows, and singing irreligious songs. Poor Anna Schimper's secluded life had not prepared her for such a shock to her

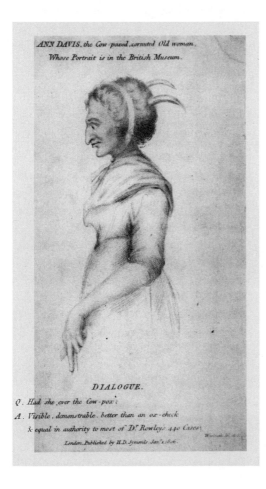

A print by Thomas A. Woolnoth of Ann Davis, a woman with cowpox and a pair of horns growing out of her head. The print was issued in London 1806. Reproduced by permission of the Wellcome Institute Library, London.

mental equilibrium: at the sight of the marauding Frenchmen, she went completely insane and had to be taken from her cell in the nunnery to another cell in the local lunatic asylum. Here, she spent most of the time banging her head against a solid table. After a number of years, the asylum attendants saw that a horn was growing from a large bump on her head, just above the right eye, where she used to pound it against the furniture. Miraculous to say, the longer and thicker this horn grew, the more Anna Schimper's clouded mind improved, and by the time she sported a thick, curved horn that almost obscured the right eye, she was fit enough to move back to the Filzen nunnery, which by this time had been restored by the German authorities. The horned nun resided there for many years, in the odor of sanctity, and was promoted to abbess in due course. In 1834, her horn had grown to such a prodigious size that she felt ashamed of it; every time she went outside the convent, she had to cover it up with her headdress. She consulted the surgeon W. Giese, who finally agreed to cut it off. It was feared that Anna Schimper might not survive this operation, but although the bleeding was quite considerable, the eighty-seven-year-old abbess soon recovered and went back to her duties at the nunnery. She died two years later, with a small horn regrowing from the thick, ulcerated skin tumor above the eye, from which the original horn had grown. A sentimental German poet wrote a lengthy epistle, entitled *The Finger of God*, to celebrate her strange life and miraculous recovery.

The largest human horn ever recorded belonged to a Mexican. Señor Paul Rodrigues was a strong, muscular fellow, who worked as a packer in a warehouse. He always kept his head covered with a large handkerchief. One day in 1820, a large barrel of sugar fell down from a pile and struck him on the head. When the bystanders removed the handkerchief from the head of the unconscious man, they saw to their horror that he had an enormous horny growth emerging from the upper and right sides of his head, not less than 14 inches in circumference. All three horns were curved, with a texture similar to that of a ram's horn. His ear could be touched through the opening between the first and second horns. The back horn had partially been knocked off by the blow from the barrel. The doctors and nurses at the Anderes hospital bandaged poor Rodrigues, and it appears as if he escaped this adventure with his life, but his secret had been exposed. Professor Cevallos, the chief medical officer at the hospital, published an account of the case, of which translation was published in the *Medical Repository*, an influential early American medical journal, along with a discussion comparing Rodrigues with some earlier cases of local interest. Mr. Scudder's Museum in Philadelphia contained a 7-inch horn taken from the head of an old woman. Not to be outdone, a certain Dr. Chatard reported that he once, in Baltimore, saw another old woman with a large horn on her nose, much resembling that of a rhinoceros.

An equally grotesque horn belonged to the widow Mme Dimanche, an elderly Frenchwoman who lived at No. 12 Rue de Bercy in Paris. At some time in the late 1830s, she was admitted as an inpatient at the Hospice de Perfectionnement of the Medical School of Paris. Mme Dimanche was quite a celebrity in Paris, where she was known as "Mère-la-Corne" or "Mother Horn." An enormous horny excrescence grew from the forehead and extended downward, shadowing her face. It was 10 inches long and 2 inches in diameter at its base. It was not implanted in the frontal bone, and its weight was fatiguing to the poor woman, who had to wear a linen sheath around her horn to support it; this sheath was fastened to the band of the night cap she always wore. Mme Dimanche was seen by many surgeons during her stay in the hospital ward and received many offers of having her horn removed by means of operation, but she always refused. Later, at the venerable age of almost eighty, having carried her grotesque horn for at least six years, she finally consented to having it cut off. Her motive was that she did not dare to meet her Maker with such a satanic ornament on her face. The operation was performed by the celebrated surgeon Joseph Souberbielle and was a complete success. According to the *Magasin Pittoresque*, Mother Horn was still alive at the age of eighty-four, without the horn regrowing. In the 1830s and 1840s, several wax or plaster casts were made of Mme Dimanche's face and the horn. In 1851, the Boston Society for Medical Improvement discussed a cast of Mme Dimanche, quoting a description of the case given by Dr. Souberbielle himself, in a letter from Paris dated March 12, 1845. The cast was described as belonging to the "College Cabinet," and a certain Dr. J. B. S. Jackson mentioned that copies of the cast of the head of Mother Horn could be found at several other American pathological museums. Indeed, copies of the model were exhibited in a number of American popular anatomy museums located in Chicago, New York, and Philadelphia. What has happened to these casts is not known, but one example of the model (perhaps the original) can still be seen at the Mütter Museum of the College of Physicians of Philadelphia. The latter specimen may well have been purchased by Dr. Mütter himself somewhere in Europe; it came into the Mütter Museum's possession as part of his original bequest in 1858. Also kept at his museum is a 12-inch (30-centimeter) horn, removed from a seventy-year-old woman who had had it for seven years. Several casts of Mother Horn were kept at various French museums; one of them was at the Musée Dupuytren in Paris in the 1930s.

❧

Some modern debunkers and rationalists have tried to cast doubt on the old cases of horned people and implied that some of them belong in the realm of the fabulous. Already Olaus Wormius doubted whether François Trouvillou's alleged "horned son" was an impostor, perhaps with some right since it seems as if this individual was merely profiting from Trouvillou's great notoriety. There should be no doubt whatever about the genuineness of François Trouvillou's own horn, however. The contemporary descriptions agree perfectly well, and the trained medical men who saw him would not have been deceived by a faked horn attached to his head. In 1935, an almost identical case was described in the *Indian Medical Gazette*: an eighteen-year-old man

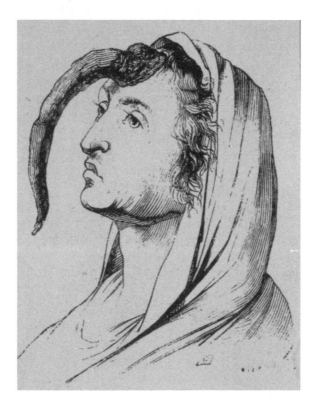

A French drawing of Mme Dimanche.

with a curved, 5-inch horn growing from the top of his bald head. This horn very much resembled that of François Trouvillou. It gave him no trouble, and the only reason why the young Indian applied to Dr. J. M. Richardson of Bilaspur was that his strange appearance had given him an unwelcome notoriety in the village, and it was impossible for him to persuade any of the local maidens to marry him! Dr. Richardson performed the operation without difficulty, and the large horn, which sprang from the aponeurosis of the occipitofrontal bone, was removed.

The exhibition of horned people for money continued well into the twentieth century. In 1930, newspapers told that a Chinese peasant with two horns on his head had been taken to Japan for the purpose of being exhibited. He was given the princely salary of two thousand pounds per year. His biggest horn was 10 inches (25 centimeters) long and 6 inches (15 centimeters) in diameter at the root. Several "horned men" have been active in American sideshows, although at least one of them seems to have been exposed as a fraud. I have seen a photograph of a Chinese man named Wang, billed as "The Human Unicorn" who had a 14-inch horn growing from the back of the head. His strange appearance certainly matched that of François Trouvillou.

Modern dermatology agrees with John Hunter and Everard Home that human horns can arise all over the body and not only on the scalp; in fact, only 30 percent of them are located on the face or scalp. They consist of concentric layers of keratinized epithelial cells; unlike true horns, they have no bony core. They are caused by a variety of skin diseases. According to a recent pathological study, 65 percent of all cutaneous horns are benign and caused by skin warts or epithelial hyperplasia. Another group of human horns (20 percent) are due to premalignant conditions, mainly solar keratosis and Bowen's disease (basal cell carcinoma). Finally, 15 percent are caused by malignant skin tumors, mainly squamous cell carcinoma. It has been noted several times that individuals with large, broad-based horns often have squamous cell carcinomata. In 1995, a Turkish woman presented with a 3-inch horn growing from the left aspect of the nose. The horn was excised by the surgeons, and the pathological diagnosis was squamous cell carcinoma. There were no signs of metastasis, and the woman recovered. In 2002, a group of medical scientists reviewed four modern cases of gigantic cutaneous horns of the scalp. One of them had grown from the scalp of a 55-year-old woman for thirty years and was 10 inches in length; it was curved and resembled that of François Trouvillou. It had never given her any pain, but she had concealed it from feelings of stigma and shame. The histology

140 in all four cases was that of a so-called proliferating tricolemmal tumor, a form of very low-malignant squamous cell carcinoma. It is very likely that some of the historical instances of horns of the scalp, such as those of Margaret Gryffith, Mary Davies, and the horned nun of Filzen, had a similar etiology.

W. H. Davies's encounter with the horned woman could have been inspired by some odd family tradition; it could also be the result of reading some popular account of Mary Davies. The biography of this horned celebrity was frequently reprinted in various nineteenth-century anthologies of *biographia curiosa*, one of which may well have been read by the young Davies. Some literary historians proposed the sixteenth-century pamphlet about Margaret Gryffith as a source for Herman Melville's account of the horned woman in *Whitejacket*, but this is extremely unlikely to have been the case. The pamphlet about her was extremely rare, and her case little known even among the antiquaries. It is also notable that Surgeon of the Fleet Cuticle actually had a plaster cast of the woman in question, and that this cast was stated to be "often to be met with in the Anatomical Museums of Europe." Only one historical case of *homo cornutus* fulfills these characteristics: it is evident that the enormous horn of Mme Dimanche was the one to have inspired Herman Melville's account of the horned woman in *Whitejacket*. It is apparent from his description that the plaster cast of Surgeon Cuticle was identical to one of the several made of Mother Horn. It is just possible that he might have seen the wax model in Dr. Mütter's collection, if it was there in 1849, or maybe one of the copies that were exhibited in various popular anatomy museums. More probably, he had seen the model of Mother Horn's head at the Musée Dupuytren in Paris. This museum was open to the public in Melville's time, although "to gentlemen only" owing to its gruesome contents. It is interesting to note that according to Herman Melville's journal entry for December 5, 1849, he went to the Musée Dupuytren and saw "Rows of cracked skulls. Skeletons & things without a name." This date was just before he finished *Whitejacket*; indeed, one of the purposes of his journey to London and the continent was to find a suitable publisher for this manuscript. The macabre sight of the plaster cast of Mother Horn is likely to have inspired him to incorporate a similar cast into his fictionalized narrative.

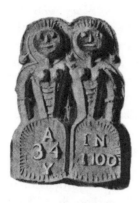

The Biddenden
Maids

O N EVERY EASTER MONDAY MORNING, THE
village of Biddenden, situated not far from Staplehurst in Kent, is
the scene of a curious old custom called the Biddenden Maids'
Charity. Through the window of a building called the Old Workhouse, tea,
cheese, and loaves of bread are given to the local widows and pensioners.
Large amounts of "Biddenden cakes," baked of flour and water, are distributed among the crowd of tourists and spectators. The cakes bear the effigy of
the Biddenden Maids, two female figures whose bodies appear to be joined
together at the hips and shoulders. A tradition of obscure and ancient origins
tells that these Maids were born in the year 1100 and that they lived joined
together for thirty-four years. The Biddenden Maids have been extensively
cited in the medical literature as one of the earliest genuine cases of conjoined (Siamese) twins on record, although some antiquaries have considered the tradition to be a mere fable, and others have suggested that the
Maids' year of birth was probably closer to 1500.

According to tradition, the Biddenden Maids, Mary and Eliza Chulkhurst, were born to fairly wealthy parents in the year 1100. Their bodies were joined at the hips and shoulders. They were naturally close friends, although one source stated that they sometimes disagreed in minor matters and had "frequent quarrels, which sometimes terminated in blows." In 1134, when the Maids had lived joined together for thirty-four years, Mary was suddenly taken ill and died. It was proposed that Eliza should be separated from her sister's corpse by means of a surgical operation, but she refused ⌐with the words "As we came together we will also go together," and she died six hours later. In their joint will, the Maids left certain parcels of land in Biddenden, a total of about twenty acres, to the churchwardens of that parish and their successors in perpetuity. The rent from these fields, henceforth known as the Bread and Cheese Lands, was to provide an annual dole for the poor. A somewhat suspect nineteenth-century account tells us that the annual income from the Maids' parcels of land was six guineas at the time of their death. Every Easter Sunday for many years, the Maids' charity of bread, cheese, and beer was given to the deserving poor. When Biddenden Church was visited by the archdeacon of Canterbury on Easter Day 1605, the custom that "on that day our parson giveth unto the parishioners bread, cheese, cakes and divers barrels of beer, brought in there and drawn" was not observed, because it was usually accompanied by "much disorder by reason of some unruly ones, which at such a time we cannot restrain with any ease." In 1645, the Rector William Horner had brought a lawsuit before the Committee for Plundered Clergymen to claim that the Bread and Cheese Lands were glebe land and thus belonged to the church rather than the villagers. The case caused quite a controversy between the rector and the churchwardens, but in 1649 the rector finally lost his case. In 1656, the persistent clergyman brought another protracted lawsuit in the Court of the Exchequer for the recovery of these lands, but again without success, and the Biddenden Easter charity continued as before. In 1681, another controversial Biddenden rector, Giles Hinton, reported to the archbishop of Canterbury that the distribution was made inside the church "with much disorder and indecency," and he suggested that the custom needed "a regulation by His Grace's Authority." The charity remained, however, although the distribution of the cakes was removed to the church porch. In the second half of the eighteenth century, the food was distributed directly after the afternoon service, and the church was filled with a large and hungry congregation. In 1770, the income from the Maids' lands was twenty guineas per annum, and a good deal of bread, cheese, and beer was distributed. Those who did not gain an entrance into the crowded church had to be content with the hard Biddenden cakes with the Maids' effigy, which were thrown out among the populace from the church roof; already in the eighteenth century, these cakes were much sought after as curiosities. According to some antiquaries, a broadsheet on the Chulkhurst sisters and their bequest was printed already in the late eighteenth century and sold outside the church during Easter. What may have been a later version of this "broadside" was printed in 1808 and sold for two pence; I have seen several copies of it, one of which is in my own collection. Furthermore, a small plaque of the Maids was made in glazed red clay in imitation of the Biddenden cake. By this time, the income from the Maids' lands had increased to thirty-one guineas and eleven shillings per annum, and as many as one thousand Biddenden cakes were baked, as well as three hundred quartern loaves and cheese in proportion.

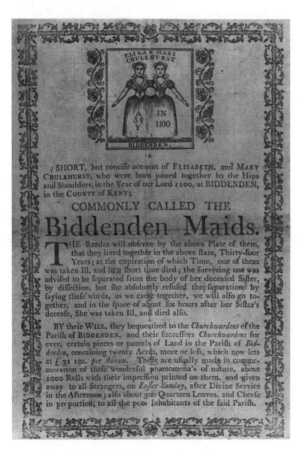

A broadsheet on the Biddenden Maids and their bequest, published in 1808. From the author's collection.

144   In the 1820s, a "new and enlarged" account of the Maids was printed, in which it was stated that a gravestone marked with a diagonal line, situated near the rector's pew in Biddenden church, was shown to visitors as the Maids' place of interment. The church floor has since been renewed, and there is no gravestone visible near the rector's pew, but it might be that it is situated beneath the organ, which now stands behind the rector's seat. It is probable that the Chulkhurst sisters were depicted on a stained glass window in the church's east wall, which has now been filled in. A poem regarding this was quoted from the old charity documents:

> *The moon on the east oriel shone,*
> *Through slender shafts of shapely stone,*
> *The silver light, so pale and faint,*
> *Shewed the twin sisters and many a saint*
> *Whose images on the glass were dyed;*
> *Mysterious maidens side by side.*
> *The moon beam kissed the holy pane,*
> *and threw on the pavement a mystic stain.*

    Thus the grave of the Biddenden Maids cannot be identified with certainty. The oldest parts of the present church of Biddenden are from the twelfth century; the impressive tower was added around the year 1400, but an older Saxon church had been standing on the same spot.

    According to the entries for March 1826 in Hone's *Every Day Book*, Biddenden was at this time completely thronged with visitors on Easter Sunday, "attracted from adjacent towns and villages by the usage, and the wonderful account of its origin." The public houses had a busy time, and the day was generally spent "in rude festivity." The increasing fame of the Biddenden Maids and their charity made the crowds that gathered in the church on Easter Sunday larger and more unruly; there were many disturbances during service, and the churchwardens sometimes had to use their long wands as weapons to keep back the hungry and impatient congregation. As a result of this, the distribution of the charitable food was moved to the Biddenden poorhouse and performed immediately after the afternoon service on Easter Sunday. In 1882, the rector of Biddenden wrote to the archbishop of Canterbury that the Easter ceremony was still disorderly as a result of excessive partaking of the beer, and he wished that it should be discontinued. The archbishop allowed it to continue, although he deprived the recipients of the beer. In April 1900, a local newspaper stated that large crowds of people

assembled in the highway at the Old Workhouse on Easter Sunday, and the
two police constables who guarded the approach to the gateway had considerable difficulties in keeping them back. Altogether 190 loaves and cheese in
proportion were distributed in that year, and the five hundred Biddenden
cakes baked for visitors were quite insufficient to meet the demand. The
Times newspaper of April 14 and 17, 1900, also gave attention to this ancient
custom and stated that actual records supported that the distribution of the
cakes, on which the Maids "were represented as united together, like the
Siamese twins," had taken place as far back as 1740, and very probably long
before that date.

In 1907, the Chulkhurst charity was consolidated with some other local
charities, in order to provide the Biddenden pensioners and widows with
bread, cheese, and tea every Easter and a sum of money at Christmas. In due
course, the Bread and Cheese Lands were sold, and today they contain a
number of cottages called the Chulkhurst Estate. This has made it possible
to extend the charity considerably. For many years, it was a custom to bake
special, very large loaves for the Easter festivity, but this ceased when the
Biddenden baker's shop closed down. The distribution of bread and cheese

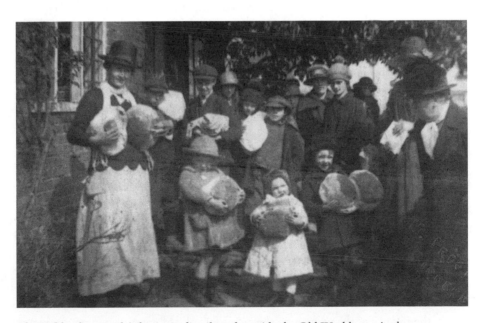

The Biddenden Maids' charity is distributed outside the Old Workhouse in the
1910s. From an old photograph in the author's collection.

146   from the Old Workhouse has been continued as a curiosity, and it is today a popular tourist attraction; every visitor may have a Biddenden cake as a memento of the ceremony. The cakes are so hard as to be almost uneatable, but they are the more enduring as travel souvenirs. At the Biddenden village green stands a wrought sign of the philanthropic Chulkhurst twins, which was erected in the 1920s.

The Antiquarian Evidence

The two best-known early sources on the Biddenden Maids are the 1775 edition of the *Antiquarian Repertory* and Dr. Ducarel's *Repertory of the Endowments to the Diocese of Canterbury and Rochester*, published in 1782. These two early accounts agree that the charity had existed for a very long time and that it had been started by two conjoined twin sisters. According to one version, they were joined together at the shoulders and "lower part of their bodies" and lived many years, while in the other, it is merely stated that they were joined together in their bodies, and that they lived in this state until they were "betwixt 20 and 30 years old." The earliest proper account of the Biddenden Maids is an anonymous article in the *Gentleman's Magazine* of 1770. Interestingly, this article stated that the Maids were conjoined from the waist down to the hips, and thus not joined at two separate anatomical sites; they lived in this way until they were "considerably advanced in years." It is specifically stated that they were not known by any particular name. In spite of the "high antiquity" of the tradition, the writer of the article did not doubt its authenticity: "An enquiry in the parish itself will procure abundant testimony, that the reality of this prodigy has always been honored with the highest credit." None of these three independent eighteenth-century accounts of the Maids mentioned two veritable cornerstones in their legend: the name of Chulkhurst and their alleged year of birth, 1100; these details were added in the broadsheet that appeared in the 1790s.

While these three early accounts of the Biddenden Maids took their existence for granted, the antiquary Edward Hasted declared the tradition to be nothing but an old fable, in his *History of Kent*. This monumental historical work, which cost its author more than forty years of labor, was published in four folio volumes between 1778 and 1799. Edward Hasted stated that the legend of the Biddenden Maids was merely "a vulgar tradition" and that the charity in reality had been initiated by two maidens by the name of Preston; the picture of the women on the cakes was the likeness of two poor widows, the most likely recipients of the Biddenden charity. He also claimed that the print of the women on the cakes had only occurred during the last fifty years (he was writing in the 1780s). Edward Hasted was an acknowledged expert on topography and genealogy, but although his conclusions about the Biddenden Maids have been largely accepted by later British antiquaries, it might be doubted whether he appreciated the ethnological aspects of the problem. Hasted's contemporary Sir Egerton Brydges described him in his autobiography as "a little, mean-looking man, with a long face and a high nose; quick in his movements and sharp in his manner. He had no imagination or sentiment, nor any extraordinary quality of mind, unless memory." Although this severe judgment of the old antiquary is probably exaggerated, some later critics have also had a low opinion of the social and biographical parts of Hasted's *History of Kent*.

Edward Hasted's harsh judgment of the Biddenden Maids tradition was uncritically accepted in several nineteenth-century British ethnological and archaeological works, and during this time there was little new information on the Chulkhurst sisters and their curious bequest. The Maids were sometimes mentioned in articles concerning the celebrated Siamese twins: a note about the Maids was added after Sir James Simpson's lecture on Siamese twins was published in the *British Medical Journal* of 1869, and in 1874, the Biddenden Maids were discussed before the Philadelphia College of Physicians. The Maids were mentioned several times in the pages of the *Notes and Queries* magazine, particularly after the original Siamese twins, Chang and Eng, had toured Europe and showed that such a malformation was certainly not incompatible with life for a considerable period of time. In a note from 1866, the editors of this journal doubted Hasted's explanation of the print of the conjoined twin sisters and the name Chulkhurst on the Biddenden cakes, and considered that the mystery of the Maids was yet unsolved and that it was "well worth the attention of some of the Kentish antiquaries" to investigate it.

This challenge remained unanswered for many years, but in 1900, the antiquary George Clinch published a thorough paper on the Maids, in which he provided a good deal of new information. He obtained plaster impressions of the molds for the Biddenden cakes and examined them closely, attempting to determine the custom's antiquity. His photographs of the three cake molds, which are reproduced here, all seem to depict the Biddenden Maids as conjoined twins. While on the broadsheet, the Biddenden Maids are depicted as handsome in feature and elegantly dressed in the costume of the time of Mary I, their picture on the oldest cake mold is primitive and bizarre. The eyes, faces, and breasts are represented only by protrusions,

148 and the wear and tear of the old mold in the baker's shop could only partially be blamed for the snoutlike expression of the faces. There are several other odd details, such as the arrangement of the hair, the presence of naked branches of trees on either side of the Maids, and a starlike object between their waists. The second type of cake differs from the first in that the design of the faces is flatter and more detailed, and the dress is more ornamental. The headdress is new to this mold, as are the large earrings. This mold was used for Biddenden cakes in the 1820s and in the 1860s; it is most probable that it was also used in 1875 and spoken of as boxwood dies cut in 1814. The third mold is the most detailed and ornamental, and certainly the latest; the semicircular top has the picture of a sun, and the tree branches from the first mold recur. The costume is not unlike that of the second mold. Another writer, the teratologist J. W. Ballantyne, spoke of two molds for Biddenden cakes being used in 1895, one being the older (probably 150 years old), while the other was made much more recently. It is likely that these were the first and third molds, respectively, of those photographed by Clinch. Today, only one cake mold is used, and this is of a much later date. According to the trustees of the Chulkhurst charity, none of the older molds have been kept for posterity.

From his examination of the lettering and costume of the molds, George Clinch considered them to be from the sixteenth century. An expert in such matters, Mr. Mill Stephenson, F.S.A., suggested that the Maids' clothing was from the latter part of the sixteenth century. However, there are strong arguments that none of the molds depicted by Clinch were actually in use before the 1780s. Specimens of Biddenden cakes from the 1770s were reproduced by Dr. Ducarel and by the anonymous writer in the *Antiquarian Repertory*; they differ markedly from those described by Clinch, which were probably nineteenth-century specimens. None of the three cakes from the 1770s record the names of the Maids or their year of birth or age at the time of their death. Clinch blamed the carelessness of the eighteenth-century engravers for this inconsistency, but this seems less likely. It is reasonable to suggest that there were in fact several older molds used during the eighteenth century: it was reported in the *Antiquarian Repertory* that the cakes were "of different fineness and forms," and drawings of two different cakes were reproduced. The pictures of the women on the Biddenden cakes from the 1770s have many details in common with those of the later cake molds, especially the oldest of these. The three eighteenth-century accounts of the Maids previously quoted do not mention their names, and it is even explicitly stated that "the Maids of Biddenden are not known by any particular

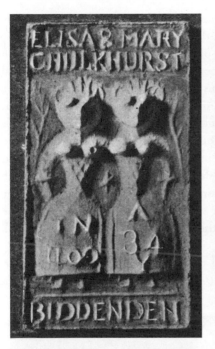

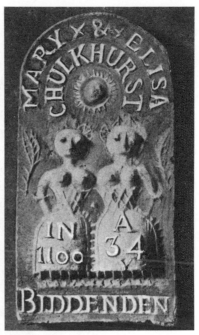

Plaster casts of the three wooden stamps for Biddenden cakes that were available to Clinch in 1900. From Clinch's article in the *Reliquary* magazine.

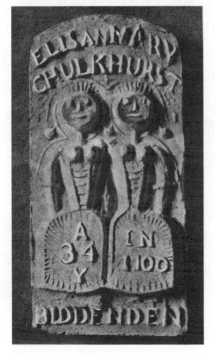

150   name." Had the cake molds photographed by Clinch been in use during this period, there would have been no difficulty in determining their proper names as well as their alleged year of birth. Clinch's arguments about the Maids' clothing may certainly be correct, since the effigy was obviously copied from the older molds. In the *Antiquarian Repertory* of 1775, it was stated that the sisters lived "as tradition says, two hundred and fifty years ago," and Clinch considered this estimate more trustworthy than the popular belief that they were born in 1100; thus their year of birth would have been in the beginning of the sixteenth century. Furthermore, Clinch's examination of the oldest cake mold led him to believe that the second numeral from the left in the date was really a slightly curved "5," and that the Maids were thus born in 1500. However, I am unable to detect any difference at all between the two first numerals in the date of this, or any other, of the Biddenden cake molds.

Several antiquaries commented on Clinch's article, usually to defend Hasted's arguments; in the *Notes and Queries* magazine, it was even stated that

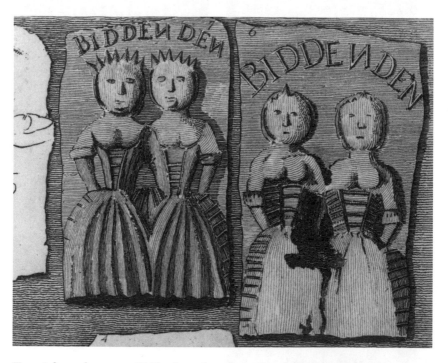

Two eighteenth-century Biddenden cakes. Reproduced from the *Antiquarian Repertory* of 1775.

"the whole story is discredited by competent antiquaries." The antiquary Arthur Hussey examined the index of wills at the Canterbury Probates Office, and found none with the name of Chulkhurst. Among the historical and ethnological writers of today, the opinions on the Biddenden Maids are divided: some agree with Hasted that the old tradition is entirely fabulous, while others favor the version that they lived in the sixteenth century. In the medical literature, however, the legend of the Biddenden Maids is uncritically accepted, including their year of birth, 1100.

The Medical Evidence

In all time, the phenomenon of conjoined twinning has fascinated both laymen and the medical profession, and the literature on this subject reaches back far into time. Normal twins are either dizygotic (70 percent) or monozygotic. Dizygotic twins are the result of the fertilization of two separate ova; monozygotic (identical) twins are the result of splitting of the fertilized ovum at an early stage of its development. In the majority of monozygotic twins (97 percent), this splitting of the ovum happens at what is known as the morula or blastocyst stages, before the development of an amniotic cavity; thus the twins will have one amniotic membrane each. If the splitting happens at a later stage, the twins will share one amniotic membrane. If the splitting is only partial, which happens in about 10 percent of monoamniotic twins, the twins will be conjoined. Thus, conjoined twins are always monozygotic and always of the same sex, share one placenta and one amnionic membrane, and have identical chromosomal patterns. The incidence of conjoined twinning is approximately one in 100,000 deliveries, but approximately 60 percent of twins are stillborn.

The conjoined (or Siamese) twins are classified by the site of connection. The most common type is thoracopagus twins, which are joined at the chest, followed by omphalopagus (or xiphopagus) twins, which are joined at the upper abdomen. Other sites of connection include the inferior margins of the pelvis (ischiopagus), the sacrum (pygopagus), and the skull (craniopagus). A major difficulty in accepting the tradition of the Biddenden Maids as entirely authentic is the nature of their malformation: in the available cakes and drawings, they are depicted as being conjoined both at the shoulders and at the hips. It is extremely rare for Siamese twins to have two separate parts of conjunction. In those few instances, two quite closely related points of fusion have been involved, such as the thorax and abdomen or lower abdomen and peritoneum. Although Professor Ian Aird, a well-known English expert on conjoined twins, did not consider such a double conjunction to be impossible, with the motivation that separate blastomeres might fuse at two different points, or that twins fused primarily at one point might obtain a secondary fusion later, very few modern teratologists would accept the possibility of a fusion at the hips and shoulders, particularly in a pair of viable twins.

In 1895, the surgeon J. W. Ballantyne, a well-known authority on obstetrics, gynecology, and congenital deformities, was the first to consider the Biddenden Maids from a teratological point of view. He suggested that they were in fact only conjoined at the hips and thus belonged to the teratological type pygopagus. Such conjoined twins each have two arms and legs, and it has often been noted that in order to walk without difficulty, they put their arms around each other's shoulders; this might have led to the Biddenden Maids being depicted in the way described earlier. The German teratologists Ernst Schwalbe and Hans Hübner agreed with Ballantyne's hypothesis, as did the French surgeon Marcel Baudouin. The teratological type pygopagus, in which the twins are joined at the sacrum, comprises about 8 percent of conjoined twins. The twins have more or less complete fusion of the rectum and other perineal structures, but the spinal cords are usually separate. The first case of pygopagi on record, living twins born in Rome 1493, was described by Conradus Lycosthenes in his *Chronicon Prodigorum et Ostentorum*. The first attempt of separating such twins was made in 1700 by the use of caustic, resulting in the death of both twins. The first successful surgical separation of pygopagus twins was performed in 1950, and in later years, several pairs of such twins were separated. The success of the operation depends very much on the extent of the conjunction between the bodies and the number of shared organs, as well as the occurrence of additional malformations of the heart and lungs.

A fair proportion of pygopagus twins are perfectly viable at birth, and several of the historical cases have reached maturity. The Hungarian Sisters, Helena and Judith, were a celebrated pair of eighteenth-century pygopagus twins; they traveled extensively through Europe and were examined by many eminent anatomists and naturalists. In 1708, at the age of seven, they were brought to England and publicly shown in London. James Paris du Plessis, the writer on monstrosities whose thoughts on pig-faced ladies were quoted earlier, had occasion to see them, as evidenced by his manuscript *History of Prodigies* in the British Library:

> They were brisk, merry, and well-bred; they could read, write, and sing very prettily: they could speak three different lan-

guages, as Hungarian, Low Dutch, and French, and were
learning English. They were very handsome, very well shaped
in all parts, and had beautiful faces. Helen was born three
hours before her sister Judith. They loved each other very ten-
derly.

Other sources agree that Helena and Judith were intelligent and beautiful,
and that their extensive tours of Europe during their most impressionable
age had made them very accomplished linguists. In later life, the Hungarian
Sisters entered a convent and died there in 1723 at age twenty-two. Among
the theologians, there was a debate about whether their souls were united
beyond death, but the question was never resolved.

Millie and Christine, pygopagus conjoined twin girls born in Columbus
County, North Carolina, in 1851, had a tempestuous early life. Their parents
were black slaves, and they were repeatedly sold, traded, and even kid-
napped by unscrupulous showmen who appreciated their value as natural
curiosities. They were later taken care of by the wife of one of their showmen, a certain Mrs. Joseph Smith, who became their guardian. They became very proficient performers, and danced, jumped, and skipped rope
during the shows. Christine could lift Millie completely off the floor and
walk or run carrying her with complete ease, without any pain or strain at

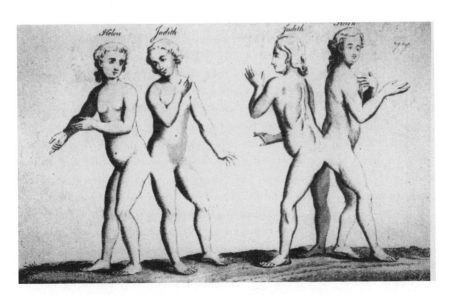

An old print of a contemporary drawing of the Hungarian Sisters. From the
author's collection.

their junction. This is likely to be because they had fused pelvises, and thus a rigid bony barrier between them. Their voices were excellent—one a soprano, the other a contralto—and their artist's name, "The Two-Headed Nightingale," took little coining. All accounts describe them as intelligent, pious, and cheerful. They had no desire to be parted by surgical means, saying that they hoped to leave this world as they came into it, together. Millie and Christine were on tour for the larger part of their adult lives and traveled to Europe several times. They were particular favorites of Queen Victoria, who received them in audience whenever they came to England. In the early 1900s, they retired from show business and bought a large house in North Carolina, which they filled with the souvenirs of all their tours. Millie became ill with tuberculosis, however, and died on October 9, 1912; Christine followed her seventeen hours later.

The pygopagus twins Rosa and Josepha Blazek were born in rural Bohemia in 1878. Their parents were much astonished by this monstrous birth and consulted the local witch, who recommended that the children be kept without food for eight days. The twins survived this cruel treatment, however, and after this impressive demonstration of resilience, even the witch agreed that they should be kept alive. Several showmen applied to Rosa and Josepha's parents to get permission to exhibit them, but the parents refused until the twins were thirteen years old. Then, a local showman took them to Paris, where they were examined by Dr. Marcel Baudouin. He thought them lively, intelligent little girls, and contrasted them to the morose stupidity of their parents, who were also present. Rosa and Josepha went on to make a career for themselves, preferring life in gay Paris to the drab existence in the Bohemian backwoods in the cabin of their rustic parents. They were called "Le pygopage du Théatre de l'age Gaité," and were a well-known attraction at the Paris stage of the 1890s; they amused the audience with singing and playing violin duets. Later, they passed out of public notice until they consulted the surgical clinic at the Prague General Hospital in 1910, after Rosa noticed a large and rapidly growing abdominal swelling. She was asked whether she might be pregnant, but denied it vehemently; her sister, who certainly was in a position to know, supported her denial. But before the investigation was brought any further, Rosa delivered a healthy son. Later, the two inseparable sisters were rumored to have married the same man. In 1922, they moved to the United States in the company of their brother; they died there later the same year, at the age of forty-three.

In the light of these three case histories, it is certainly not unlikely that the Biddenden Maids might have lived as long as thirty-four years. Nor it is impossible that one sister survived the other for six hours. At the deathbed of the original Siamese twins, Chang survived Eng for at least two hours, despite the fact that their livers were connected, and in a French case, one conjoined twin survived the other for more than ten hours. The German teratologist Hans Hübner quoted several similar cases, including that of a pair of omphalopagus twins of which one individual survived the other for seven hours.

Evidence from Historical and Teratological Chronicles

Due to the mystery and fascination of congenital malformations, the annals of teratology stretch back far into the dark ages. The "monsters" and strange births were considered as portents of war and misery, or frightening signs of Divine displeasure. Although the old prodigy books and chronicles of strange events are unreliable sources, it was considered of interest to examine some of the old standard works of teratology, as well as some English historical chronicles, in order to look for early references to the Biddenden Maids. Due to Clinch's argumentation about the Maids' time of birth, both the twelfth century and the fifteenth and sixteenth centuries were taken into account. It turned out that the Maids were not mentioned in any of the major teratological works of the sixteenth and seventeenth centuries, such as those by Aldrovandi, Liceti, Paré, Schenckius, and others. Nor were they noticed in the *Philosophical Transactions* or any other British collection of teratological descriptions. This is an argument against the opinion that they lived in the sixteenth or seventeenth century, since most other remarkable conjoined twins that reached maturity occasioned much publicity in the popular and scientific works of this period. For example, both the Scottish Brothers, who had only one pair of legs but two perfect bodies from the waist upwards, and Lazarus Colloredo, who had an imperfect parasitic twin, Joannes Baptista, hanging from his epigastrium, created much interest among men of learning. There were also several notable early English cases. In 1552, ischiopagus conjoined twin girls were born in a village near Oxford; they lived for eighteen days and were much admired by the country people. The births of stillborn conjoined twins at Plymouth in 1670 and at Petworth in 1677 were recorded in the *Philosophical Transactions*, and the omphalopagus twins born at Isle Brewers in 1680, who lived for two or three years, were also well described both in the medical literature and in popular broadsheets. Conjoined twins who lived for thirty-four years were quite a sensation, and it is reasonable to presume that if the Biddenden Maids had lived in the sixteenth or seventeenth century, they would certainly have been mentioned in the annals of teratology.

There is a remarkable accumulation of reports of English conjoined twins in the beginning of the twelfth century. Ballantyne observed that Lycosthenes, in his *Chronicon Prodigorum et Ostentorum* from 1557, stated that there were conjoined twin brothers born in England in 1112, and that their bodies were joined at the hips and "ad superiores partes," like in the popular descriptions of the Biddenden Maids. Even more interesting is that a medieval historical chronicle, the *Chronicon Scotorum*, told of a woman who gave birth in A.D. 1099 to "two children together, in this year, and they had but one body from the breast to the navel, and they were two girls." In the Irish chronicle *Annals of the Four Masters* is an almost identical description, although the conjoined twin girls were stated to have been born in 1103; in the *Annals of Clonmacnoise* their year of birth is given as A.D. 1100. These ancient descriptions are unreliable in details and probably dependent on each other, but in spite of this, they add some credibility to the old tradition that the Biddenden Maids were really born in 1100. It should be added that in this year, there was a strange happening that excited popular imagination: King William Rufus was found dead in the New Forest with an arrow either of a hunter or of an assassin in his breast. Several prodigies were said to have preceded the death of this sinful and extravagant monarch, and at Pentecost, blood was seen to gush up from the earth like a fountain. Conjoined twins born this year might well be regarded as another strange prodigy foreboding the king's death, and thus be much noticed both in the chronicles and in folk tradition.

Another unexpected source on the Biddenden Maids was pointed out in 1869 by a certain Mr. R. H. Cresswell, in a letter to the Reverend James Boys, rector of Biddenden; this letter is now kept by the Biddenden Local History Society. Mr. Cresswell had read an obscure three-thousand-line medieval poem entitled *De contemptu mundi*, written in the first half of the twelfth century by Saint Bernard of Morlaix, an English monk in the monastery of Cluny. One section dealt with a strange birth in England at this time, which the pious monk considered a portent of the day of judgment:

> *In geminum egrediens apud Anglia rura*
> *Faemina prodiit ipsaque finiit in duo crura.*
> *Crura quidem duo, sed sibi bis duo brachia stabant,*
> *Hanc duo pectora, quatuor ubera, mirificabant.*

Vos volo credere, me vera dicere, scribere rerum
Par erat actio, par via, sessio par mulierum
Ex mulieribus, immo sororibus, o stupor istis,
Altera transiit, atque superfuit altera tristis.
Post breve denique, pars ruit utraque, morte soluta
Utraque pars ruit, hans obitu fuit illa secuta.

In a free translation, this corresponds to:

Two twin women in the English countryside
Having, between them, only one set of legs,
But wondrous to tell, both of them had
a trunk, two breasts, two arms to themselves.
If you wish to believe what I say and write,
that when one of these united women, or sisters even,
who had spent their lives sitting next to each others,
was finally released by death from her bondage,
the other followed her shortly after.

The rector believed that this poem proved without doubt the existence of the Biddenden Maids, but this was a somewhat hasty conclusion. Although the sex and geographical location agree with the legend of the Maids, the nature of the malformation in question does not agree with the early descriptions of the Maids.

In many books and articles on conjoined twins, the Biddenden Maids are stated to be the earliest case of such a malformation in the history of mankind. However, this is quite untrue, and there are several earlier examples of such monstrosities. The first of these cases is from Constantinople of the tenth century: conjoined twin boys from Armenia were taken to this city in 945 to be exhibited for money. They were both fully developed, with all members complete; their bodies were connected from the umbilicus to the lower part of the abdomen. They were residents of Constantinople for a long time and were admired by many until the superstitious townspeople had them expelled for being a bad omen. They returned during the reign of Constantine VII; when one of them died, skilled doctors were audacious enough to attempt a surgical separation, but the surviving twin died after three days. This is the first known attempt of surgical separation of conjoined twins; the first successful operation was performed by the German Dr. König in 1689 on a pair of omphalopagus twins, by tightening a ligature around the rather slender connecting bridge of fibrous tissue.

Concluding Remarks

The old legend of the Biddenden Maids has many elements of truth. Several events in the Maids' story, such as their living joined together for a considerable time, their refusal to be separated, and one of them living for some hours after the other had died, are likely to have had a great impact on popular imagination. The old tradition is teratologically quite possible, providing that the hypothesis of Ballantyne, that the Maids were pygopagus conjoined twins, is accepted; this interpretation has support from the earliest description of the Maids, and it is possible that the idea that they were joined in two places derives from a later misinterpretation of the figures on the Biddenden cake. The historian Edward Hasted's attempt to discredit the old legend seems less convincing, and some of his statements have been proved wrong. The antiquary Robert Chambers supported Hasted's arguments and presumed that the ignorant villagers invented the story of the conjoined twin sisters, after the real origin of the charity was forgotten. However, it is impossible to find a reasonable motive for the eighteenth-century Biddenden villagers to make up such a story, and it would certainly have been beyond their capacity to make it teratologically correct.

The Biddenden Easter charity can be traced back into the first years of the seventeenth century, and the mid-seventeenth-century legal documents from Parson Horner's unsuccessful lawsuit about the Bread and Cheese Lands stated that it had existed for many years. Furthermore, the depositions of witnesses among these documents inform us that these lands had originally been given by "two Maidens that grew together in their bodies." This important finding proves that already in the 1650s, tradition stated that the Biddenden Maids were conjoined twins. Thus Edward Hasted's unsupported claim to the contrary can be disproved with certainty. It is remarkable that these depositions of witnesses do not contain the names of the benefactors, neither Chulkhurst nor Preston; because the twin sisters' name was stated to be unknown also in the reliable eighteenth-century accounts of the tradition, the names Mary and Eliza Chulkhurst must be suspected to be a later invention. It should be noted, though, that the International Genealogical Index reveals that a family with the uncommon name of Chulkhurst lived in Biddenden in the seventeenth and eighteenth centuries, and that no natives of this district had the family name Preston at that time.

Of the two earlier writers on the Biddenden Maids, the teratologist J. W. Ballantyne favored the traditional version of the legend that they were born in 1100. The antiquary George Clinch suggested that in fact they had lived in the fifteenth or sixteenth century, but his arguments concerning the cake molds do not stand up to a critical examination. Furthermore, it would seem odd that the only pair of British conjoined twins to reach maturity would have gone totally unnoticed in the popular and scientific literature, if they had lived at this time of great interest in the study of congenital malformations. Instead, there is a remarkable accumulation of old records concerning the birth of conjoined twins in the early twelfth century; the old legend that the Maids were born in 1100 cannot be dismissed.

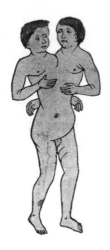

The Tocci Brothers,
and Other Dicephali

O N JUNE 12, 1668, SAMUEL PEPYS VISITED THE
village of Norton St. Philip, situated in Somerset, not far from
Bath. He decided to walk to the church, hoping to see the very ancient tomb of a knight templar. He also saw an old tombstone on which there
were only two heads, and no other text or ornament, and made inquiries
about its meaning. He was told, in a manner he described as fully credible,
that there lay buried "the Fair Maidens of Foscott, who had two bodies upwards, and one belly." More than one hundred years later, the Reverend
John Collinson wrote a brief description of Norton St. Philip and its church
in his *History of Somersetshire*. The much-mutilated stone portraitures of the
united twin sisters were on a tombstone in the floor of the nave of the
church. They were called "the Fair Maidens of Foscott" in local tradition.
Foscott (or Foscote) had once been a neighboring village, but it had become
depopulated by Collinson's time. According to tradition, the twins were born
conjoined in their bodies, but nevertheless grew to mature years. Collinson

160

wrote that when one of them died, "the survivor was compelled to drag about her lifeless companion till death released her of the horrid burden." It is clear from Collinson's account that the Fair Maidens of Foscott must have lived a long time before he came to Norton St. Philip: not only was the village of Foscott, their place of birth, depopulated, but the stone portraiture of them on the tombstone in the nave of the church was severely mutilated through many years of wear and tear.

In the 1890s, the writer James John Hissey visited Norton St. Philip, which he described as a thoroughly old-world place, looking the same as it must have looked many generations ago. The church, although ancient, did

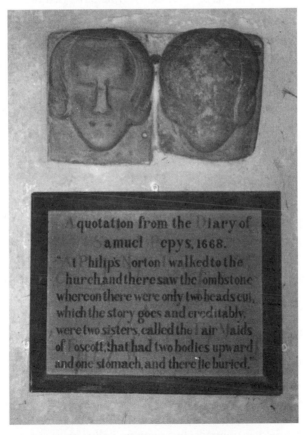

The stone portraiture of the "Fair Maidens of Foscote."
From a photograph by Mr. Tony Day, Churchwarden of
Norton St. Philip, reproduced by permission.

not appear to him very noteworthy architecturally, but a garrulous local old woman he met in the street pointed it out as "very curious" and promised to fetch a book on the history of the building. She returned with "an old and much-thumbed book" in her hands and particularly recommended Hissey to see "the heads of the two ladies" on the top of the cupboard under the tower. When they reached the cupboard in question, however, nothing was there, and the old lady declared herself astonished, since the heads of the ladies had been there as long as she could remember. When the puzzled Hissey asked for further particulars about these mysterious "ladies," the woman brought out her book, in which there was a chapter (or perhaps rather a bound-in pamphlet), amounting to about twenty pages of small print, giving "a true account of the twin maidens of Foscote." It transpired that the tombstone of the twin maidens, with their heads carved in stone with hair down their sides, had once been in the floor of the chancel of the church, beneath which they were buried. They had two heads and only one body.

Posterity would have been better served if Hissey, instead of regaling his readers with another ten pages of vapid travelogue in his *Through Ten English Counties*, had made a proper reprint, or at least an abstract, of this curious old pamphlet. Not a single copy of it seems to be extant today, either in the British Library or in any local collection. It is particularly unfortunate that the exact age of the monument, and thus the twin sisters' date of death, is unknown, but from Pepys's description, it is likely to have been before the early seventeenth century. The remains of the tombstone, with the mutilated portraits of the heads of the twin sisters, is now mounted on the wall of the entrance hall of the Norton St. Philip church, where I saw it in 1997.

ॐ

If the brief descriptions of the Fair Maidens of Foscott are trustworthy, they are one of the earliest examples of live-born conjoined twins belonging to the group *dicephalus*. These twins have what is known as rostral duplication, which means they share one pelvic girdle and one pair of legs, but have a variable degree of duplication of the upper body. In the subcategory of dicephalus twins known as *dicephalus tetrabrachius*, the bodies divide above the waist: there are two torsos, four complete arms, and two heads. These dicephalus twins are the most likely to be viable, as evidenced by both historical and modern instances; it is not unlikely that the Fair Maidens of Foscott, with their "two bodies upwards, but just one belly" belonged to this group. In another subcategory, known as *dicephalus tribrachius*, there is just one torso, with one arm to each side and a third, sometimes atrophied, arm between the two heads. Finally, in the most extreme subcategory, *dicephalus di-brachius*, the twins have one torso, two arms, and two heads and necks situated next to each other.

The perpetual wonder and fascination of conjoined twins have ensured that they are often mentioned in ancient chronicles; the dicephali, with two heads and just one lower body, were considered the most remarkable of all these prodigies of nature. Higden's *Polychronicon* and Capgrave's *Chronicle of England* agree that in A.D. 375, a two-headed boy was born in the castle of Emaus. Higden wrote that this boy was "divided from the navelle upwarde, havenge 2 brestes and 2 hedes, with wittes dividede, in so moche that the oon slepynge or eitenge, that other did not eyte neither did slepe." The twins died when two years old. Roger of Wendover's *Flowers of History* mentioned another pair of medieval dicephali reaching adulthood, this time in Gascony, France. A woman in these parts had two heads, four arms, and everything double down to the navel, but two legs and feet.

When one twin laughed, ate, and talked, the other wept, fasted, and

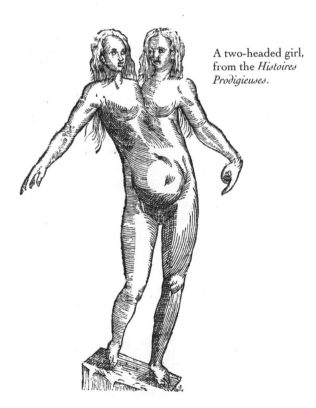

A two-headed girl, from the *Histoires Prodigieuses*.

kept silence. What they ate with two mouths was expelled through a single orifice. According to Higden's chronicle, they both died within the space of two days, but Roger of Wendover added some lurid details, presumably of his own invention. One of the twins died, and the other had to carry the dead carcass on her back for nearly three years, until she herself died from the oppression and stench of the corpse.

By far the most fascinating of these early instances of dicephalus conjoined twins are the famous Scottish Brothers, who were born near Glasgow in 1490. Like the twins described earlier, these brothers were two complete individuals above the waist, with two heads and four arms, but had only one set of lower extremities; like them, they belonged to the type dicephalus tetrabrachius. According to the historian George Buchanan, the Scottish Brothers were taken to the court of King James IV of Scotland at an early age. Just as Henri II of France wanted to study hairy little Petrus Gonzales as a curiosity, King James ordered that these unique children were to be carefully brought up and educated. They had a particular talent for music and learned to sing and to accompany themselves on various instruments of music. Another Scottish historian, Robert Lindsay of Pitscottie, who had probably heard them perform, wrote that they "became very ingenious and cunning in the Art of Musick; whereby they could sing and play two Parts, the one the Treble, and the other the Tenor; which was very dulce and melodious to hear." The Scottish Brothers were also very proficient linguists, and the king took care to educate them: By the time they were twenty years old, one or both of the twins could speak English, Irish, Latin, French, Italian, Spanish, Dutch, and Danish. They could stand up and even walk, and used all four upper extremities with dexterity. It was observed that they often differed in opinion and sometimes quarreled; the inseparable brothers were also prone to chide others for various "disorders in their behaviour and actions." George Buchanan wrote that "in their various inclinations the two bodies appeared to disagree between themselves, sometimes disputing, each preferring different objects, and sometimes consulting for the common pleasure of both."

The Scottish Brothers died in 1518, during the regency of John, duke of Albany; they were then twenty-eight years old. The majority of chroniclers did not notice anything remarkable about their death. George Buchanan, who was himself twelve years old when the Scottish Brothers died, pointed out that at the time he was writing his history, there were many people of undoubted veracity still alive who could vouch that his description of them contained no exaggerations. Lindsay of Pitscottie added some details that were probably the remnants of a medieval popular legend about conjoined twins. One of the Scottish Brothers died long before the other, Lindsay asserted, and when the living twin was requested to sing and be merry by the courtiers, he replied:

> 'How can I be merry, that have my true Marrow as a dead Carrion about my Back, which was wont to sing and play with me. When I was sad he would give me Comfort, and I would do the same to him: But now I have nothing but Dolour of Bearing so heavy a Burden, dead, cold, and unsavoury, on my Back, which taketh all earthly Pleasure from me in this present Life: Therefore I pray to Almighty God, to deliver me out of this present Life, that we may be laid and dissolved in the Earth, wherefrom we came.'

This fanciful addition, which is medically quite impossible, still does not undermine the veracity of the main part of the story of the Scottish Brothers.

The *De Monstris* of Fortunio Liceti, a valuable early chronicle of strange births published in 1665, does not mention either the Fair Maidens of Foscott or the Scottish Brothers, but this is probably due to Liceti's lack of knowledge about British sources. He was much better read in the European annals of monstrous births. In Florence, there was at this time an ancient monument, rather like that in the church of Norton St. Philip, depicting a pair of conjoined twins born in 1316. It was an effigy placed in a stairway of the Ad Scala hospital in Florence, with an epigram from Fransisco Petrarca's *De Rebus Memorandis*. The twins were named Peter and Paul, and they lived thirty days. Liceti's illustration depicts them with two heads, four arms, and two torsos, but just one pair of legs. The German naturalist Johannes Schenck von Gräfenberg wrote that when he was just seven years old, his father showed him a picture of the monument to Peter and Paul, which had been sent to him by a burgher in Florence. The boy was told to contemplate this hideous monster and to promise one day to show the picture to his own children. In Professor Luigi Gedda's *Twins in History and Science*, a picture of what may well be the original monument is reproduced from a bas-relief in the San Marco museum. If that is the case, Liceti was wrong, since the twins are depicted with three legs; thus they are an example of ischiopagus tripus conjoined twins rather than dicephali.

Fortunio Liceti also depicted the dicephalus twins born in Esslingen in Schwaben in 1512. They were named Elsbeth and Elisabethen in a broadsheet issued in the same year; it is illustrated with a crude portrait of the twins, and the arms of the families involved. According to a German historical chronicle, Schedel's Weltchronik, "this horrible monster" died just an hour after birth. None less than Albrecht Dürer left a compelling, if somewhat fanciful, drawing of these twins. Some art historians claimed that Albrecht Dürer never even saw the twins, and that his drawing was inspired by the aforementioned broadsheet. Like in the broadsheet, he depicted them

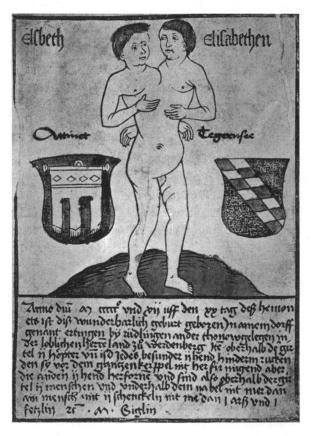

A re-engraving of the handbill about the German dicephali born in 1512. From the author's collection.

standing up, which is manifestly impossible. The anatomy and proportions of the twins were perfectly illustrated, however, and Dürer's drawing was to remain the best illustration of dicephalus twins for many years to come. Five years later, in 1517, another pair of dicephali were born not far away, in Landshut an der Donau in Bavaria. The right twin died just half an hour after birth, and the other soon also died, but the mother survived. The twins were dissected by the local surgeon, who marveled that from the navel upward, they were two complete children, from the umbilicus downward just one. They had two hearts, two livers that were united in the middle, two pair of lungs, two stomachs, and two spleens. It is remarkable that they were not considered as a portent or even a "horrible monster," but instead were called "these beautiful twins" and a marvelous prodigy of nature. The reason is probably that they were not described by a chronicler or theologist, but by a certain Dr. Wilhelm Rosenzweydt, surgeon and anatomist, who was capable of seeing beauty in God's creation, even in an unusual form.

Gould and Pyle, in their *Anomalies and Curiosities of Medicine*, abstracted two curious sixteenth-century reports from Bateman's *The Doome* in the British Library. One concerns a "double-headed male monster" in Switzerland. Observed in 1538 at the age of thirty, each head possessed a beard, and the faces resembled each other. The two bodies fused at the umbilicus into one single lower body. The twins had one single wife, with whom they were said to live in harmony. Bateman also described a German woman with two heads, who begged from door to door. One of the heads was deformed, and her countenance was altogether so frightening that she was given her expenses to leave the country, as it was believed that women would miscarry or receive dreadful "maternal impressions" at the sight of her. Other writers on monstrosities also mentioned this Bavarian woman, thus providing much-needed additional credibility to Bateman's account.

Liceti and other seventeenth-century writers on teratology reported several contemporary cases of dicephalus conjoined twins, all of them stillborn or less viable. Dr. Andreas Emmenius described two of the most interesting instances in a thesis entitled *Abbildung und Beschreibung zweier Wunder-geburten*, published in Leipzig in 1627. One pair of dicephalus twins, baptized Sara and Anna, lived for just half an hour. They had three arms, one on each side and a third between the two heads. At autopsy, the two hearts were found to lay close to one another, in a common pericardium. Another four-armed pair of dicephali, named Justina and Dorothea, actually lived six weeks. They died in an attack of seizures without previously seeming unwell. Autopsy

168   showed that their hearts were separate and distinct, but the right one was malformed.

Probably the most curious illustration of a dicephalus in all times is the Turkish Archer depicted in an old German print. This striking-looking individual is clearly an adult; he is said to have been captured by the troops of Doge Morosini in 1697, in the Peloponnesian war between the Austrians and the Turks. In contrast to the living dicephali described earlier, he has only two arms, and the two necks are attached to a common trunk. He is thus a dicephalus dibrachius. There is no other mention of this Turkish archer in the late seventeenth-century literature on monstrosities, however, and some scholars have presumed that he was a product of early wartime propaganda, aimed to show the Turks as monstrous, subhuman creatures. In that case, it is amazing that the artist produced the portrait of a teratologically fully correct dicephalus rather than some fanciful imaginary creature.

In the nineteenth century, there was a great upsurge in interest and knowledge in both normal and abnormal human anatomy. This was the heyday of scientific teratology, particularly in Germany and France. In addition to dissecting every malformed infant that came into their hands, the pioneer teratologists reviewed the old annals of strange births to discover historical cases of rare malformations. By this time there had been several dissections of stillborn dicephali, one of the most detailed ones, by the obstetrician Dr. Bland, was described in the *Philosophical Transactions* of the Royal Society of London in 1781. Although some of the earlier dicephalus twins, like the Scottish Brothers, had been capable of prolonged extrauterine life according to the original sources, many of the skeptical teratologists tended to doubt the veracity of this ancient tale, particularly as there had not been a single eighteenth- or early-nineteenth-century instance of viable dicephalus twins.

All of this would change when "Ritta-Christina, l'Enfant Bicéphale" appeared in Paris in October 1829. These little girls had been taken to Paris for exhibition when they were just six or seven months old. They were born in Sassari, Sardinia, and their mother, thirty-two-year-old Maria Teresa Parodi, had previously given birth to eight other children. Like the Scottish Brothers, Ritta-Christina shared a common waist, one pelvis, and two legs, but had two upper bodies, four arms, and two heads. It was soon noticed that the right twin, Ritta, was weaker and more delicate than her sister Christina; as the twins grew older, this difference increased. Christina seemed like a vigorous and healthy child, but Ritta, who had the smaller ap-

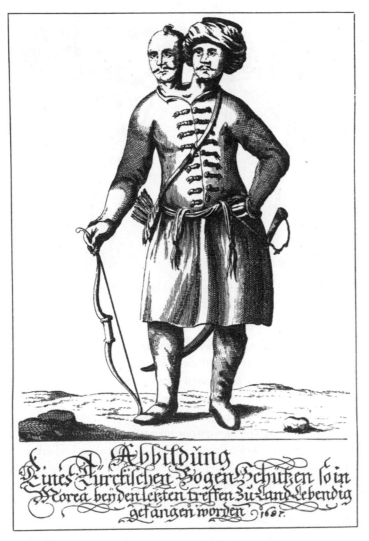

A print published in 1697 of the two-headed Turkish archer.

petite of the two, was pale and sickly. At times, she had alarming attacks of cyanosis and difficulties in breathing. The parents of Ritta-Christina were desperately poor. Much impressed by the great interest in their extraordinary twins, from both the medical profession and the general public, they decided to make money from the children while they still could. After a brief tour of some Italian cities, they set out for Paris.

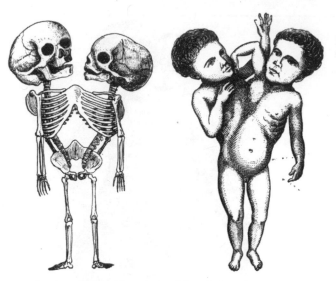

A print of Ritta-Christina and her skeleton. From a
plate in the author's collection.

The civic authorities were averse to such a degrading monster show,
however, particularly as the children were of a tender age, and after some
deliberation, the magistrates decided to shut the show down. The parents,
still in dire financial straits, had to move to a derelict house in Paris, where
they clandestinely showed the twins, for a fee, to journalists and members of
the medical profession. The newspaper men wrote flippant articles, inquiring
whether this monster was really one or two children, and whether they had
one or two immortal souls. Several Parisian lovers of curiosities urged the
authorities to allow the parents to put Ritta-Christina on show again, but
while the magistrates debated this issue, the health of the twins rapidly deteriorated. For want of money to purchase coal or firewood, their parents had
to put the twins' cot into a room without a fire, during a cold winter evening.
Christina withstood this exposure to the elements without ill effects, but
Ritta developed acute bronchitis and was soon in a critical state. The medical
men were amazed to see that when Ritta was in extremis and gasping desperately for breath, her sister was playing and laughing. These doctors may
have been benevolent enough to have offered their professional assistance
for nothing, but rather sinisterly, there is no mention of this in either the popular or the medical press; instead there was much speculation on what the

autopsy would show and what museum would get the skeleton of such an anatomical rarity.

On November 23, 1829, three days after Ritta had taken ill, she finally gave her final gasp for breath, after a long struggle. At the same instance, her sister, who had previously appeared completely unaffected, gave a cry, let go of her mother's hand, and died. The twins were then eight months and eleven days old. The local *curé* had barely had time to finish his duties when a deputation of members of the Academie Royale de Médécine came in with a large cask of plaster of Paris, to make a cast of the tiny corpse. According to a newspaper report, dated the day after the demise of Ritta-Christina, the distraught father had not yet decided whether he would allow the anatomists to dissect his daughters. The next day, he was prevailed upon by the distinguished anatomist M. Isidore Geoffroy Saint-Hilaire, who had seen Ritta-Christina alive more than once. It is, again sinisterly, reported that Geoffroy Saint-Hilaire arrived in the company of the police, and that later the same day, his assistants transported the remains of the twins to the amphitheater of the Jardin du Roi. According to another account, which the *Times* obtained from the *Courier Français* newspaper, Ritta-Christina's father "refused for a long time to suffer the monster to be dissected, but the solicitations of M. Geoffroy Saint-Hilaire, and the injunctions of the Police, overcame his repugnance, and the bicephalic infant has been taken to the Theater of Anatomy of the Jardin du Roi." Exactly by what means the father was persuaded (threats or bribes?) is not stated; it is unlikely that the wretched man was moved by zeal for the science of teratology. At any rate, the anatomists had won, and "ce produit monstreux" was prepared for dissection. An exulting medical journal promised, "Nous ferons connaitre cette autopsie curieuse"—We will know the result of this curious autopsy.

There was a good deal of bickering in the French newspapers about who was to blame for the premature death of the two-headed phenomenon. Ritta-Christina's parents were blamed for putting their children on show, and there were lurid rumors that the twins' death was due to overexposure and a too fatiguing exhibition schedule. The doctors and anatomists involved, particularly a certain Dr. Martin Saint-Ange, were also roundly criticized for their callous attitude, and it was asserted (probably with some right) that they had been more interested in the girls' anatomy than in caring for their well-being. Dr. Saint-Ange retorted that in fact, Ritta-Christina's condition had deteriorated for a considerable period of time. Furthermore, had the parents been allowed by the magistrates to put Ritta-Christina on show before the (paying) multitudes eager to see the twins, this would have solved their financial difficulties and enabled them to keep their children warm and well fed.

The autopsy of Ritta-Christina was performed by a certain Dr. Manel, in the presence of Baron Dubois, Isidore Geoffroy Saint-Hilaire, Dr. Etienne Serres, Baron Cuvier, and many other French medical luminaries. After all, this was the first dissection of viable dicephali in several hundred years, and the occasion had certainly been well advertised in the newspapers. The autopsy showed that the twins were each other's mirror images: all Ritta's internal organs were transposed. The two hearts were situated next to each other within a common pericardium. Ritta's heart was severely malformed: there were two ascending cavernous veins leading to the auricles of the heart, and the septum between the auricles was perforated in three places. This must have led to a considerable admixture of arterial and venous blood, to a degree that might actually have been fatal in a normal child. Christina had a perfectly normal circulatory system, however, and large branches of the twins' iliac arteries were connected, thereby ensuring that oxygen-rich arterial blood from Christina could be shunted into Ritta's circulation. The defective appetite of the ailing Ritta was compensated for by the fact that the twins had a common large intestine, from which the partly digested food eaten by Christina could be absorbed also by Ritta. The liver was common, with a central furrow, and there were two gallbladders. The twins each had a stomach, spleen, pancreas, and larger part of the small intestine. The two spinal columns fused into a common pelvis. There were two uteri, one of them imperforate, but both with its normal appendages, but only one set of external genitals. The anatomist Etienne Serres, who published a lengthy study on the anatomy of Ritta-Christina in 1833, was amazed that the larger uterus of the twins appeared to be fully functional. If the twins had survived to a mature age, he speculated, conception might have occurred, and a single child would have had two distinct mothers. The major part of Dr. Serres's three-hundred-page article attempted to prove, using a novel system of teratology of his own construction, that Ritta and Christina were two persons with fused lower extremities. The same system of teratology led him into some absurd reasonings, and he even stated that in a dipygus monster—an individual malformed in exactly the opposite way as Ritta-Christina, with double lower bodies, four legs, and only one head—the single brain must share the combined thoughts of two personalities. In contrast to his theoretical reasoning, Dr. Serres's anatomical description of the twins is excellent and illustrated with beautiful plates. The skeleton of Ritta-

Christina, figured on one of them, was for many years exhibited among the skeletons of animals at the Musée d'Histoire Naturelle. It made a lasting impression on no less an observer than Stephen Jay Gould, when he saw it there in 1982.

In his novel *Une fille d'Ève*, published in 1838, Honoré de Balzac described the strictly religious education of two sisters with the words: "Cette sévère et religieuse éducation fut la cause des mariages de ces deux sœurs, soudées ensemble par le malheur, comme Rita-Christina par la nature." Such had been the fame of "La fille bicéphale" that even nine years after their death, Balzac did not need to explain this reference to his readers. It is very likely that he had read Isidore Geoffroy Saint-Hilaire's *Histoire générale des anomalies de l'organisation*, which was completed in 1836, and seen the illustration of Ritta-Christina in the atlas volume of this famous work. Geoffroy Saint-Hilaire marveled that dicephalus twins could live as long as eight months. He proposed that this certainly gave an appearance of truth to some of the older tales of viable dicephali, the Scottish Brothers in particular. Less than fifty years later, another pair of dicephalus twins would prove him right.

∿

The most celebrated pair of dicephalus conjoined twins of all times, the brothers Giovanni Baptista and Giacomo Tocci, were born in Locana, a town in northern Italy, on October 4, 1877. Their father was the thirty-two-year-old workman Giovanni Tocci and their mother, nineteen-year-old Maria Luigia Mezzanrosa. Unlike the situation for the majority of other conjoined twins, the labor was easy, as the twins were very small and the mother's pelvis wide. The head of one twin presented first, followed by the other head and upper body, and finally the lower body and legs, with one umbilical cord and placenta. The midwife, who had practiced in Locana for many years, gave a shriek of horror and astonishment when she saw the twins, whose bodies seemed to blend together at the level of the navel—was this one or two children? Poor Signor Tocci was affected even worse: he fainted dead away when his first-born children were held up before him. One source stated that he had to be restrained in a lunatic asylum to gather his wits after this shock to the system. The twins had two heads, two necks, and four perfect arms, but only one lower body and one pair of legs. The two upper bodies fused into each other at the level of the sixth ribs, to give the impression of just one lower body underneath a double thorax.

Having recovered from the nervous attack, Signor Tocci decided to make his extraordinary children the family breadwinners: when they were

174   just four weeks old, he took them to Turin to exhibit them for money. They
became quite an attraction in show business, as they should have been, being
absolutely unique in the world. When the Tocci brothers were one month
old, they were examined by Professors Fubini and Mosso from the Turin
Academy of Medicine. In spite of their deformity and small size, the twins
appeared vigorous; they only weighed 8 pounds together. Using a stethoscope, Fubini and Musso established that the boys had two separate hearts,
which were beating independently: one with a frequency of 152 heart
strokes per minute, the other with a frequency of 154. Importantly, they
make no mention of hearing any heart murmur. The pulse in each leg was
synchronous with the heartbeat on the same side. Their movements of respiration were not synchronous, indicating that each had a pair of lungs. Fubini
and Mosso were doubtful whether the Tocci brothers would live long: they
knew the tragic story of Ritta-Christina, and thought that these tiny twins
were as unlikely to survive.

In May 1878, the twins were exhibited in Paris, and in October that
year, when they were just one year old, they came to Lyons. Here, two local
doctors described them thoroughly in the *Lyon Médical* magazine. Some of
their attention was apparently usurped by the charming Signora Tocci,
whom the doctors approvingly described as being "une belle et vigoureuse
femme, brune comme une Italienne, parfaitement constituée." The twins
were vigorous and agile, with blond hair and grayish blue eyes. Giovanni
Baptista was a little smaller and more slender than his brother. Although
small at birth, they had grown into strong and healthy-looking children: the
doctors attributed this to the nourishing effects of the milk of a sturdy wet
nurse employed by Signor Tocci. The doctors did not hesitate to declare that
their general development, both bodily and intellectually, was well in line
with that of a normal infant of the same age.

Throughout the 1870s and 1880s, Signor Tocci and his wife toured Europe with their extraordinary children. They visited most larger cities in
Italy, France, Switzerland, Poland, Austria, Germany, and perhaps also
Britain. They were always on the move, and the exhibition schedule was
hard, with the twins on show almost every day of the week. According to
one account, Signor Tocci had been very much affected by Fubini and
Mosso's opinion that his children would not live long. He had decided to get
as much money as possible out of them while they were still alive. All accounts agree that the Tocci family made considerable sums of money and
could live in relative luxury. In August 1879, the twins were demonstrated
before the Swiss Society for Natural Science in Bern. A certain Dr. Grün-

wald described the twins and agreed with the French doctors that they looked healthy and likely to live. He was much amused when both twins eagerly tried to grasp a spoonful of food held out between them, and had this scene drawn as an illustration for his article.

In 1881, the Tocci twins were exhibited in Vienna. They were billed as "The Greatest Wonder of Nature," and in the exhibition handbill, Dr. Richard Hescht, professor of pathological anatomy in Vienna, affirmed that they were genuine united twins and probably unique in the world. They were on show in the sessions room of the Vienna Gardening Society, from 10–12 AM and 1–5 PM every day of the week. A visiting English doctor bought a large photograph of the twins, on the back of which he made some notes about their development. At the time they were on show in Vienna, the twins were three years and four months old. Both spoke Italian, but while Giovanni Baptista, the right twin, seemed clever and alert, poor Giacomo was described as "somewhat idiotic." The doctor was amazed that each child could see, hear, feel, think, eat, drink, and cry, and that their mental activity

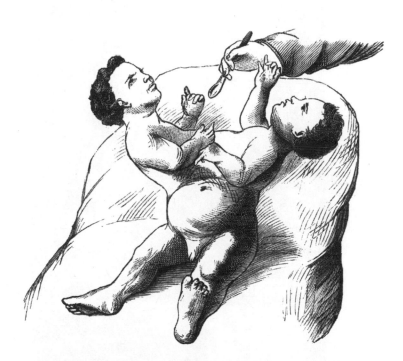

The Tocci brothers in 1879. From the article by Dr. Grünwald in *Virchows Archiv* of that year.

176   was completely independent. Two heartbeats were heard with the stethoscope, and again there was no mention of any heart murmur. The breathing of the twins was also distinct, and in swallowing each moved his individual thorax half, indicating two separate diaphragms. One twin might vomit while the other sucked, so there must have been two stomachs. The intact penis and anus served for both children; posteriorly, there was a rudimentary second male sexual organ.

In 1886 and 1891, the celebrated pathologist Rudolf Virchow saw the Tocci brothers and left a very good description of them. Shaming the gloomy prophesy of Fubini and Mosso, the twins appeared healthy and strong and gave every indication that they would live to an advanced age. In 1891, the Tocci brothers were hired by a German impresario, who exhibited them at the Panoptikon in Berlin. Rudolf Virchow was interested to note that by this time, the Toccis had several other children. Signor Tocci was a thin, swarthy

A photograph of the Tocci brothers in 1881. From the author's collection.

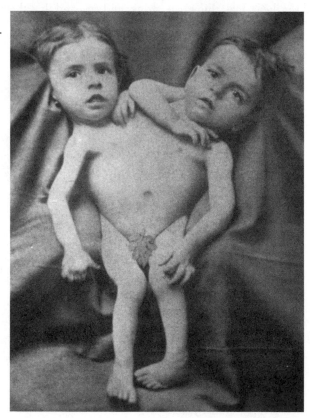

man with typical Italian features. His thirty-three-year-old wife, who had
been admired by the French doctors just thirteen years earlier, was described as a very robust-looking, corpulent woman. A contemporary photograph verifies this unflattering description, and it is clear that her several
childbirths, and the free access to calory-rich food allowed by the family's recent affluence, had destroyed whatever good looks she had once possessed.
The Toccis' other children were perfectly normal; one of them, a sturdy boy,
was exhibited together with the twins.

Each of the Tocci brothers had control of the leg on his side. Both legs
were weak from want of muscular training, and Giacomo's foot had so-called
talipes equinovarus, a form of clubfoot that prevented him from resting it
flatly on the floor. Thus the twins could not stand up independently, unless

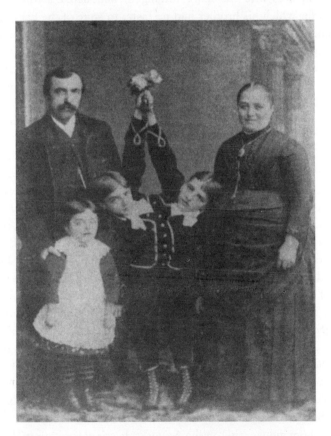

A photograph of the twins in Berlin 1891, featuring their
parents and sister. From the author's collection.

they supported themselves with their arms or were held by some other person. They could also stand up using a ring perambulator, but the lack of coordination prevented them from walking. All available photographs of them as adolescents represent them standing supported by a chair, which they grip with the hands of their outer arms; their inner arms are stretched up over their heads to hold a nosegay or a toy. All accounts agree that the twins were amiable and eager to please. They willingly replied to questions from their audience, and in addition to their native Italian, could speak French and German. They both had a liking for music and readily learned to read and write. When young, the twins were quite alike, but as they grew up, it was noted that their mentality and external appearance varied a good deal. Giovanni Baptista was the stronger and better formed, with a more alert expression; he was also the more intelligent and had a natural talent for drawing, for which his brother had no taste. In spite of the harsh judgment of the English medical man quoted earlier, Giacomo was by no means idiotic. The German showman H. W. Otto, who saw the twins in 1886, considered their mental condition to be perfectly normal. Although the Tocci brothers normally got along quite well, they had their regular disputes, which they sometimes settled using their fists.

Late in 1891, the Tocci brothers came to America, where a showman had planned an extensive tour for them. They were promoted as "The Two-Headed Boy," as "The Wonderful Blended Twins," or even as "The Greatest Human Phenomenon Ever Seen Alive." They were reputedly paid not less than one thousand dollars a week. In Philadelphia, they were examined by Dr. Robert P. Harris, a leading obstetrician and pediatrician. He already knew about the Tocci brothers from the European literature and considered them "the most interesting of all the double monsters in the world." Since the Tocci brothers were decidedly top heavy, and their legs weak, Dr. Harris predicted that they would never be able to walk. Like Rudolf Virchow, he deplored that the parents were always on guard at the exhibition, and that they did not allow any thorough medical examination of the twins, from a misguided belief that this would diminish their extraordinary children's attractiveness in show business. Actually, the medical press did its best to advertise the exhibition of the Tocci brothers. Apart from Dr. Harris's article in the *American Journal of Obstetrics*, no less a periodical than the *Scientific American* called them "probably the most remarkable human twins that have ever approached maturity."

The anonymous writer in the *Scientific American* went on to describe the twins, who were now fourteen years old. He had probably been expecting some repulsive, idiotic freaks, and was amazed that Giovanni Baptista and Giacomo were actually good-looking young lads, with bright, intelligent faces. They lived on excellent terms with each other and seemed "unconscious of any misfortune in their condition." They sometimes spoke to visitors through an interpreter and signed their names as souvenirs. Photographs of the twins were for sale at the exhibition for two dollars; one is still kept at the New York Academy of Medicine, and several in private collections. The account in the *Scientific American* confirmed the earlier observations of the twins' independent minds and actions. They could dress and undress themselves and were able to stand, but could not walk a single step. Their locomotion consisted of crawling about on the floor, using all six extremities. Giovanni Baptista liked beer and drank it in considerable quantities, but Giacomo preferred mineral water. Giovanni Baptista was also very fond of drawing, and maybe some American sideshow enthusiast retained one of his sketches of visitors to the show. Giacomo was less bright than his brother, but the *Scientific American* writer found him the more talkative and voluble of the twins. When he found some fault in his brother's drawing, he kicked it off his knee, to the amusement of the spectators.

An old sideshow buff, Mr. Charles E. Davis, saw the Tocci brothers exhibited in Hartford in 1891 and later wrote an article about them in the *Hartford Daily Courant* of March 27, 1932. Charles Davis was one of the few people who actually spoke to the twins, through an interpreter, and they told him that far from delighting in traveling and earning lots of money, they were often sad and downhearted and minded their abnormal condition very much. He described them as pathetic and added that although they were able to stand up or sit down by themselves, they could not walk a single step. In March 1892, the twins went to New York. They were advertised as the marvelous two-headed boy who spoke French with one head and German with the other, and induced so much curiosity among the single-headed, simple-minded New Yorkers that their stay in town was extended to three full weeks, before they were succeeded at the theater by Jo-Jo, the Russian Dog-faced Boy. Under the management of Mr. Frank Uffner, the Tocci brothers then went on to Boston, where a three-page exhibition pamphlet entitled *Tocci, The Wonderful Two-headed Boy (Giovanni and Giacomo). The Greatest Human Phenomenon ever seen alive* was published to advertise them; a copy is still kept in the Boston Public Library. An illustration depicts them standing up and waving their bowler hats. The pamphlet writer firmly regarded them as one individual, whether out of ignorance or as an advertising gimmick is not known. An interesting observation is that "Tocci usually eats with both mouths, although one can provide nourishment enough for the entire organism." Signora Tocci by this time had not less than nine other children, all living and healthy. In October 1892, the *Million* newspaper reported that the Tocci brothers had arrived in Chicago.

The writer Samuel Langhorne Clemens, better known as Mark Twain, one day saw "the picture of a youthful Italian freak" on exhibition in the sideshow and decided to write a short story with a two-headed man for a hero. Mark Twain called the conjoined twins in his story Count Angelo and Count Luigi Capello, and put them through many ludicrous adventures, all described with his particular kind of heavy-handed humor. In the story, these twins insisted on being paid for two when they did any work, but traveled on the railway with just one ticket. A typical incident involves the twins kicking a man and being brought on trial for assault. They are defended by a lawyer named Pudd'nhead Wilson, who manages to get them acquitted with the argument that it is impossible to say which twin did the kicking, and that the guilty one could not be punished without wrongfully incarcerating his innocent brother. This element of the story was probably originated by an incident in the lives of the original Siamese Twins, Chang and Eng. Mark Twain had written a sketch about them in *Packard's Monthly* in 1869. He also paralleled their lives by making one of his twins a smoker and drinker, and the other one a teetotaler. At the end, Mark Twain decided to take the part about the conjoined twins out of his novel *Pudd'nhead Wilson*, and make them ordinary identical twins; he also published the original farcical concept under the title *Those Extraordinary Twins*. I personally find both these stories rather tedious, and the one about the twins somewhat repulsive, knowing the details of the true existence of the Tocci brothers. Both *Pudd'nhead Wilson* and *Those Extraordinary Twins* have been the subject of much admiration, however; they are hailed as great American classics, have Internet pages dedicated to them, and have been "analyzed" to bits by earnest sociologists and literary historians.

In November 1893, the arduous U.S. tour of the Tocci brothers took them back to New York, where they performed at the Harlem Museum. Billed under them were Ad Carlisle's Dog Circus and the Boxing Kangaroo. They then were at Huber's Theater for two weeks in mid-December, sharing the stage with Tattooed Mac, The Turtle Boy, and Mlle Vallette and her Dancing Goats. They remained active in U.S. show business well into 1894, and probably longer than that. According to the German circus historian H. W. Otto's book *Abnormitäten*, their original contract was for a one-year tour of the United States, but demand was so great that they toured the country for five full years. In 1897, at the age of twenty, they decided to retire for good. They had had enough of the degrading sideshow, and their mother and father, whose love of money had got the better of whatever parental affection they still nourished toward the family breadwinners, no longer had any legal control of them or their earnings. Giovanni Baptista and Giacomo returned to Italy and bought a pretty little villa near Venice. This villa had a garden surrounded by very high walls, to enable them to avoid the gaze of intrusive curiosity seekers. In 1900, H. W. Otto reported that the brothers were alive and well, but living as recluses in their villa, determined never to be exhibited for money again. In 1904, their names again appeared in the French and Italian newspapers, after it was revealed that although they possessed only one single set of genitals, the Tocci brothers had married two separate women. There was a light-hearted debate in both the newspapers and the medical journals about the legal implications of this extraordinary marriage. Who of the twins was legally the father if one of the wives conceived a child, and how should the Tocci brothers' inheritance be divided if there are several children? The famous French teratologist Marcel Baudoin speculated that each twin was the legal owner of one of their testicles! A book, memorably entitled *La vie sexuelle des monstres*, by a certain Dr. A. P. de Liptay, was inspired by this controversy. This bawdy-minded author queried whether the Tocci brothers, when copulating, would actually enjoy "une *double* sensation voluptueuse." He also speculated what the result, physical and psychological, would be in an "accouplement" between dicephali of different sexes, like the Tocci brothers and Ritta-Christina. Leaving no lewd avenue of thought unexplored, he even discussed the desperate situation that would ensue if one brother was "alright" and the other one a homosexual! Some newspaper correspondents found the marriage of the Tocci brothers too disgusting to speculate on further, and their wives were blasted as vulgar curiosity seekers, particularly as most medical experts were of the opinion that the Tocci brothers were impotent. The simple explanation that the twins felt a need for human company in their lonely life, after their long and dismal career as sideshow monsters, does not seem to have entered anyone's mind.

It is not known how the Tocci brothers fared in their marriage, but if they had vowed to keep a veil of secrecy around the remainder of their lives, they certainly succeeded. From 1904 onward, there was hardly any mention of them, in either the popular or the specialist press. In 1906, the French teratologists Lesbre and Forgeot actually announced that the Tocci brothers had died, but other writers insisted that they were still living. The German teratologist Hans Hübner affirmed that in 1911, they were still residing in

182   their villa in Venice. The French teratologist Maurice Gille, writing in 1934, claimed that as far as he knew, the Tocci brothers had still been alive in 1912. They were still married and "had, it appears, children"! According to another version, in the French writer Martin Monestier's *Human Oddities*, they died childless in 1940, at age sixty-three.

✎

The frequency of conjoined twins being born is between one in 50,000 and one in 100,000 of all deliveries. The dicephalus variety is by no means one of the rarest types: it encompasses 11 percent of all conjoined twins, with a slight female preponderance. The mechanism is that complete splitting of the fertilized ovum occurs only in the cephalic region. In the two- or three-armed subtypes, this fission occurs at a higher level than in the four-armed subtype. Of all three subtypes of dicephali, the vast majority are stillborn or less viable. This is most often due to heart and lung malformations in the right twin. The Tocci brothers demonstrated to the world that four-armed dicephalus twins can live for a prolonged period of time. In 1912, the German teratologist Hans Hübner postulated that while four-armed dicephali might well be viable, the two- and three-armed varieties are more poorly organized and have a higher incidence of malformations of the heart and lungs. In a series of papers published between 1929 and 1931, the German teratologist Professor Georg Gruber disagreed. From autopsy studies, he argued that three-armed dicephalus twins might well be sufficiently well organized to reach adult life. The level of conjunction was relatively random in between types, and that the twins had four arms and two torsos did not exclude severe anomalies of the hearts; at the same time, a two-armed dicephalus might have two normal hearts and no obvious defects in the lungs and circulatory system. It is interesting to note that conjoined twins that could not be surgically separated were legally considered as *one* person in Germany at that time. The parents of one pair of dicephalus twins objected to this reasoning, and Professor Gruber wrote a certificate to support them, with the argument that the children were two independent individuals; this was not enough to impress the rigid German bureaucrats, however, and the parents had to feed both mouths of their hungry infant with a single support from the *Kinderkasse*.

The majority of early twentieth-century instances of dicephalus twins were stillborn or less viable. More than one medical thesis or article on dicephali recommended that no attempt to treat or resuscitate the "two-headed monster" should take place; this kind of "mercy killing" of dicephali occurred as late as the 1960s, if not even later. Indeed, the English-language literature on the subject was more devoted to techniques of cutting one head off the "monster" to facilitate labor, than to the study of the anatomy and viability of dicephalus twins. According to a brief press report, a two-headed Russian girl was born in the 1930s. The two heads were baptized Ira and Galya, and she lived to be one year and twenty-two days old. Another, more lurid news-paper story told that some decades later, during the Cold War, a two-headed girl was kept in a Russian research institute, where she was subjected to var-ious experiments. This may or may not be the same twins described in *Life* magazine in 1966 and on an Internet site. These Russian girls were called Masha and Dasha and were born in Moscow in 1950. Their anatomy was identical to that of the Tocci brothers, except that they had a short, vestigial third leg; thus, by definition, they were ischiopagus tripus twins just like the Florentine twins of 1313, but shared many characteristics with the four-armed dicephali. Interestingly, Masha and Dasha walked quite well al-though each twin controlled one of the legs. They were still alive, and in good health except for "psychological maladjustment," at the age of sixteen. According to the aforementioned Martin Monestier, they were the wards of the Soviet state and permanently confined to a physiological research insti-tute, circumstances not conducive to mental well-being in any person, whether a conjoined twin or not.

In 1953, four-armed dicephalus twins were born near Petersburg, Indi-ana. Named Danny Kaye and Donald Ray Hartley, the twins very much re-sembled the Tocci brothers in structure, but they had apparent weaknesses in cardiac function, and the right twin was almost continually cyanotic. In spite of this, they developed well and were discharged from the hospital into the care of their parents. The parents were poor, but nevertheless refused all the intrusive attempts from the media to capitalize on the twins. They even turned down an offer of one thousand dollars a week—the same rate as for the Tocci brothers sixty years earlier—from a leading American showman. At the age of four months, the twins developed pneumonia and died soon after from acute cardiac dilatation. Interestingly, the description of these twins in a medical journal stated that surgical separation of these twins was but briefly considered: it was well-nigh impossible with the surgical tech-niques of the 1950s, and the moral and ethical problems involved were daunting.

The birth of another pair of viable dicephalus twins did not take place until 1977. These twins were of the three-armed variety (dicephalus tri-brachius) and referred to the Arkansas Children's Hospital a few hours after cesarean section delivery. It was soon clear to the doctors that the right twin had severe heart malformations and that the extent of shared organs made it impossible to surgically separate the twins with both surviving. The technical problems of surgically separating dicephali were daunting, and no such operation had been previously attempted. The parents wanted separation at all costs, however, even if this meant that one twin should die. The surgeons began to explore the possibility of amputating the right twin to save the left one. They first had to contact the county prosecuting attorney and the state attorney general, to ensure that no criminal prosecution would result from the death of the right twin. When the dicephali were eighteen days old, the right twin had a prolonged episode of severe cyanosis, and the heart rate of the left twin slowed down. It was decided to operate at once. The surgeons sawed through the right spinal column and spinal cord and divided the junction between the right twin's small intestine and the common large bowel. The connection between the atria of the right and left hearts was divided. The chest wall was closed by wiring the ribs together. Seven weeks after the operation, the left twin also died, before being weaned from the ventilator. Even if the left twin had survived the ordeal, she would have been a one-armed, one-legged invalid, with multiple other defects, including an imperforate anus, severe scoliosis, and considerable cosmetic problems secondary to the chest wall closure.

Katie and Eilish Holton, three-armed dicephalus conjoined twins born in Ireland in 1989, have been well described in two television documentaries. Their anatomy was quite different from that of the Tocci brothers, and their conjunction more extensive. The twins had one lower body, a shared thoracic cavity, and a short third arm between the two heads. In many respects, they were like the Arkansas twins born in 1977. In spite of their deformity, they seemed healthy and viable. The Irish pediatricians did not consider it possible to separate them surgically, nor did, at least initially, the parents desire separation. The twins grew and developed well, although it was known that Katie, the right twin, has some kind of heart malformation. In 1992, at the age of three, they were surgically separated at the Great Ormond Street children's hospital in London. No description of the case or the surgical procedures used has been published in the medical literature, but the operation must have been a formidable one. Katie, the weaker twin, died three days after surgery. Eilish, who was still alive in 1995 at the age of six, had learned to walk with a leg prosthesis.

The most remarkable modern instance of dicephalus conjoined twins involves Abigail and Brittany Hensel, born in the American Midwest in 1990. Like Katie and Eilish, they were three-armed dicephali, but only had a short, deformed arm between the two heads. This rudimentary arm was amputated when the girls were three months old. In 1996, at the age of six, Abigail and Brittany were the subject of large articles in *Time* and *Life* magazines, as well as a television documentary. The twins have developed remarkably well, both physically and emotionally. Since the operation to remove the third arm, they have required no further specialist medical attention. Although one twin controls the arm and leg on each side, they are remarkably agile, and can not only walk, but also run, swim, and ride a bicycle. Probably due to highly advanced tactile and proprioceptive capacities, developed during their six years together, they coordinate their movements perfectly. The excellent general health of the twins rules out any severe heart malformations, although their shared liver indicates quite a high level of conjunction of the inner organs. It is interesting that one of the magazine articles mentioned that Abigail has by far the greater appetite of the twins; this is likely because she has the larger stomach, like many other left dicephalus twins. The twins share the large bowel and probably parts of the small bowel as well, and the food eaten by Abigail also nourishes her sister. At their small local school, the twins became well adapted. Just like the Tocci brothers, they have differing characters and personalities, but although they sometimes tended to quarrel, their schoolteacher used them as a model to show the other children the advantages of teamwork in solving various problems. The parents of Abigail and Brittany never even considered the option of surgically separating the twins, but instead accept them as they are and give them a loving home. In one of the television documentaries about Katie and Eilish, the commentator criticized the Hensel family roundly for their "eccentric" decision not to have their children cut apart, but the parents fortunately chose to ignore such ill-judged advise. At the time of writing, the twins are alive and well, and still united. They are lucky not only in that the random conjunction of their inner organs happened in a way that made them fit for prolonged life, but also in that they were born into a particularly harmonic family in a small rural town. Had they been the children of a "dysfunctional" urban family, in which one or both parents had an entrepreneurial spirit and a thirst for money resembling that of Signor Tocci and his wife, their lives might well have paralleled that of their famous nineteenth-century counterparts, with the money-making media circus beginning when they were in the crib.

∾

In view of the Hensel twins and their development, it is possible to re-evaluate some of the historical cases of dicephali. For example, the spectacle of the Turkish Archer no longer appears as extraordinary and impossible as before.

The nineteenth-century teratologists disbelieved the evidence from historical chronicles that the Scottish Brothers could walk, but the Hensel twins have shown that this is definitely possible. The failure of the Tocci brothers to walk has most often been blamed on Giacomo's clubfoot and the twins being decidedly "top heavy." The main reason is likely to have been the boys' poor muscular development, however. This, in turn, was caused by too much bed rest and too little activity. The exhibition schedule was too demanding for the boys to get the exercise they needed, and their parents might actually have decided, at a later date, that it was advantageous to keep the boys immobilized, since this made the exploitation of them much easier. Their failure to walk diminished their quality of life immeasurably.

It is also clear that Professor Gruber was right when he postulated that dicephali of any of the subcategories can be capable of prolonged life. The main predictor of survival is the degree of conjunction, and deformity, of the hearts. The stillborn majority usually have cardiopulmonary malformations that are incompatible with extrauterine life. In other instances, like Ritta-Christina and the 1952 U.S. twins, the left twin has a functional heart, but the right twin's heart is malformed. In a few cases, like the Scottish Brothers and the Tocci and Hensel twins, there are two fully functional hearts, as evidenced by the absence of cyanosis and heart murmurs and by the prolonged survival of the twins.

The fact that a pair of dicephalus conjoined twins may live for a prolonged period of time — sixty-three years in the case of the Tocci brothers — has importance for the issue of whether surgical separation of dicephali should be performed. As we have seen, the separation of several other types of conjoined twins is a well-established procedure and enjoys considerable success. It is clear, from all standpoints, that it is desirable to separate less extensively conjoined twins, like the pygopagus and omphalopagus types discussed earlier, and that the children's quality of life is definitely much improved. In dicephali, and also in certain more extensively conjoined types of twins, like the thoraco-abdominopagus variety, the anatomical structure is often such that it is unlikely that both twins could survive an attempt at separation. This has led to the introduction of the concept of "sacrifice surgery": one twin is deliberately killed to save the other, and used as a donor of shared organs. By 1996, sacrifice surgery on conjoined twins had been performed nine times. A much publicized case was that of the extensively conjoined Lakeberg twins, who had a common liver and a shared, six- chambered heart. Nevertheless, the parents pressed for an operation. One of the twins was "sacrificed" by the surgeons, but the operation was still a failure;

the surviving twin died before her first birthday, having been hospitalized and ventilator dependent her entire life. The Lakeberg case triggered an unprecedented debate about the ethical issues involved. It was reasoned that the only way to justify taking one life to save another was by informed consent: one twin must voluntarily give his or her life to save that of the other. Since newborn twins cannot speak for themselves, the assumption is that the parents will make this choice on behalf of their children. At various times, Protestant, Roman Catholic, Rabbinical, and Islamic theologians have been consulted in these difficult cases: they have agreed that sacrifice of one twin to save another is ethical.

If a decision had been made to separate, at all costs, a pair of dicephalus twins like Abigail and Brittany Hensel, the extremely unlikely best-case scenario would be that after a lengthy course of operations and years of hospital stays, a mobile, vigorous body with two minds would be changed into two one-armed, one-legged invalids, with half a pelvis each. They were both likely to be sterile, probably incontinent, with grossly deformed thoracic cavities, extensive scarring, and vast cosmetic defects. It is unlikely that both twins would survive, and quite likely that neither twin would survive the attempt. Sacrifice surgery surely would be unethical in a pair of equally strong, viable twins, but if the decision were to sacrifice one twin as an organ donor to the other, the odds of survival are unlikely to improve greatly. In none of the nine such operations performed up to 1996 did *any* of the twins survive to be discharged from the hospital or weaned from the ventilator. A danger in all advanced, high-technology medical procedures is the attitude that all that *could* be done also with necessity *should* be done. There is good reason to doubt, based on both medical and ethical reasons, that surgical separation of dicephalus conjoined twins should be attempted at all, except in a situation in which one twin is clearly dying. In such a situation, both medical and ethical issues should be considered before surgery is attempted, and the situation with regard to the quality of life of the survivor of the operation should be given as much (if not more) consideration as the quantity of life. In the 1977 Arkansas case, the surgeons actually stated as one of the arguments to operate that the twins might survive for a prolonged period of time, but this attitude that life as a conjoined twin is literally a fate worse than death is highly questionable. Although an adult person would find it intolerable to be linked for life to another individual, things are very different when the conjunction is present from birth. Many of the historical cases discussed in this book, like Helen and Judith, Rosa and Josepha Blazek, and the original Siamese Twins Chang and Eng, would hint that the twins themselves would not agree that their lives were a complete, utter misery — many of them grew up to be stable, socially well-adjusted people. They knew no other life than to be a conjoined twin and accepted its limitations; in fact, both Millie-Christine and Rosa-Josepha Blazek themselves refused to be separated.

The life story of the Tocci brothers is a more tragic one, however. Until they were twenty years old, they knew no other life than that of an interesting object on show before the curious. Already at the age of four weeks, their father took them to Turin for exhibition, and they had few holidays since. According to their Austrian handbill, the brothers were on show six hours every day, seven days a week. To spend one's teenage years as a "freak" in the American sideshow of the 1890s is unlikely to be an uplifting experience. Every day, goaded by their possessive and avaricious parents, the boys were put on show before a coarse, unfeeling audience of carnival "rubes." They were not cute little children any more, like a funny little two-headed puppet, but had grown up to be a near-adult, humanoid monster with whom people could identify. Like their contemporary, the original "Elephant Man" John Merrick, they must have been sickened by people exclaiming in horror "What a monster!" "What a freak!" After this kind of experience, their decision never to be seen by a stranger again seems quite rational. John Merrick asked his benefactor Frederick Treves if he could be sent to a solitary lighthouse or a blind asylum; the Tocci brothers had ample money from their tours, and they put it to good use. It is hoped that at the end of their lives, living in their villa in Venice, Giovanni Baptista and Giacomo found some happiness.

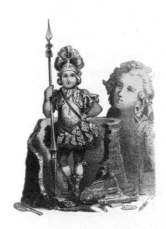

The King of Poland's
Court Dwarf

DROTTNINGHOLM CASTLE, AN IMPOSING baroque building situated on the island of Lovö facing the lake Mälaren just outside central Stockholm, is the permanent residence of the Swedish royal family. It was built in the 1660s, from a design by the architect Nicodemus Tessin the Elder. About ten years ago, I visited Drottningholm Castle to see the remains of Queen Lovisa Ulrika's private museum, originally founded in 1750, which I planned to describe in a book on various remarkable seventeenth- and eighteenth-century museums of natural history. As things turned out, this book was never written, but the beautifully designed, but now empty and somewhat dilapidated museum rooms were nevertheless a remarkable sight. In 1803, the museum was dissolved, and various university institutions and museums helped themselves to the more attractive preparations. Only one of its major original specimens remained: an astonishingly lifelike wax statue of the once-famous court dwarf Nicolas Ferry, alias Bébé, said to have been a present to Queen Lovisa Ul-

190   rika of Sweden from King Stanislas Leszynski of Poland. It is possible that as an act of reverence toward the late queen, the statue was kept at her old museum and not taken away; for 197 years, this statue of the king of Poland's court dwarf has guarded the empty museum rooms like a bizarre sentinel, standing in a niche in the wall.

There is a story that Empress Catherine the Great of Russia once posted

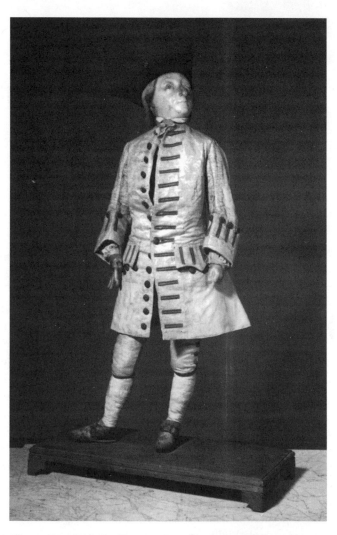

The statue of Nicolas Ferry at Drottningholm Castle.
Reproduced by permission of the National Museum of Sweden.

a sentry to stand guard over a particularly beautiful garden flower in one of the royal parks. As time went by, the purpose of the posting of this sentry was forgotten, but this does not mean that the practice was discontinued: many years after the flower had withered, a sentry still stood guarding the flower bed where it had once grown, as the orders of the empress could never be questioned. In some strange way, the statue of Nicolas Ferry has suffered a similar fate. The sight of it standing in the near-empty museum rooms inspired me to investigate the life story of Nicolas Ferry, alias Bébé, and the circumstances under which his statue had been taken to the royal castle in Stockholm.

In the early eighteenth century, it was fashionable among European royalty to build up private museums or cabinets of curiosities. More often than not, these museums contained valuable natural history specimens. About the year 1750, Crown Prince Adolf Frederick and Crown Princess Lovisa Ulrika of Sweden each founded a private museum. Whereas Adolf Frederick soon lost interest, Lovisa Ulrika extended her museum considerably. She was the sister of Frederick the Great of Prussia and at least initially resented being married off into the Scandinavian outback. She was a snobbish, supercilious woman who wholly lacked the common touch. Drottningholm Castle was among the few Swedish buildings she considered at all inhabitable. Her pro-German sentiments did not deter her from lavishly spending the ample funds allocated to her by the Swedes. She was a possessive character, much given to collecting, and a fair proportion of her income was spent on purchases of coins, paintings, minerals, and natural history specimens for her museum. According to none less than Carl Linnaeus, who was used as an agent to procure new specimens, her copious purchases of corals, shells, and dried insects caused a great boom in the European marketplace for natural curiosities. Some of Linnaeus's fellow naturalists complained that they could no longer afford to enrich their own collections, because the wealthy princelings, smitten by the current craze for natural history exhibits, bought everything that was worthwhile.

Queen Lovisa Ulrika housed her museum in three rooms in the newly built north wing of Drottningholm Castle: the cabinet of natural history, the cabinet of minerals, and the cabinet of coins. Carl Linnaeus was summoned by the queen to arrange her collection of natural curiosities, since she herself had little knowledge on how to do it. To begin with, Linnaeus accepted this assignment with alacrity, since the queen's collections of shells and dried

192   insects were the finest he had ever seen. The daily social intercourse with the royal family was flattering at first, but Linnaeus soon tired of court life. The king was a stupid, henpecked bore, and the queen haughty, imperious, and conceited to a degree remarkable even among eighteenth-century royalty. In a letter to his friend Abraham Bäck, written in 1753, Linnaeus likened himself to a wretched prisoner on the island of Drottningholm who could not be released without a royal pardon. In a later letter, he wrote that the mere mention of the name of the royal residence sent a shiver down his spine!

Although Queen Lovisa Ulrika lost some of her enthusiasm for her museum in the late 1750s, she kept adding new specimens, some of which had been presented to her as gifts by other royal personages. An Egyptian mummy, an ostrich's egg, a little stick said to have belonged to Julius Caesar, and a cast of the hand of the giant Bernhard Giglio were all deposited in her museum. After the succession of her son King Gustav III in 1771, the museum became increasingly neglected, however, as the young king had no interest at all for his mother's collections. Lovisa Ulrika lived on at Drottningholm Castle, which was her private property, but her son cut her allowance. Since she kept spending lavishly, she was soon in dire financial straits. In 1777, she had to declare herself bankrupt, and the only way for her to settle her enormous debts was to sell Drottningholm Castle and all its contents, the museum included, to the Crown.

The wax statue of Nicolas Ferry is 3 feet 5 inches tall, including the cocked hat and the sturdy oak fundament; the figure itself is slightly less than 3 feet tall. It is dressed in Nicolas's own clothes, an elegant suit of pale blue silk, with white stockings and a cravat. The nose is quite black, as many museum visitors have taken the liberty to pinch it. It is not known exactly when the statue was taken to Drottningholm Castle. The earliest mention of it is in the 1788 castle inventory, and two less detailed inventories made in 1764 and 1777 do not record its presence. There is a tradition, however, that the statue had once belonged to Queen Lovisa Ulrika, and that it had been a gift from King Stanislas Leszynski of Poland, Nicolas Ferry's original patron. Although this hypothesis cannot be proved with certainty, it is supported by the fact that King Gustaf III took little interest in his mother's museum, and that very few specimens were added after 1771. In 1796, the statue was thoroughly described in a book by the castle warden, Mr. Anders Björklund, who pointed out that it was a life-size model of Bébé, wearing a suit of his own clothes. A later guidebook added that the face was a wax impression of the famous court dwarf's own. There are fewer records of the statue after the rest of the museum's contents were removed in 1803. The castle was open to visitors, and the writer of a laudatory poem, in 1819, pointed out the statue of Bébé and the hand of the giant Bernhard Giglio as two of Drottningholm's foremost attractions.

❧

Nicolas Ferry, whose statue was to reside at Drottningholm Castle for many years, was born on October 14, 1741, in the little village Champenay, situated in the Principality of Salm in France. His mother, who was seven months pregnant according to one account, and had gone full term according to another, suddenly and unexpectedly went into labor. Before the midwives and neighbor women could be summoned, she rapidly gave birth. She was horrified to see the diminutive size of the infant: the boy was only 8¼ inches (21 centimeters) tall and weighed 22.3 ounces (625 grams). Despite his minuscule stature, he was well shaped and beautifully proportioned, like a precious little bibelot. When the neighbors finally bustled in, they cried out, "Un vrai petit Jésus!" According to the village gossips, the pregnant mother of little Nicolas had spent much time praying, in the local church, before a small statue of the infant Jesus in the crib. They supposed that this gazing at the statue had induced a sinister "maternal impression," and that her unborn son had assumed the same size as this diminutive statue. The boy screamed at a particularly shrill, thin note, which was likened to the squeaking of a mouse. The village know-alls considered this feeble cry, along with his particularly low birth weight, a clear indication that he would not live long. Even the local *curé* seemed to agree, since he decided to postpone the baptismal ceremony.

Nicolas Ferry's mother was determined that he should live, however. Instead of a crib, she put him in a wooden shoe lined with straw. His mouth was too small to allow him to suckle her breast, but it was possible to make him drink small amounts of goat's milk from a diminutive feeding bottle. Later, he suckled the family goat, which was soon well trained enough to come running, on its own accord, whenever it heard the boy crying. The parents of Nicolas, the young farmer Jean Ferry and his wife, thirty-five-year-old Anne Baron, were not very poor people, nor were they particularly wealthy. They were both in excellent health and would later have two normal children. In 1883, the French antiquary A. Benoît reported to the *Société Philomatique Vosgienne* that he had traced Nicolas Ferry's place of birth. The house, which was still standing, was one of the oldest buildings in the village, and over the front door was the date 1712.

When he was exactly one month old, little Nicolas was put on a plate covered with hemp and carried to the Plaine village church, where the *curé*, M. Sebastien Pelletier, baptized him with much ceremony. Both godparents were illiterate, but they marked their signs on the certificate of baptism, as was the custom. At the age of three months, Nicolas developed smallpox, and again his life was feared for, but he survived, with two large pockmarks on the forehead remaining as the only indication of his illness. As the years went by, Nicolas grew slowly but steadily, but compared to children of the same age, he developed in a retarded fashion. For several months, the goat's milk had been his only sustenance, but later, his customary diet was the typical food of the Vosges laboring man: milk, potatoes, vegetables, bread, and lard. Not until he was eighteen months old was Nicolas able to utter some words in the local patois; it would be many years before he could express himself fluently. When two years old, he walked without any support; before that time, he crawled swiftly on all four limbs to rejoin his foster-mother, the goat. At this time, his first shoes, which were only 1½ inches (4 centimeters) long, were presented to him by the local shoemaker.

The word about this fantastic dwarf boy spread rapidly, and already when Nicolas was just a few months old, the curious thronged to see him. Although he was never formally put on show, it is not unlikely that his parents were given sums of money by various affluent spectators. In 1746, some noble ladies from the court of King Stanislas of Poland, who was also the duke of Lorraine and Bar, were passing through the region of Champenay. They visited the Ferry family to see little Nicolas and were vastly impressed; they later described his appearance before King Stanislas, who was at once particularly interested. King Stanislas Leszynski was married to the daughter of King Louis XV of France. He had twice been king of Poland, the second time after King Charles XII of Sweden conquered Poland and made him tributary king; twice he had been dethroned by fierce political opponents and expelled from his kingdom. In the later part of his life, King Stanislas was content to spend much time in affluent idleness in his French duchies. His close relationship with King Louis kept him well supplied with money, which he spent lavishly on his own amusements; his habits were regal and his court opulent. There were noble courtiers, beautiful, high-born ladies, and well-mannered servants aplenty; King Stanislas only lacked a court dwarf.

In July 1746, the king sent one of his court physicians, M. Kast, to Champenay, to examine little Nicolas and determine his usefulness as a court dwarf. The now five-year-old boy had become a little more than 2 feet tall and weighed 10½ pounds. His bodily proportions resembled those of an adult, and M. Kast proposed that it was unlikely that he would grow any more. This was an ill-judged speculation, however, since Nicolas later grew nearly another foot. Nicolas Ferry's body was slender, agile, and well shaped. His face was handsome except for a large, protruding nose; his eyes were dark brown and the hair a silvery blond. His voice was thin and shrill, like that of a newborn. Nicolas was lively and animated throughout M. Kast's examination; he did not rest for a moment, and when his interest once became captivated by any object, he could not be distracted from it. M. Kast concluded that even for a five-year-old, Nicolas seemed slow-witted and dull; his memory was weak, and his command of the French language showed much to be desired.

M. Kast described Nicolas Ferry before King Stanislas, who ordered that the boy be taken to Lunéville without delay, so that the king himself could see him. Jean Ferry was overjoyed when the royal messenger knocked on his door at Champenay to explain his business. Without any delay, he harnessed his donkey cart, put little Nicolas on the platform normally used for vegetables, covered him up with a tablecloth, and drove off toward the castle of Lunéville. King Stanislas and Queen Katarina Opalinska were much impressed by the lively, pretty little boy, and the king suggested to Jean Ferry that Nicolas reside permanently at his court and be brought up and educated there. Jean Ferry accepted this offer with alacrity; either because he was pleased that the boy would be provided with a superior education for nothing, or because he had the (misguided) belief that he himself would stand highly in royal favor. As evidenced by later events, King Stanislas apparently considered that Nicolas was now his own property, purchased just like one buys a puppy or a kitten. Jean Ferry had left home in such a hurry that he left his wife behind. When she came to Lunéville fifteen days later, to say farewell to her beloved son, he did not, at first, seem to recognize her. The courtiers sniggered and gossiped that Nicolas was an imbecile, but when his mother left, a few hours later, the little boy wept bitterly.

Nicolas Ferry's life changed completely when he moved to King Stanislas's court. He was admired by the courtiers and flunkies, treated as an interesting little pet, handed around to be fed bonbons by the ladies, and generally spoiled rotten. On the queen's birthday in 1747, King Stanislas gave Nicolas to her as a present; whether he was wrapped up in a parcel or not is not known. She gave him the name Bébé (Baby), by which he was to be known for his remaining days, just as a puppy is renamed Fido by its new owner. To be fair, the queen seemed to have taken good care of her court dwarf. On her deathbed, later in 1747, she bequeathed him to her cousin, the Princess de Talmont. The princess admired Bébé's pretty looks and became genuinely fond of him. She proposed to King Stanislas that Bébé receive a superior education, and the king agreed. Competent teachers of reading, writing, arithmetic, music, dancing, and good manners were employed to instruct him. In her spare time, the princess herself attempted to give him lessons, but in spite of all her esprit, she was unable to develop any intelligence in Bébé. Her grand scheme of educating the wretched little boy failed miserably, and after some years of bravely struggling, the distinguished pedagogues reported to King Stanislas that Nicolas was almost completely uneducable. Although he slowly but steadily learned to speak good French, they could not, by any means, induce him to read or write a single word or to add two numbers together. As an illustration of his level of intelligence, they told an anecdote: Bébé had once strayed into a meadow with high grass and weeds; he thought he was lost in a forest and desperately cried out for help. The eminent clergymen charged with explaining the mysteries of the Christian faith to Bébé could only report that the boy was wholly impervious to all kinds of religious thought. He had a certain ear for music: although unable to play any instrument, he liked to beat time on a small drum. He could be taught to dance, but his long-suffering dancing master had to explain every movement many times to his bumbling little protégé before Bébé was able to reproduce the dancing steps in question. After many years of tutoring, Bébé was finally able to perform a dancing show when a troupe of Italian comedians visited Lunéville in 1754.

In a corner of one of the great halls of the Château de Lunéville, King Stanislas ordered a wooden dwarf house to be erected for his novel acquisition. It was somewhat more luxurious than a dog's kennel, but then Bébé had a much higher standing at court than the king's favorite dogs. The dwarf house had an entrance hall, a bedroom, a drawing room, and a dining room, all in a scale to suit Bébé perfectly. The house is reported to have been so small that even a dog could not enter it; this was probably to the benefit of little Nicolas, who was thus safe from being pulled out of his bed by a playful hound the size of a prize bull.

Bébé's wardrobe contained a large variety of costly suits and costumes, made at the orders of King Stanislas. The dwarf house also contained a large number of birdcages, and Nicolas was amused by the song and antics of a large number of caged birds: warblers, siskins, and goldcrests. There were also two snow-white miniature turtledoves, a gift to Bébé from the empress of Russia. When Bébé quarreled with his royal master, he used to withdraw to his house and sit sulking for hours. When King Stanislas sent a footman to knock at the door, Bébé opened a window and haughtily called out, "Vous direz au Roi que je n'y suis pas!" — Go tell the King that I am not at home!

King Stanislas was much amused when his court dwarf was up to mischief, and the spoiled, naughty little rascal seldom disappointed him in this respect. The stolid, dignified headwaiter bringing a plate of delicacies to the king's table had to keep a wary eye out for the horrid dwarf, who might be lurking under the table, ready to kick his shins or trip him. The fragile old lady walking in the galleries at Lunéville lived in fear that Bébé should dart

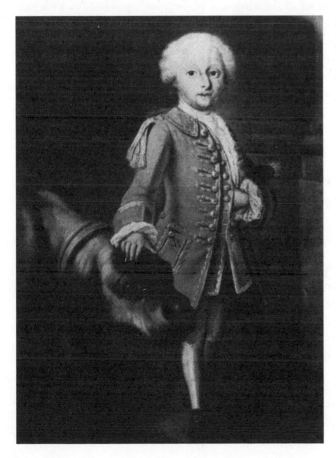

An early-nineteenth-century engraving of a portrait of Nicolas Ferry together with a large dog, by an unknown artist. From the author's collection.

in under her long skirts and do her some unspeakable mischief. The scatter-brained, hyperactive court dwarf had the run of the castle and was perpetually on the move. He darted through the staterooms and corridors, shrieking with his shrill, penetrating voice. The king indulged him in everything, and he was a perpetual nuisance to the elderly, staid, and nervous people residing at Lunéville.

Bébé was never punished in any way; even after the worst outrages, the king just gave a merry laugh at the discomfiture of the horrid dwarf's victim. Nicolas had terrific temper tantrums, to which he freely gave way whenever he was refused anything: a bonbon, a piece of cake, or a new suit of clothes. He screamed, kicked, and broke vases and china. When reproached, he sullenly walked back to his dwarf house to sulk for hours. King Stanislas even tolerated the mischievous behavior of the little fellow when he jumped up onto the gaming table while the king was playing backgammon, to kick the pieces down onto the floor. The king was much worried that Bébé would one day walk out of the castle grounds and then not have sense enough to return the same way, but instead stray onto some forest and be lost forever. Several times, the entire staff of the château had to be commandeered to search for the missing dwarf in the surrounding woodlands. After a long and futile hue and cry, the dirty, exhausted menials trudged back to the castle, to face the anxious king, who feared that Bébé had drowned in a pond or that he had been caught and eaten by some wild beast. The next moment, Bébé jumped out from his hiding place with a piercing cry: as usual, he had hidden deliberately, for the pleasure of seeing the others look for him. There was no risk that Bébé would be punished even for this dire offense; indeed, the king was overjoyed and fed him sweets.

Bébé was always immaculately dressed, according to the fashion of the time. The Princess de Talmont took pride that he should at least look like the perfect little gentleman. His long hair was powdered and arranged by a footman each morning. In spite of his appetite for cakes, chocolate, and bonbons, Nicolas remained lean and agile. He liked to drive about in the garden of the château in a specially built, beautifully decorated little cart, harnessed with four white goats; it must have been a remarkable sight to meet his unique equipage being whipped forth, with enthusiastic yells and screams, on some secluded garden path. Another of Nicolas Ferry's interests was military drill, and he liked to watch the training of the royal guards on the barrack square.

The king had a full grenadier's uniform made in Bébé's size, and the court dwarf for once proved a willing pupil: the king could soon amuse his court by drilling Bébé, who stood on a high table, dressed in his uniform and brandishing a miniature rifle.

At one of the court banquets at Lunéville, the dessert was a huge pastry in the shape of a military fortress, decorated with towers, guns, and battlements made of sugar and confectionery. It was much admired by the guests, who ate and drank well during the sumptuous banquet. The king had a surprise in store for them, however. Without warning, Bébé jumped up from the pastry's interior, fired two pistols at the roof, and whirled a sword around threateningly. A young nobleman, the Chevalier de Vintimille, was so frightened that he tipped his chair backward, shrieking out with fear and alarm, and ran out into the garden.

During the heyday of Nicolas Ferry's reign as the court favorite of King Stanislas, many people were appalled by the bad character of this horrid dwarf, who had nevertheless been brought up by cultured, educated people and indulged in everything. Bébé was choleric, selfish, and jealous to a marked degree. Once, when he

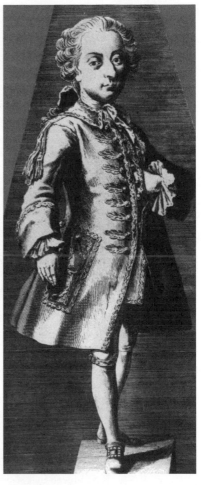

A print of a contemporary engraving of Nicolas Ferry. From the author's collection.

observed the Princess de Talmont sitting with a little dog on her lap, he ran up to her, snatched the lap dog, and threw it out the window with the words, "Pourquoi l'aimez-vous plus que moi?"—Why do you love this dog more than me? He was a petty tyrant who savored his privileged position and relished ordering the court pages and servants about. Despite his many failings, Bébé remained the great favorite of King Stanislas. His fame had spread like wildfire across Europe, and all the king's guests at Lunéville wanted to meet

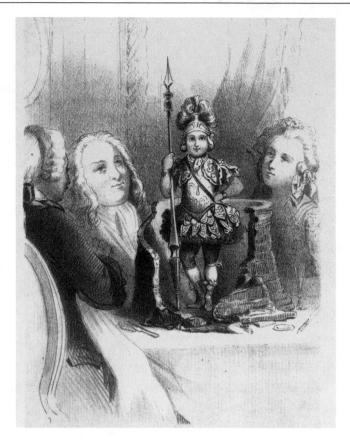

A tinted lithograph from Maison Aubert, after A. Géniole, of Nicolas Ferry standing in the remnants of the pastry he had been "served" in, before the admiring eyes of King Stanislas. Reproduced by permission from the Wellcome Institute Library, London.

him. Celebrities like Duke de Richelieu, the Count de Clermont, and the Prince de Condé were entertained by the king and his faithful Bébé, and a few years later, they were visited by Voltaire and Mme du Châtelet.

In 1759, Nicolas was severely shocked when a rival for his royal favor arrived. The Countess Humiecka, one of the ladies in waiting at the court of King Stanislas, who knew well the elderly monarch's penchant for midgets, brought a twenty-year-old Polish dwarf named Joseph Boruwlaski to

Lunéville. He was just 2 feet 6½ inches tall, and thus more than an inch shorter than Bébé. While poor Nicolas's attempts at conversation quickly palled, Joseph Boruwlaski, whom King Stanislas renamed Joujou in his usual manner, was quick-witted and amusing, with the polite manner of a courtier. When the two court dwarfs were formally introduced, Boruwlaski politely apologized for being the shortest of the two. The confused Bébé merely replied that he himself had been ill and that he soon would grow up and become tall. He then retreated to sit sulking in his house. A certain M. Durival wrote in his diary that Bébé "choked with fury when eclipsed by another little man, and was livid with rage when he saw the king and his court caress and flatter the newcomer, while he himself was ignored." The king, who had previously showed Bébé much patience, now started to reproach him for his morose stupidity. On one occasion, King Stanislas put a series of questions to his two court dwarfs. The toadying little Boruwlaski provided witty and apposite replies, but poor Nicolas was as scatter-brained as ever. The king then turned to his old favorite and pointed out the difference between the two: Joujou was merry, amusing, and well educated, but Bébé was just "une petite machine." Nicolas received this deadly affront in silence, but as soon as the king left the room, he crept behind his rival, seized hold of him, and dragged him across the room toward the open fireplace, where a large bonfire was roaring! Boruwlaski gave a great yell when he felt the clutches of the furious court dwarf. Fortunately, the king heard this outcry and returned just in time to save him. Although Boruwlaski begged for mercy for his rival, the king decided that for once, Bébé was to receive a sound thrashing, which was immediately administered by some sturdy menials. The wretched court dwarf was so mortified by this novel experience of corporal punishment that he did not speak for several days.

If he had wanted to, Joseph Boruwlaski could easily have usurped Bébé's position at King Stanislas's court. But although the king was rapturous about the new court dwarf he had discovered, Boruwlaski was less impressed by King Stanislas and his court. He was shrewd enough to appreciate that his minuscule stature, coupled with a ready wit, could make his fortune among the many noble and wealthy curiosity seekers of Europe. He realized that he had to remain his own master and not settle down as court dwarf. In late 1795, Boruwlaski left Lunéville for Paris, and to his great relief, Bébé gradually reclaimed his position as the royal favorite. Joseph Boruwlaski later made a brilliant career as an itinerant performer; he was received at most European courts and made a small fortune. At the age of sixty, he retired from show business, settled in England, and purchased a life annuity, at favorable terms, from a foolish man who did not think that this little fellow could live much longer. Joseph Boruwlaski proved him wrong, however, since he lived to be ninety-eight years old; he survived the money lender, whose relatives had to keep paying the annuity for many years. As befitting a man of his wealth and social position, Joseph Boruwlaski is buried in Durham Cathedral.

~&

Several of the physicians attached to the court of Lunéville were interested in Bébé and tried to figure out what was the cause of his abnormal growth. A certain Dr. Sauveur Morand several times spoke to and examined the court dwarf, while preparing a lecture before the Academie des Sciences. His opinion of Nicolas Ferry's intellect was very low. He wrote that the celebrated court dwarf's mind was generally clouded and confused, and that his capacity did not exceed that of a well-trained dog. A distinguished nobleman, Louis Elizabeth de la Vergie, Comte de Tressan, who was grand marshal at the court of King Stanislas, also took an interest in Bébé. The count was actually a member of the Academie des Sciences, and in 1760, he read a paper comparing the accomplishments of Bébé with those of Joseph Boruwlaski. This comparison was highly unflattering for poor Nicolas. Comte de Tressan wrote that in spite of the king's unceasing attempts to educate him, Bébé remained a complete imbecile. He could not read or write a single letter and was incapable of doing any useful work.

Count de Tressan continued with the words:

> Bébé can really be brought forward as a better proof for the theories of Descartes about the souls of animals, than a monkey or a poodle . . . . I must confess that I have never cast an eye on Bébé without feeling repugnance and secret horror, inspired by this vile caricature of human nature.

Some individual, perhaps the count himself, was unfeeling enough to read these very severe censures out loud to the unfortunate Nicolas, who cried out in horror: "If this be true, I am nothing—the king will never care for me any more!" The Princess de Talmont was appalled by the count's actions, and she wrote a pamphlet to avenge her poor Bébé. In this publication, she reproached the cruel count for his invectives against Nicolas and claimed, with some reason, that far from being like a dumb animal, he was quite capable of reasoning and was by no means an imbecile. Although vain and conceited — "il connatit le prix de la petitesse de sa figure" — and easily won over by flattery, he was also capable of understanding reproaches and trying to better himself. Nicolas was sincerely attached to the king and herself. Without urging, he distributed alms among the poor country people, often giving them pieces of silver instead of the customary small copper coins. Once, the well-to-do court dwarf gave a piggy bank crammed full of money to his younger brother Louis, who thereby became the wealthiest inhabitant of the village of Champenay.

❧

Until he was sixteen years old, Nicolas Ferry was healthy and agile; he never complained of illness, and his limbs, although small, were strong and supple. But in his later teens, the celebrated court dwarf began to age prematurely. His back gradually became stooped and one shoulder hunched; his legs weakened, and he walked in a weak, tottering manner. The head bent forward and the toothless chin dropped; his already prominent nose became monstrously huge and beaklike as the rest of his face wasted away. Nicolas also lost his cheerful, mischievous personality and became a dissatisfied, complaining valetudinarian. In 1759, Count de Tressan predicted that Bébé would die of old age before he was thirty years old; whether the nobleman told poor Nicolas about this sinister prophesy is not known. In 1760, when Bébé accompanied King Stanislas to Paris, he was seen by the encyclopedist Diderot, who was much struck by the nineteen-year-old court dwarf's premature aging: his back was much stooped, and his complexion a sickly gray.

King Stanislas let his court physician, the Swede Kasten Rönnow, examine Nicolas, and several other physicians and surgeons were consulted later. Their diagnosis was that Bébé's premature senility was caused by puberty; this process disrupted the balance of the tissues of his small body: his blood became thin and depleted, and the nerves desiccated. The wicked Count de Tressan added that Bébé's sexual excesses were likely to have accentuated his aging process further. The vast majority of contemporary chroniclers have disagreed with the insinuating count on this point, but several other sources agree that Bébé did consort freely with the young ladies at King Stanislas's court. It was frequently gossiped at the time that King Stanislas was an elderly libertine, and that the moral tone at his court was deplorably low. There were rumors that the king put Bébé up to rush in under the wide crinolines of the ladies, and to make a detailed report of his observations to his delighted royal master. The ladies did not at all appreciate these intimacies, and sometimes — wittingly or unwittingly — the victim put down her pointed heel on the foot of this inquisitive little fellow, who let out a great howl that echoed under the wide skirts, before he crawled out, purple with rage, and limped away to tell the king about the indignity he had suffered.

Another rumor was that in the late 1750s, Nicolas proposed to a normal-sized young lady residing in Lunéville, but her parents, who did not want a court dwarf for their son-in-law, refused him in no uncertain terms. In 1761, King Stanislas thought of a novel idea of amusing his court. He arranged a grandiose dwarf's marriage between Bébé and the equally diminutive Mlle Thérèse Souvray, another native of Lorraine. Although they had never met, both were initially agreeable to spend the remainder of their lives in holy matrimony. Thérèse was delighted to marry the wealthy young court dwarf, and Bébé had seen her pretty portrait and was happy to get a wife after his earlier rebuff. But after viewing her prospective husband, whose ill health was unlikely to improve his temper and character, Thérèse Souvray asked the king's permission to remain single, which was granted. Nicolas Ferry's reaction to this disastrous course of events is not known, but his flagging spirits can hardly have been revived by the indignity of being rejected once more. There was indeed a rumor that Bébé "entra dans une violente colère" after being jilted, and that the amorous dwarf rapidly fell into a decline and died, like the heroine of some French novel. This was an after-construction, however, since it is well known that Nicolas had been ill for several years before being rejected. His intended fiancée never married, and at some stage of her career as an actress and performer, she actually called herself Mme Bébé, to exploit the legendary court dwarf's notoriety. As late as 1819, at the age of seventy-three, she performed in a play titled *Bébé, ou le nain du Roi Stanislaus*, accompanied by her sister Barbe, who was a little taller than her and an accomplished singer and dancer.

Later in 1761, Nicolas Ferry enjoyed his final triumph as a court dwarf, when Louis XV's two sisters, Princesses Adelaide and Victoire, visited King Stanislas in Lunéville. As a surprise, Stanislas had arranged a military parade in which the uniformed "Capitaine Bébé" led the grenadiers and the citizen's cavalry past the royal party. The next year, when he was twenty-one years old, Nicolas Ferry fell into a lethargy and became bedridden. He was incontinent and could not even stand up without support. The doctors were again consulted, but they had no worthwhile suggestions at all, except to emphasize the uniqueness of Bébé's case. They were probably already whetting their autopsy knives and corresponding with various scholarly journals likely to publish a paper on the famous dwarf, complete with the necropsy findings.

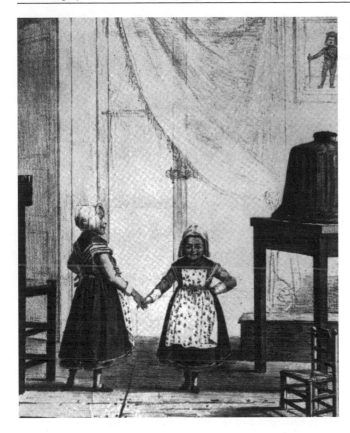

A print published in 1819 of Thérèse Vouvray, the alleged Madame Bébé. From the author's collection.

To their disappointment, Nicolas rallied after a couple of months and was again able to totter about on his own. A weak, frail, grumbling invalid, he could not even walk one hundred steps and had to be carried upstairs. He always complained of being cold and could not abide a drafty room; the only thing that would raise his spirits was when the servants carried his stretcher out into the garden on a warm and sunny day. In May 1764, Nicolas caught a cold, which was followed by lengthy fever spells, ague fits, and excessive weakness. He could not eat or move from his bed; when someone he knew spoke to him, he tried to reply but could not. On June 5, he seemed a little stronger and was again able to speak; to the astonishment of those present, the ailing court dwarf now displayed more knowledge and reason than he had ever done during his previous life. Although he had never before appeared to understand religion, he now confessed his sins to one of the court chaplains, partook of the Holy Communion, and received the extreme unc-

206   tion. The next day, the emaciated, exhausted dwarf again seemed on the brink of death, and at eight o'clock in the evening of June 8, he finally died, at the age of twenty-two years and seven months.

~&

When King Stanislas received the news of the death of his favorite, he wept bitterly. At first, he was unwilling to have Bébé autopsied, but Count de Tressan managed to persuade him, with the argument that it would be a great loss to medical science if such a curious *jeu de nature* was not properly anatomized. He also promised the king that he could keep Bébé's mounted skeleton as a souvenir; just like he used to have his favorite dogs stuffed after death.

The autopsy was performed by the court physician, the Swede Kasten Rönnow, assisted by the court surgeon, M. Perret, and the junior surgeon, M. Saucerotte. The inquisitive Count de Tressan was present as a spectator. When Nicolas Ferry's corpse was measured, it proved to be 35 inches (89 centimeters) tall. His inner organs were in good condition, except that there was a small amount of fluid in the pleural cavities and certain pleural adherences; neither of these findings is of much significance. The curvature of the ribs was greater on one side, due to the scoliosis of the back. Count de Tressan specifically mentioned that the genital parts were normal. The official autopsy report mentioned nothing further, but the surgeon Saucerotte published an addition in 1768. He stated that a spongious, reddish tumor was situated between the parietal bones. This tumor pressed directly against the brain. The insides of both parietal bones were covered with a similar substance, and the bony structures in this area seemed brittle and diseased.

After autopsy, Kasten Rönnow boiled Nicolas's skeleton and put the bones in a large box, kept in the royal library of Lunéville. Despite Count de Tressan's promise to King Stanislas, it was never mounted. King Stanislas himself followed Bébé into the grave two years later. His way of death was an unusual one. One evening, as the elderly, corpulent monarch stood warming his backside before a roaring fire, his dressing gown suddenly caught alight. A party of servants and courtiers were summoned by the king's cries, but a loyal gendarme, posted outside the bedroom door with strict orders from the king that no one was to enter and disturb his sleep, held them at bayonet point even when thick smoke started to billow out underneath the door! When they finally managed to force their way in, the king was too badly burned to survive, a victim of his own predilection for court etiquette.

After the death of King Stanislas, Bébé's skeleton was taken to the Cabinet du Roi in Paris, where the celebrated George Louis Buffon personally examined it. He mounted the skeleton and measured all the bones. It was apparent to him that Bébé had suffered from bilateral genua valga (bandy-legs), as had been described already during his lifetime. This was due to early-onset osteoarthritis of the knee joints, affecting the medial compartment of the joints much more than the lateral one. Nicolas also had had a severe, left-convex scoliosis (curvature of the spine). Poor Bébé did not have a single tooth at the time of his death. Only one alveolar process was observed in the lower jaw, and the upper jaw was in even worse condition. Old Kasten Rönnow had boiled Bébé's skeleton far too long and thus destroyed all traces of muscles and tendons, which made Buffon's work more difficult. Another odd matter was that two ribs were missing; Buffon suspected that they had either been lost or taken as souvenirs. The latter hypothesis seems quite likely and is further supported by the fact that several bones from Bébé's hands were also missing; Buffon had to procure suitably sized replacements from the museum's repository of children's skeletons. It is by no means unlikely that Count de Tressan and other curiosity seekers who had known Bébé during his lifetime had taken some of these bones as mementos of the famous court dwarf.

The remains of Nicolas Ferry's body were buried, with much ceremony, in the Église des Minimes at Lunéville. A mausoleum was built over the grave, with an ornate urn, and the inscription:

> *Hic jacet*
> *Nicolaüs Ferry, Lotharingus,*
> *Naturæ ludus,*
> *Staturæ tenuitate mirandus,*
> *Ab Antonio novo dilectus,*
> *In juventute, ætate senex,*
> *Quinque lustra fuerunt ipsi*
> *Sæculum.*
> *Obiit nonà die junii MDCCLXIV.*

This means:

> Here rests Nicolas Ferry of Lorraine, a jest of nature who was admirable for his small build, and who pleased the novel Anthony. In midst of his youth, he became an old man, and twenty-five years was for him the same as a century. He died on June 9, 1764.

The "novel Anthony" mentioned in the inscription was a flattering reference to King Stanislas himself. The Minimes church was destroyed during the French Revolution, but Nicolas Ferry's mausoleum was saved; it is today exhibited at the Musée du Château de Lunéville. Another, lengthier inscription, adding that not the skeleton, but only the innards, had been put into the grave, was quoted in an engraving at the Cabinet des Estampes.

Throughout his stay in Lunéville, Bébé was a European celebrity. The people who had once seen him did not forget him in a hurry, and he remained famous long after his death. He was frequently mentioned in the contemporary chronicles of court life and in the many volumes of eighteenth-century society memoirs, as well as in several medical treatises on human anomalies. Many museums still treasure various mementos of the famous court dwarf. Foremost of them is his skeleton, which was later moved from the Cabinet du Roi to the Musée d'Histoire Naturelle in Paris, where the wretched dwarf's skeleton was put among the skeletons of animals in the department of zoology; the harsh and unjust censures of Count de Tressan were thus confirmed through the irony of fate. In the twentieth century, Nicolas Ferry's skeleton was finally moved to the Musée de l'Homme.

King Stanislas spared no expense to equip Bébé with splendid clothes and hats, and the dwarf house was kept well stocked with beautiful handcrafted furniture, porcelain, and cutlery. A few of these objects are still kept in museums or in private collections. In 1883, the French antiquary A. Benoît published an inventory of "les souvenirs de Bébé." The Musée d'Unterlinden had a hat, a pair of breeches, a costume in blue silk, and a short rapier made especially for Bébé. M. Gilliot, a master printer residing in Savenne, had a pair of white socks, a pair of breeches, and two 4-inch shoes. Another pair of breeches "dans un triste état de conservation" were at the Musée de Lunéville. The Benedictine monks at Senones treasured another pair of Nicolas Ferry's shoes. Bébé's drinking goblet was at the Musée d'Amiens, and his easy chair was kept in a private collection.

Bébé's elegant little carriage pulled by four goats had an interesting history. It reappeared in a noble family in Lunéville, where it was used as a toy by generations of children. When it was in derelict condition, it was sold to a poor mason, who used it to transport his harvest of vegetables. The architect M. Joly, a historian of the Château de Lunéville, saw it in the 1850s. In spite of its prosaic use, there were still traces of gilding on its ornaments, and the philosophical M. Joly paused to meditate on the change of fortunes for Bébé's "voiture de gala"; it would have been better if he had given the mason a few francs for this unique vehicle, to save it for posterity.

Today, several of Nicolas Ferry's clothes are kept at the Musée Historique Lorrain in Nancy: his cap, spats, and dressing-case, among other objects. Several drawings, and a beautiful oil painting of Nicolas Ferry with a large dog, are also at this museum. The Musée Municipal at the Château de Lunéville has two other oil paintings, and a fourth is in the private collection of a French nobleman. The latter museum also owns a unique life-size porcelain statue of Nicolas Ferry dressed in the uniform of the Polish hussars. It was made in 1746, when he was six years old and had just joined the court of King Stanislas. It has the inscription "Portrait.naturel.dvn.enfant.age,de six ans/NP fecit/de.lanee/1746."

❧

It is apparent that wax statues of Nicolas Ferry were made on several occasions. When Dr. Morand went to lecture about him at the Academie des Sciences, he brought with him a life-size wax dummy of Nicolas, dressed in a suit of his clothes. This statue had been made in 1759, when Nicolas was eighteen years old, by M. Jeanet, a surgeon of Lunéville. Some of Bébé's fine coiffure had been cut off to provide it with hair, and its face was carefully molded to resemble his own. It is not unlikely that another statue was made during Nicolas's lifetime, by a certain Francois Guillot, a specialist molder of statues, who had his workshop in Nancy. Finally, at least one statue was made after death, probably at the Cabinet du Roi. To get the proportions right, every bone in the skeleton was measured, and the resulting wax statue was "superbement habillé" in a suit of Nicolas's own clothes.

The statue at Drottningholm Castle is by no means unique. Surprisingly many wax statues of Nicolas Ferry have survived wars and revolutions and are now treasured exhibits in various museums. At the Musée Orfila in Paris is a statue that has been at various Parisian anatomical museums since at least the 1830s. It was a well-known and familiar sight for thousands of medical students. One of them, Dr. Liegey, who later read a paper on Bébé before the Société d'Émulation des Vosges, saw it in 1832, "vêtu à la mode Louis XV," and standing on a window sill. This statue is dressed in a light blue coat with lace cuffs, a long gray waistcoat, red breeches, gray stockings, and a black cocked hat. This statue is less detailed than that at Drottningholm Castle: the face is quite unlike that of Nicolas Ferry, and the hair very sparse. The few remaining strands may well be Nicolas's own, however. Furthermore, the proportions of the stocky, ungainly figure do not resemble those of Nicolas Ferry. It is possible that the statue has sunk somewhat; indeed, the stockings are sagging quite badly, which would support this theory. Several authors have identified this statue with the one made in 1759, which Dr. Morand took with him to the Academie des Sciences in 1764. It is just under 2 feet tall, which would support this hypothesis, since Bébé grew almost 8 inches during the latter part of his life.

Another statue of Bébé is at the Musée Historique Lorrain in Nancy. Like the others, it is mounted on a wooden fundament and dressed in one of Nicolas's most splendid suits of clothes. The face is stated to be "moulée rigoreusement authentique" and resembled that of Nicolas more than the Paris statue did. The luxuriant hair is likely to be a wig; otherwise, poor Nicolas's head would have had to be completely cropped to provide the statue with hair. Its position is somewhat unlike that of the statue at Drottningholm Castle, and it lacks the hat. Another wax statue of Nicolas Ferry is at the Musée

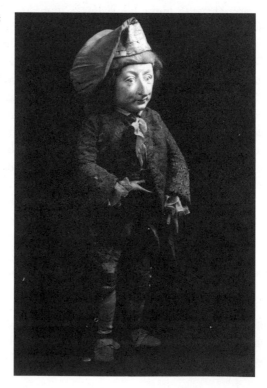

The wax statue of Bébé at the Musée Historique Lorrain, Nancy. Reproduced by permission, copyright musée Lorrain, Nancy/photo G. Mangin.

Municipal at the Château de Lunéville; it was deposited there in 1985 by the Musée d'Unterlinden in Colmar.

Yet another wax statue, wearing a suit of Bébé's own clothes, is at the Herzog Anton-Ulrich Museum in Braunschweig. Its history is of some interest, since it seems as if it originally belonged to the Duke Anton Ulrich of Braunschweig's private museum. It was made in France and arrived at Braunschweig before 1806. Its proportions, with an elongated torso and short legs, are very unlike those of Bébé; nor does its face resemble his. A similar statue is kept at the Hessisches Landesmuseum in Kassel.

∿❧

Already Dr. Morand and Count de Tressan discussed what kind of obscure disorder had made Bébé into such a remarkable *lusus naturae*. Neither of them were particularly well read in the contemporary medical literature, however, and even if they had been, there was much confusion, at the time, concerning how to classify cases of extreme nanism. Dr. Morand distinguished two categories of dwarfs: the deformed and the nondeformed. The former category must have encompassed the chondrodystrophies and those suffering from rickets; Bébé belonged to the latter category, also called "les véritables nains." In the early nineteenth century, other diagnostic suggestions were put forth, but without much ground being gained. A certain Dr. Virey suggested that Nicolas Ferry had suffered from both rachitis and an unspecified "maladie de foetus," and some other French obstetricians proposed that his mother's placenta had been insufficiently developed to nurture the growing fetus.

In 1890, the French obstetrician Dr. Porak made a novel suggestion in a lecture before the Société Obstetrique et Gynecologique in Paris. He had showed Nicolas Ferry's skull to Professor Fournier, a distinguished venereologist, and the professor unhesitatingly pronounced that the appearance of the parietal bones indicated that Bébé had been a victim of gummous periostitis of the skull, a manifestation of congenital syphilis. Professor Fournier knew well that children with congenital syphilis often were of a short stature, and he considered the famous court dwarf an extreme example. To those unconvinced, Dr. Porak handed around Bébé's skull as evidence.

Seven years later, the teratologist L. Manouvrier re-examined Nicolas Ferry's skull at the Musée de l'Homme. Like Porak and Fournier, he found changes in both parietal bones speaking in favor of what he called an "Ostéo-periostite," but he did not speculate about what disease had origi-

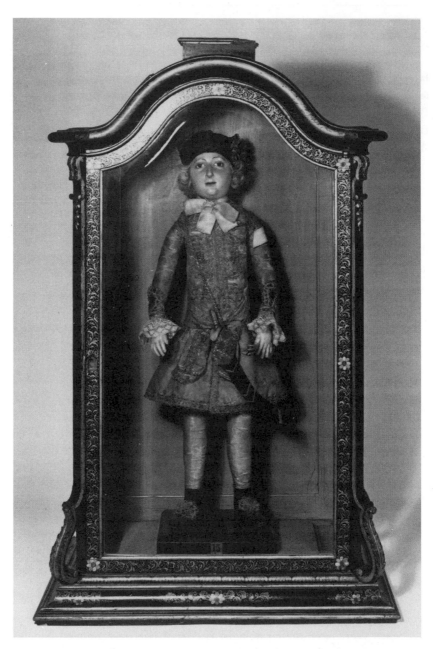

The wax statue of Nicolas Ferry at the Herzog Anton-Ulrich-Museum in Braunschweig. Reproduced by permission.

nally caused these changes. Among later authors, there have been differing opinions regarding whether Nicolas Ferry really had syphilis and whether this disease could really explain his remarkable growth retardation and premature aging. The discovery of the surgeon Saucerotte's autopsy report in an obscure publication has made it clear that Bébé really had some kind of lesion on the inside of the skull, just as Porak and Fournier had assumed from the appearance of the bones. It was not only situated on the parietal bones, however, but also between them, and this reddish tumor even pressed against his brain.

From the overall clinical picture, it is extremely unlikely that Nicolas Ferry had congenital syphilis. His parents and siblings were reported to be strong and in excellent health, and Nicolas himself never showed any of the typical signs of congenital lues (Hutchinson's triad). It may be that he caught a venereal contagion at some later date, but although the gossipy court chronicles hinted that he was sexually active, it is unlikely that the frail, sickly dwarf was capable of any exertions of this kind, at least during the latter five years of his life. The court physicians, who knew him well and who reported his failings without any concern for the privacy of their patient, mentioned nothing about any venereal disease, and at autopsy, his genitals were normal.

In 1911, the British surgeon and teratologist Sir Hastings Gilford re-examined Nicolas Ferry's case. He quoted the contemporary French diagnosis of "syphilis, microcephaly and infantilism, ending in senilism," but did not agree with it. In particular, he found it impossible to accept that Nicolas Ferry's remarkable intrauterine and postnatal growth retardation could be the result of congenital lues. Instead, Hastings Gilford compared Bébé with some other cases of "ateleiosis," a syndrome of symmetrical dwarfism with "delay in growth and development," and found several common characteristics. In particular, Bébé's skeleton, and the portraits of him during life, showed the same nanocephalic, or "bird-headed" profile as several other cases, with a large, beaklike nose and a feeble, receding chin.

In the mid-twentieth century, several geneticists understood that the old syndrome of ateleiosis was in fact a heterogeneous group of conditions. In 1960, the American geneticist H. P. G. Seckel reconsidered Nicolas Ferry's case. In a detailed monograph, he gave Bébé the diagnosis "bird-headed dwarfism," or as it is now called, Seckel's syndrome. This autosomally recessive condition is characterized by a variable degree of intrauterine growth retardation, severe proportional postnatal dwarfism, and a characteristic "bird-headed" profile with a large beaklike nose, a weakly developed chin, a receding brow, and a small cranial cavity. Professor Seckel made an extensive search of the older literature and rightly concluded that Bébé had had the lowest recorded birth weight of any "bird-headed dwarf."

In modern clinical genetics, it has become apparent that the old term "bird-headed dwarfism" is an uncouth as well as an imprecise denominator, and that primordial microcephalic dwarfism is quite a heterogeneous condition. For example, when I described the case of Caroline Crachami, one of the best-known historical cases, in 1992, it did not take long for some experienced pediatricians to discover similar modern instances. The so-called Caroline Crachami syndrome is today a recognized subgroup within the spectrum of primordial microcephalic dwarfism.

Nicolas Ferry had many characteristics in common with the typical individual with bird-headed dwarfism: his microcephaly, mental retardation, large nose, hyperactivity, thin shrill voice, and extrovert personality are all recognized features of this condition. In his youth, his facial configuration, with a broad forehead and well-developed mandible, was quite unlike that of a patient with Seckel's syndrome, however. What particularly distinguishes Nicolas Ferry from the vast majority of individuals with primordial microcephalic dwarfism is his premature aging. After the age of eighteen, he developed a typical bird-headed facies with a grotesquely large, beaklike nose and a receding chin. In his original monograph, Professor Seckel wrote that "senile features are virtually unknown in bird-headed dwarfs," but this may, on good grounds, be doubted. Six of Seckel's original fifteen cases died between the ages of five and twenty-three years. One of them had evidence of cardiomegaly and generalized atherosclerosis. In his teens, an American patient developed, as had Bébé two hundred years earlier, alopecia, graying of the remaining hair, a stooped posture, and considerable accentuation of his bird-headed appearance; his growth retardation was much less pronounced than that of the famous eighteenth-century court dwarf, however.

There is a condition called progeria, or the Hutchinson-Gilford syndrome, in which the main symptom is premature aging. Already in their early teens, the sufferers of this loathsome disease develop a wrinkled, wizened appearance, alopecia, osteoporosis, and pronounced arteriosclerosis; they are unlikely to survive their twenty-fifth birthday, and die as bedridden invalids. Someone who has seen one of these individuals is unlikely to forget the encounter. It is interesting to note that patients with progeria often are of a short stature, and that individuals with the related Werner's syndrome, or progeria adultorum, sometimes gradually develop a bird-headed appearance. Considering the case of Nicolas Ferry, and a few others, it seems reasonable to suggest that there is a progeroid variant of osteodysplastic primordial dwarfism, with more or less pronounced intrauterine growth retardation.

∽❧

During Nicolas Ferry's lifetime, medical men and other observers consistently had a very low opinion of his intelligence and character. He was likened to a trained dog or monkey, and described as highly selfish, jealous, choleric, and sensuous. Like the majority of the victims of osteodysplastic primordial dwarfism, Nicolas was definitely mentally retarded. It should be noted, however, that the degree of mental retardation is not related to the size and birth weight of the individual, as evidenced by the famous "Sicilian Fairy" Caroline Crachami. This girl's birth weight was only 16 ounces (450 grams), second to Nicolas in the annals of this syndrome. At the age of eight, a time when poor Nicolas could hardly make himself understood in French, Caroline Crachami learned to express herself fluently in a foreign language and gave witty and apposite replies to questions.

Some of the anecdotes about Nicolas Ferry would imply that he was far less mentally retarded than Dr. Morand and Count de Tressan had claimed. Furthermore, the person who knew him best, the Princess de Talmont, was outraged by the count's accusations. It does not seem unreasonable that the spiteful count, who seems to have loathed the spoiled, scatter-brained, irritating court dwarf, let his detestation cloud whatever scientific judgment he may have possessed. After all, it is rare, even in France, to find a trained dog or monkey expressing itself fluently in French.

Nicolas Ferry's contemporaries were much impressed by his triumphant career at the court of King Stanislas, and he was called the happiest of dwarfs. A local dignitary, President Hérault, ridiculed Bébé's simple-minded mother, who persisted in having masses said for her son to grow and be tall; was it not his dwarfism that had made his fortune? In fact, King Stanislas probably did Nicolas a great disfavor when he removed the boy from his parents. Voltaire was not the only observer to question the moral tone at Lunéville, and it was certainly a very improper place for an impressionable young child to grow up. Instead of leading a harmonic, rural life with his parents and siblings in Champenay, he was spoiled, overindulged, and treated as an interesting little pet trained to perform a few tricks before distinguished visitors. The ladies at court dressed him in splendid clothes like a

216   little doll, and he had his own doll's house to live in. A popular epigram
about King Stanislas said:

> *Voilà les trois jouets d'un roi cher aux Lorrains*
> *Griffon son chien, son singe et Bébé son nain;*

The King's dog, monkey, and court dwarf were often taken for a walk
together in the garden. Although his disease had a genetic origin, environ-
ment rather than heredity caused Nicolas Ferry's bad character.

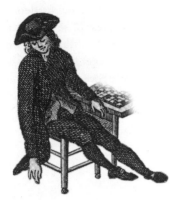

Daniel Cajanus,
the Swedish Giant

O N FEBRUARY 5, 1734, A LARGE CROWD OF
spectators had gathered to see *Cupid and Psyche* at the Drury Lane
Theatre in London. Earlier performances of the same play had
been little heeded by critics and audience alike, but there had been rumors
that something extraordinary was afoot, and that this particular show would
indeed be worth seeing. The play was enacted just as usual until the character of Gargantua was to appear: at that instance, a trapdoor opened, and a
gigantic figure, 7 feet 8 inches (234 centimeters) tall, suddenly appeared on
the stage "to the no small Admiration of the Spectators."

This was the theatrical debut of that legendary figure, Daniel Cajanus,
the Swedish Giant. He had come to London early in 1734, to earn money by
exhibiting himself. The theatrical directors got the bright idea of recruiting
the giant to their own show, and Cajanus was not unwilling to make his
debut as an actor, particularly as their offer was most generous. On February 22, a handbill announced that "this is the last time of Mynheer Cajanus,

the Tall Man's Appearance on the Stage," but the giant was persuaded to stay in London for another couple of weeks "at the Request of several Persons of Distinction." He appeared again on February 28, March 2, and March 5, to a total of twenty plays in all on the London stage. In his *Epilogue Spoken by Monimia*, the poet Aaron Hill gave the gigantic Swede a fitting poetic tribute:

> *What thinking face will any praise ordain us,*
> *Whose climbing eyes have scal'd* — Mynheer Cajanus!
> *Give place, Great Alexander!* — *Go, retire* —
> *We have enroll'd a* Hero — *Three foot higher!*

⁘

Daniel Cajanus was born in Paldamo, Finland, in 1704. At this time, Finland was still a province within the kingdom of Sweden. His father was Anders Cajanus, a theological graduate from the University of Turku. In 1694, Anders Cajanus was ordained curate of Paldamo, the Finnish town in which the family lived. Their family was quite a distinguished one. In the late sixteenth century, Admiral Nils Svensson of Hevonpää, a Finnish gentleman who had risen to high command in the Swedish fleet, was raised to the peerage by King Eric XIV. He assumed the name Gyllenhierta (Golden Heart), and his coat of arms was a red heart surrounded by golden flames. One of the admiral's grandsons, Anders Eriksson Gyllenhierta, was governor of the province of Kajana in Finland. Three of his sons became clergymen, advancing to become rectors in large Finnish parishes. These scholarly gentlemen all assumed the name of Cajanus, thus denouncing their noble descent. One of them was murdered by the Russians in 1713, when they burned his church in Kajana, where he was the rector. The other two lived to an advanced age and had numerous children and grandchildren; several branches of the Cajanus family are still flourishing in Finland. Another son of Anders Eriksson Gyllenhierta was Jeremias Gyllenhierta, who never went to the university and thus felt free to keep his father's noble surname. He became the sheriff of Paldamo in Finland. His eldest son Alexander succeeded him as sheriff and had several children, who took the name Cajanus; it was his second son, the clergyman Anders Cajanus, who was the father of Daniel the giant.

Anders Cajanus married the daughter of a fellow cleric, Miss Anna Sculptorius. He was a stubborn, difficult character, continuously at loggerheads with his clerical superiors and his parishioners alike. He was finally defrocked in 1710, on account of his quarrelsome nature. It was an aggravating circumstance that he had been caught red-handed affixing certain

pagan, magic amulets to his fishing nets to improve the catch! When learning the shocking news, the bishop rightly decided that such a curate would
not be the right person to teach Christianity to the rough farmers and trap-
pers in the Finnish outback. The last official act of Anders Cajanus was to
curse, from the pulpit, his cousin and superior, Eric Cajanus, rector of Paldamo; he solemnly hoped that every evil spirit of Hell would infest the rector's house and make his life an utter misery.

Daniel Cajanus had five brothers, two of whom became clergymen, and
two sisters. He received a reasonably good education and attended both "low
and high school," as he later put it, but never went to a university. His youth
coincided with the time of the Great Nordic War, waged by King Charles
XII of Sweden against King August of Poland, Czar Peter the Great of Russia, and King Frederick of Denmark. Finland bore the full brunt of this
lengthy war, which lasted from 1700 until 1718. In the late 1710s, the Russians invaded Finland and plundered and ravaged the countryside. Daniel
thus grew up during a great famine in Finland, but nevertheless, he attained
a great height already during his teens. In 1723, the records tell that Daniel
Cajanus paid the taxes along with his father Anders and their family and servants. The erring curate had been reinstated in 1713 and allowed to lead the
life of an itinerant preacher who roamed the Finnish villages just outside the
territory of his cousin Eric. The year 1723 was the last time the giant's name
appeared in the lists of Finnish taxpayers, however, and it is likely that he
decided to leave his native country in the mid-1720s.

❧

There was a tradition in Sweden and Finland that Daniel Cajanus went to
Prussia, where he visited the court of King Frederick Wilhelm I. He intended to enlist in this king's "giant guard," a troop of particularly tall soldiers, and the king was more than willing to accept him. When he became
aware that Daniel was a head taller than the other soldiers, he declined the
giant's offer to join his guard, however, as this colossus would put all the
other soldiers to shame. Before Daniel went away, the king ordered his portrait to be painted and hung in one of the galleries of Potsdam. According to
tradition, Daniel Cajanus remained in Prussia for some time. One day, a celebrated strong man challenged him to a bizarre duel: they would in turn slap
each other's faces until one of them was out cold. Although he was a man of
peace, Daniel accepted this challenge. The Prussian won the toss-up and delivered the first, resounding blow. Daniel nearly fell backward but did not
pass out. Infuriated, he dealt the Prussian such a tremendous box on the ear

that the man fell dead to the ground. Since this strange duel was illegal, Daniel had to flee Prussia, to seek his fortune elsewhere.

The reliable later sources on the life and journeys of Daniel Cajanus do not mention any stay in Prussia, but it may be that he himself did not want his exploits there to attract any notice. In 1911, the Finnish antiquary J. R. Aspelin contacted a German colleague to try to find out whether there were any traces of the giant's Prussian career, but none could be found: although portraits of several giant guardsmen were still kept, Cajanus was not among them. The Potsdam military archives, which might have provided a clue, were destroyed by enemy action in 1945. The tales of the Swedish Giant's dramatic experiences in Prussia thus rely on hearsay alone.

It is certain, however, that Daniel Cajanus spent a considerable period of time at the court of King August II of Poland. This king was a colorful, eccentric character, known as August the Strong, and famous for having a great number of concubines and illegitimate children. He was also elector of Saxony, under the name Frederick August I; it is possible that a careless historian may have confused him with Frederick Wilhelm I of Prussia. During his stay in Poland, Daniel Cajanus was employed as a cornet in the Polish cavalry. He obtained a Polish military uniform and often wore it during his later travels. He spent much time at King August's court in Dresden, and a letter written by him in 1731 was mailed from this town.

It is not known whether Daniel Cajanus visited other European courts before coming to London in 1734. King August the Strong had died in 1733, and it may be that his successor did not see the point of having a resident giant lounging about his court. It is not unlikely that Cajanus had stayed some time in Germany, since the actor and playwright Theophilus Cibber spoke of him as "a Fellow of an enormous Height" who came to London from Germany "to be shewn for a sight." The earl of Egmont, who saw Cajanus at Drury Lane on February 22, 1734, described him in his diary as "the tallest man of all I have ever seen. He is seven feet ten inches and half in height, a German by birth." Daniel Cajanus may also have been staying in Holland, since he was frequently referred to as "Mynheer Cajanus" in the London newspapers. The details about his height varied considerably: some advertisements said that he was 7 feet 8 inches tall (this was probably his true height); some that he was 8 feet tall and thus surpassed the German Maximilian Miller who had exhibited himself in London some years earlier. When Cajanus was in an expansive mood, he even claimed to be 8 feet 8 inches tall; this figure has been quoted in some ill-researched modern books, but has no foundation in fact.

Daniel's success induced one of his elder brothers to come to London to join him in his theatrical career. It is recorded that a certain Mynheer Cajanus Senior, billed as "the Brother to the famous Tall Man who lately appeared at Drury Lane" performed the part of Captain Bully in *Britannia* at Goodman's Fields in the spring of 1734. The fact that he repeated the performance at least thirteen times would imply that this Finnish cleric, who apparently shared his gigantic brother's excellent command of the English language, did not lack talent as an actor. Another London actor, John Rich, capitalized on Daniel Cajanus's popularity by acting the part of "Mynheer Cajanus's sister, the Tall Woman" in a burlesque play.

During his visit to Britain in 1734, Daniel Cajanus was later employed as a porter by John, duke of Montagu, who inhabited Boughton House in Kettering. During this time, two life-sized portraits of the Swedish Giant were painted by the artist Enoch Seeman. These portraits were at Dalkeith Castle, Scotland, in the 1760s, and later belonged to the dukes of Buccleugh. In 1911, one of them was owned by Admiral Lord Charles Scott, of Boughton House. In 1975, it was sold to the National Museum of Helsinki, where this huge portrait of the Swedish Giant has found a fitting home. It measures not less than 12 feet by 7 feet 9 inches (3.64 by 2.34 meters), the frame included. This portrait depicts the thirty-year-old Daniel Cajanus as a pleasant-looking young man, dressed in his usual Polish uniform, with his cavalry sword at his side, and wearing a turban and a great fur coat. Unlike most other portraits of giants and dwarfs, there is no normal-sized person in it as a contrast, and the only indication that Cajanus is actually a giant is the inscription on a stone tablet in the picture: "Caianvs, born in Lapland who was in London 1734 his hight is 7 foot and 10 inc. Ae 28. E Seeman pinx. 1734." The other Seeman portrait, which is very similar to that in Helsinki, was sold at Christie's in 1977, and is still in private ownership.

❧

After he left London late in 1734, Daniel Cajanus settled in Amsterdam. He took up residence at the Blauw Jan, a large inn situated in the Kloveniersburgwal. This remarkable establishment was the meeting place for dealers in exotic animals and natural curiosities from all over Europe. Carl Linnaeus came there several times to deal with his friend Albert Seba, who had a large, resident collection of stuffed animals, skeletons, dried insects, and other natural history specimens. Next to the inn was a small zoological

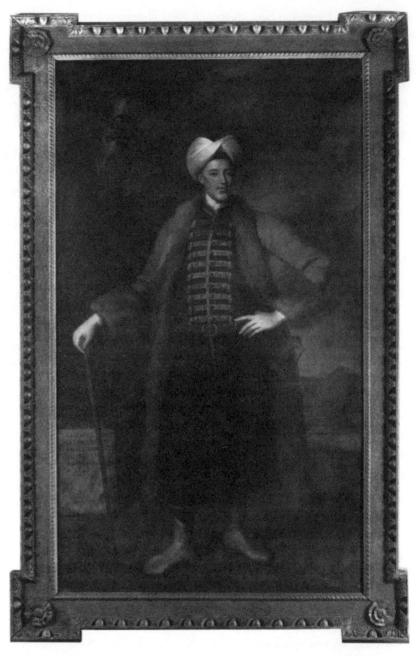

Enoch Seeman's portrait of Daniel Cajanus. Reproduced by permission of the National Museum of Finland, Helsinki.

garden with monkeys, lions, leopards, and exotic birds. In 1735, Daniel Cajanus visited Paris, where he astounded everyone when he walked along one of the main avenues, his head towering over those of all passers-by. For fifteen days, he stayed at the Hôtel de la Porte Royale and exhibited himself before large audiences from nine to twelve o'clock in the morning, and one to seven o'clock in the afternoon. He was even honored by King Louis XV, the queen, and the dauphin, who met him in a private audience at the court in Versailles.

The owner of the Blauw Jan, Evert Metz, encouraged Daniel Cajanus, among other human curiosities—dwarfs, Eskimos, pygmies, and conjoined twins—to reside permanently at his inn for exhibition purposes. Daniel stayed at the Blauw Jan from 1735 until 1741. He liked to play chess or checkers in the main hall of the inn, sitting before the great blazing fire. Friend and foe alike acknowledged him as a skillful player. Once, after he was defeated at checkers by a visiting gentleman, Cajanus slapped his opponent's shoulder so hard that the man screamed out in agony. This story was repeated as evidence that the giant did not know his own strength; one wonders, however, whether he was not just a bad loser! Daniel Cajanus was a remarkable sight as he sat on a chair that seemed designed to suit a small child, playing chess before an admiring crowd of spectators. His arms were so long that they almost touched the floor when he was sitting down. He could easily pick up a checkers piece that had fallen off the board without bending forward, as depicted in the drawing by a Dutch artist, engraved in an obscure publication, the *Almanak tot Nut van 't Algemen* of 1802. The Dutch doctor and writer Wilhelmus Greve published a book on giants and dwarfs in 1838 that contains some valuable observations of Daniel Cajanus, made by Dr. Greve's father one hundred years earlier. Cajanus had been a particular friend of Dr. Greve's father, and they often met at the Blauw Jan. Daniel was a polite, entertaining, and well-spoken man who was very popular among the Blauw Jan habitués. He was a masterly player at checkers. He was good-looking, and his body well proportioned, except for his prodigiously long arms. He was well thought of among the Amsterdam burghers and often asked to parties and dinners. When traveling to these festivities, he used a special carriage, from which the front bench had been removed to give him adequate leg room.

In 1737, a certain Antony Bergmeyer and his wife took over the Blauw Jan. Daniel Cajanus remained on the payroll of this establishment for several years to come, however, as evidenced by an illustrated poster. Although Daniel Cajanus suffered the indignity of being underbilled to a pair of ostriches, a young lion, a couple of tigers, some cassowaries, and the dwarf Wybrand Lolkes, he was still one of the main attractions of the Blauw Jan. One suspects that he rather enjoyed life at this busy inn, where he could come and go as he pleased and eat and drink at the expense of the house. Amsterdam was a pleasant city then as well as today, and Daniel Cajanus gradually began to consider himself a Dutchman. Quite a few foreign naturalists regularly came to the Blauw Jan to trade specimens, and Daniel is

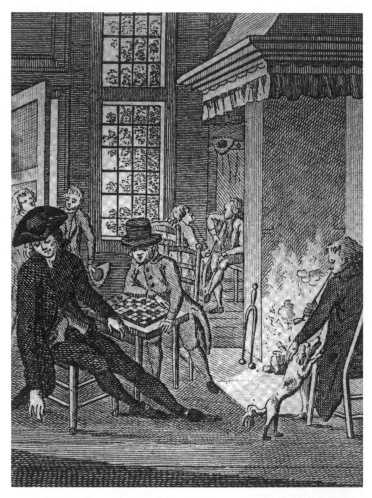

A contemporary drawing, later published in the *Almanak tot Not van't Algemen* of 1802, of Daniel Cajanus playing draughts at the Blauw Jan.

likely to have been seen and admired by them. Carl Linnaeus, a frequent visitor as stated earlier, probably saw his gigantic countryman there. In 1745, Linnaeus wrote a commentary to the Swedish Academy of Sciences, stating that he had, some years earlier, seen a three-year-old, enormously fat boy being exhibited at the marketplace in Amsterdam. His mother called him "Little Cajanus," and even had the effrontery to tell Linnaeus that Cajanus was really the child's father. After some investigation, Linnaeus concluded that it was unlikely that Cajanus had ever seen this woman. Little Cajanus weighed 133 pounds (7 lispounds; 60 kg) and was so fat that he could not stand up without having his legs placed widely apart. His corpulence was probably due to his mother's habit of nourishing him entirely on sweet beer; Little Cajanus always had a jug of beer near him, and Linnaeus saw him swig from it thirstily.

Daniel Cajanus had come to Amsterdam a wealthy man, having saved money from his successful tours of Poland, Germany, Britain, and France. He decided to invest this money by setting himself up as a moneylender. Several Dutch businessmen borrowed money from him. A certain Willem Pelgrom borrowed three thousand guilders from Cajanus, at an annual interest rate of 7 percent. This gentleman made his annual repayments in good order, but the brothers Metz, unscrupulous Haarlem innkeepers, soon refused to pay their half-yearly interest. This was apparently not due to lack of money but to some clauses in the "fine print" of the lending contract. After a legal wrangle lasting more than three years, from 1738 until 1741, Cajanus managed to recover the bulk of his money from these scoundrels, but none of the interest. A certain Anthony van Eck, an Amsterdam merchant who had borrowed nine thousand guilders from Cajanus, went bankrupt shortly afterward, and the giant could only recover five thousand guilders from the executors.

෴

After these disastrous experiences as a usurer, Daniel Cajanus decided to return to London and once more put himself on show. He was thirty-eight years old and wanted to provide for old age. In October 1741, he made a contract with his Dutch friend Roelof Sweris, who arranged to provide him with a showroom in London and to see that the Swedish Giant was well advertised. Cajanus was to receive three-fifths of the profit, and Sweris, who had to pay all the expenses, the remaining two-fifths. Daniel Cajanus did not neglect to take care of his property in Holland: according to another contract, two of his friends were charged with the responsibility of maintaining

226   his various investments and carrying on the lawsuit against the Metz brothers. Daniel Cajanus was advertised in the papers in a similar way as in 1734:

> This is to acquaint gentlemen and ladies, that that prodigy of
> nature, the Living Colossus, or Wonderful Giant of Sweden, is
> now to be seen, at the Lottery Office, next door to the Green
> Man, Charing Cross. It is humbly presumed that of all the nat-
> ural curiosities which have been exhibited to the publick, noth-
> ing has appeared for many years so extraordinary in its way as
> this surprising gentleman. He is near a foot taller than the late
> famous Saxon, or any person ever yet seen in Europe, large in
> proportion; and all who have hitherto seen him declare,
> notwithstanding the prodigious accounts they have heard, that
> he far exceeds any idea they had fram'd of him.

Daniel Cajanus later rented himself to an English showman for six
months for two hundred pounds, and was taken on a tour to Oxford and
then back to London, where he lodged in an apartment facing the Mansion-
house. A later advertisement in the *Daily Advertiser* revealed that Cajanus had
been indisposed for five weeks because of a violent fever, which had caused
a rumor that he had actually died. Daniel Cajanus recovered from this disease, however, and was again on show at the sign of the Mansion House and
French Horn, between the Poultry and the Royal Exchange, at the usual
price of sixpence per person, from nine o'clock in the morning until eight at
night. The advertisement concluded by asserting that he was the same giant
who was on show previously, as some malicious individuals had evidently
started a rumor that Cajanus had died and that his manager had procured a
replacement giant to "let the show go on"!

At the meeting of the Royal Society of London on January 21, 1742,
Daniel Cajanus was introduced as an instance of "gigantic Size of the human
Body." He was seen by, among many others, such medical luminaries as
James Douglas, James Parsons, and William Nourse. Cajanus stood at one
of the pillars at Crane Court and had his height marked on it: he was 7 feet
4¼ inches tall, but the heels of his shoes were about an inch. Daniel Cajanus
could reach within the architrave between two pillars, 10 feet above the
ground, with the greatest ease. He told the Fellows present that his father
was 6 feet 6 inches tall and his mother 6 feet 3 inches; his usual daily meal
was about 4½ pounds of meat. Cajanus also told the blatant lie that he was

actually *the brother* of the giant with the same name who had visited London a few years earlier. This was apparently something that had been planned beforehand, for him to keep his novelty and attract also those lovers of curiosities who had already visited him back in 1734. But several Fellows of the Royal Society had apparently seen him before, since they objected that the giant's features were certainly very like those of his presumed brother. The Reverend Dr. Pearse, who had also seen Cajanus in 1734, disagreed, however. He observed that although in 1734, he had been unable to reach higher than the "brother's" forehead, he could reach about an inch higher than the forehead of this man. The president of the Royal Society of London, the antiquary Martin Folkes, ordered that Cajanus was to be given a present of two guineas.

A week later, while Martin Folkes was reading the minutes concerning "the tall Finlander," he added that the painter William Hogarth and others had informed him that this giant was undoubtedly the same man who had appeared in London some years earlier, and not his brother. Folkes told the earl of Egmont, who had seen Cajanus in 1734, that the giant had now seemed feeble and unwilling to stand up for a long time. Another nobleman, the earl of Pembroke, had taken the giant's measurements by the method used to measure men in the army and found that he was 7 feet 4⅞ inches; no mention was made as to whether Cajanus was wearing shoes and how high his heels were.

Later during the Swedish Giant's stay in London, a certain Thomas Boreman published his biography, *The History of Cajanus, the Swedish Giant, from his Birth to the present Time.* Boreman was an author and publisher of children's books who could often be seen displaying his works from a stand near Guildhall; he sold enough to stay in business for nearly a decade. His most famous work was a set of miniature children's books called the *Gigantick Histories*, each volume of which was the size of a matchbox. One of these volumes contained the life of Daniel Cajanus. According to Boreman, Daniel had once aspired to marry a young lady in his native village in Finland, but her parents did not want a giant for their son-in-law. After this rebuff, he decided to set out on his voyages. At the time Thomas Boreman knew him, Daniel's contract with the English showman had run out, but he stayed on in London to have a look at the town. Boreman helped to guide him among the sights of the metropolis; in particular, he recommended that the Swedish Giant should see the statues of the legendary giants Gog and Magog in Guildhall, near his own bookstall. Daniel Cajanus had read about them in a previous volume of the *Gigantick Histories*, and one day, he turned up at the Guildhall to see these huge statues, twice his own height. Then, according to Boreman,

> the people began to gather around the strange Giant from all parts of the Hall; but he, not caring to be stared at too much, strides gently up to the Bookseller's, next to the Giants, looked at his books, then turns himself round, and without saying one word, takes two or three colossus strides across the Hall, into the coach, and away he goes.

The previous volumes of the *Gigantick Histories* had been popular among British children and had even found subscribers in the American colonies. But at the time of his encounter with Cajanus, Thomas Boreman had run into hard times, and only 106 children subscribed to the Swedish Giant's biography. To build up a reserve stock, Boreman added "Giant Cajanus" to the list of subscribers and put him down for one hundred volumes, but in spite of this, the biography of Cajanus is a very rare book indeed, the vast majority being quickly read to rags and thrown away. In 1932, the American bibliophile Mr. Wilbur Macey Stone announced that what he believed to be the only complete set of the *Gigantick Histories* was in his ownership, and to date, no one has been able to disprove him, particularly since the Cajanus volume is so very scarce. The Guildhall Library had eight of the ten volumes, lacking the Cajanus and one of the two volumes dedicated to Westminster Abbey. Today, copies of the Cajanus volume are kept at the Houghton Library, Harvard University, and at the Library of the Society of Antiquaries in London.

In 1745, Daniel Cajanus settled permanently in Haarlem, where he bought himself a small house in the so-called Proveniershuis. This was a combined hotel, hospital, and old people's home, where invalids and old soldiers could purchase a small house or apartment, along with free meals and access to medical attention. The Haarlem Proveniershuis is still extant and looks not unlike it did in Cajanus's time. To be allowed to stay there for life, Daniel Cajanus paid the considerable sum of twenty-eight hundred guilders. He became a popular public character in his new hometown and made it his habit to walk through the streets every day, dressed in his blue Polish uniform, a periwig, and a large, gold-braided hat. After all the years of being on show, he apparently liked to walk in public, letting every person see him for free. The Dutch writer Jan Marchant, who saw Daniel Cajanus in Haarlem, wrote that the giant's head and shoulders were above the heads of the people thronging near him, and that he almost resembled an ordinary-sized man riding on horseback. He could easily light his pipe from one of the street lanterns. In 1747 and 1748, Daniel Cajanus again visited Amsterdam, where he stayed at the Blauw Jan. The main purpose of this was probably not to put himself on show again, but to demand repayment of some of his bad loans to various insolvent Amsterdam businessmen.

Jan Marchant, in his account of Daniel Cajanus in 1746, mentioned that the giant walked with difficulty. This corroborates the evidence from the Royal Society of London that all was not well with Cajanus's health. Indeed, in June 1746, he drew up a will at the notary's office in Haarlem. He was apparently well aware that his health was failing, and thought it prudent to arrange his affairs. He was particularly worried that his corpse might be indelicately treated after death, and insisted that he wanted to be buried in as secure a fashion as possible. Daniel Cajanus was a Lutheran, and in his will, he bequeathed one thousand guilders to each child of Jacob de Wijs, vicar of the Evangelical Church of Haarlem, and also a legacy to the Lutheran Poorhouse. Whatever remained of the giant's fortune was to be equally divided between his own brothers and sisters; his wretched father, who had once more been defrocked, had died in the 1730s. Three weeks after notarizing the will, however, the giant came stomping back to the notary's office and changed his will completely. He had apparently quarreled with his Lutheran brethren, and the poorhouse and the children of Jacob de Wijs were left nothing at all. Instead, Daniel Cajanus left his old friend Roelof Sweris, who had accompanied him to London in 1741, a legacy of one thousand guilders, on condition that he remained living in the Proveniershuis (to act as Cajanus's servant?) and that he repaid all his debts to Cajanus before the giant's demise. Various other friends were given smaller legacies, and Daniel Cajanus again insisted on having a particularly grand funeral in the Groot Sint Bavo Kerk, with a long parade and an ornate carriage to transport his coffin.

Not the least remarkable fact about Daniel Cajanus's later life in Haarlem is that he actually became a published poet. In 1747, he wrote a long valedictory poem to the prince of Orange, likening himself to the legendary Dutch giant Klaas van Kieten, who had fought for the counts of Holland, just as Cajanus himself was honoring one of their descendants in verse. Another poem, in the same style, was published a year later. Both Daniel

230 Cajanus's poems contain overblown tirades in the manner of the valedictory ode of the time, but their rhymes are impeccable, and it would take no little talent to compose such poems in a language not his own. Jan Marchant wrote that Cajanus, although a quiet, laconic man by nature, was much more clever than one might suppose, as proved by his literary endeavors.

In March 1748, Daniel Cajanus moved to house no. 25 inside the Proveniershuis square, next to his friend Roelof Sweris in no. 24. He also agreed to pay an extra three hundred guilders to the Proveniershuis for the privilege to have his food served at his own table. A few months later, the ailing giant rallied somewhat and relinquished this privilege; the three hundred guilders were repaid, and he again took his meals in the common dining room of the Proveniershuis. An inventory of Cajanus's effects made in 1749 shows that he was quite well off. His house was no larger than the others in the Proveniershuis square, and its fitted "cupboard-bed" was so small that the giant could not use it. Instead, he moved his huge bed into one of the rooms upstairs. His furniture was of excellent quality. He had a large, gilt-edged mirror, some giant-sized leather easy chairs, two tables, and an elegant cupboard. On his bookshelf were two rusty birdcages, a Bible with the Augsburg Confession, a catechism, three Lutheran religious tracts, and six other books. His wardrobe contained several costly garments, including his blue and red Polish uniform and a red silk coat from Tours.

On February 27, 1749, the forty-six-year-old Daniel Cajanus died in his house in the Haarlem Proveniershuis. He must have been ill for some time, as two physicians, two surgeons, and an apothecary sent in their bills. All the Dutch papers of importance, particularly the local *Opregte Haarlemsche Courant*, published his obituary. A short obituary notice also appeared in the *London Magazine*, in which it was claimed that he had been 7 feet 8 inches tall, and that his pulse rate, as measured by Dr. Bryan Robinson during the giant's late stay in London, had been fifty-two beats per minute. The funeral was particularly grand, just as Cajanus had wanted. It was compared with that of a statesman or a wealthy noble, except for the obvious fact that the coffin was nearly twice the size of a normal human being. Two horses with black horse cloths pulled a large ornate hearse, and on the black hearse cloth were, on one side, Daniel Cajanus's huge, silver-hilted sword, and on the other, his enormous gloves. The funeral ceremony was one of the most magnificent ever witnessed in Haarlem. The hearse and coffin, with its sixty-five pairs of pallbearers, were seen by several thousand spectators. An eloquent

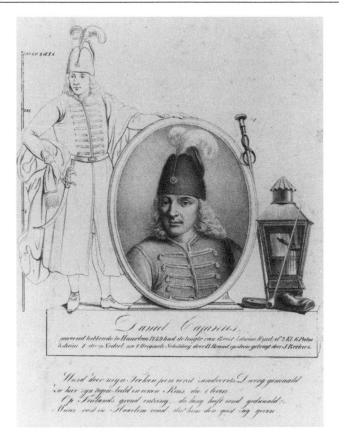

A Dutch engraving made in 1749 to commemorate Cajanus. Reproduced by permission of the Gemeentearchief of Haarlem.

poem celebrating the life and death of the goliath of Haarlem was handed out according to the custom of the time; its final part can be translated as:

> *There he lies now, Mortus, dead;*
> *His future poems will remain unread.*
> *There lies the second Klaas van Kieten,*
> *Whose memory remains unbeaten.*
> *Great CAJANUS, now that you have left us, we must have something to*
> *remember you from,*
> *We will make a statue of you in metal or marble to put in the city hall,*
> *and your huge picture will be there for generations to come*
> *to say: That was him, whose mind was as artless as his body was tall.*

The Swede C. G. Gjörwell wrote that Daniel Cajanus had died very rich, and that he left legacies of twenty thousand Dutch guilders to a Lutheran orphanage and other charities. This statement was believed well into the twentieth century, but turned out to be complete fantasy. In the 1970s, the Dutch antiquary Dr. B. C. Sliggers managed to trace Cajanus's will and the inventory made after his death. Daniel Cajanus had many valuable belongings and quite a treasure of English gold guineas; his estate was valued at eight thousand guilders. But he also had quite a few debts, and after the cost for his lavish funeral was deducted, his estate had only a little money left: just two thousand guilders were finally distributed between his brothers and sisters. A certain Pieter Langendijk wrote that although Daniel Cajanus had earned considerable sums on his tours, he was a bad businessman and unable to invest his money shrewdly. He was simply too kind, and incapable of seeing through the lying scoundrels who applied for loans that they had no intention of repaying. Langendijk suspected that Cajanus had actually feared poverty in his old age when he bought himself into the Proveniershuis.

Daniel Cajanus had paid fifty-three guilders for the privilege to have his grave in a vault inside the Sint Bavo church itself; this was twice the cost for an ordinary tomb. As indicated by his will, the main reason for this was that he wanted his body to rest undisturbed. He was probably well aware of the risk that his corpse might be stolen by grave robbers and later preserved by some unscrupulous collector in a museum of natural curiosities. Any grave robber would have found it difficult to break into the giant's grave inside the church, however, particularly because Cajanus ordered that his gravestone have neither ornaments nor inscription to indicate where he was buried. But in spite of all the Swedish Giant's precautions, his grave did not remain undisturbed for long. In the late eighteenth century, it is recorded that Cajanus's vault "came into the possession of the Hodshon family." The exact circumstances of this transaction were not explained further. A charitable interpretation is that the giant had been careless, as usual, in his business transactions, and that he had secured the vault only for a certain number of years, not for life. A more sinister version is that the authorities knew that Cajanus had no descendants in Haarlem that could plead his cause, and that they resold the giant's vault and had his skeleton taken to the Museum of Natural History in Leiden. This latter version is supported by the fact that in the early nineteenth century, parts of Cajanus's skeleton turned up at various Leiden museums. Today, the Swedish Giant's pelvis, thighbones, legs, and feet are on exhibition in the Leiden Museum of Anatomy. It is intriguing that

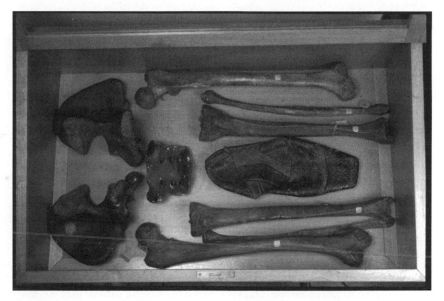

The skeletal remains of Daniel Cajanus at the Anatomical Institute of Leyden.
Photography by J. Lens, copyright Leiden Museum of Anatomy.

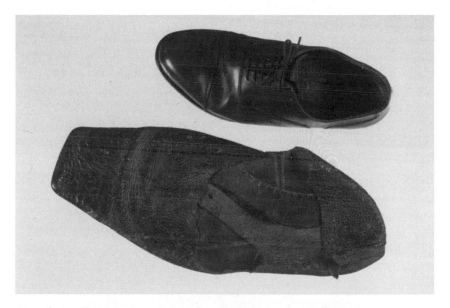

One of Daniel Cajanus's enormous shoes, together with one of ordinary
dimensions. Photography by J. Lens, copyright Leiden Museum of Anatomy.

234   most of the bones are actually high-quality nineteenth-century casts of the originals, whose whereabouts are unknown. This museum also owns two of Cajanus's huge shoes. Three more shoes and Daniel Cajanus's linen shirt are at the Teylers Museum in Haarlem.

There is no question whatsoever about the cause for Daniel Cajanus's tremendous growth: he must have suffered from pituitary gigantism. In this disease, a pituitary adenoma produces an excess of growth hormone; if this adenoma is present from an early age, the individual will grow to an enormous height. Such a pituitary tumor is benign and does not metastasize, but it can grow to compress the chiasma of the optic nerves; this was fortunately not the case in Daniel Cajanus, as there is no record that he had any visual symptoms. Some pituitary adenomas cause hypopituitarism by compression of the remaining functional pituitary tissue or by secondary hypothalamic involvement; whether this was the case in Cajanus is difficult to say. Although Boreman's story of the young Daniel Cajanus wooing a village maiden may have been true, the giant showed little interest in the opposite sex during his adult years, something that might well have been due to hypogonadism secondary to hypopituitarism during adolescence. The fact that Daniel Cajanus had what is known as eunuchoid bodily proportions, with prodigiously long arms, supports this notion. It is of some interest that several of Daniel Cajanus's relatives may also have suffered from pituitary abnormalities. The Swedish writer C. G. Gjörwell courteously stated that Daniel's surviving sister Agneta, who came to Haarlem to collect what remained of his estate, "could by no means be considered as a short-statured woman." In Tor Carpelan's dictionary of Finnish biography, this same lady is described as "extremely tall." Israel Cajanus, the grandson of Daniel's first cousin Gustaf, who was sheriff of Pyhäjoki, was well known in Finland for his enormous hands and feet. There is sometimes a hereditary tendency to develop pituitary adenomas of this kind, and although the clinical data are insufficient, it is tempting to suggest that Agneta Cajanus also had pituitary gigantism, and that Israel Cajanus had acromegaly. The latter condition results from a growth hormone–producing pituitary adenoma developing in adult life, when the epiphyseal junctions are closed. Thus, the individual's height no longer increases, but the overproduction of growth hormone leads to soft tissue growth, resulting in enormous hands and feet and a coarsening of the facial features.

Another puzzle concerning Daniel Cajanus is that of his exact height. In the Sint Bavo church in Haarlem is a pillar indicating the contrasting heights of the two foremost local human curiosities, Daniel Cajanus and the Friesland dwarf Simon Jane Paap. The Swedish Giant is stated there to have been 8 feet 4 inches tall, and from such clerical authority, this figure has been widely quoted in both historical and medical works, thereby granting Cajanus a place among the tallest men that ever lived. Even the German Professor R. Martin, author of the influential *Lehrbuch der Anthropologie*, accepted the myth that Cajanus was 9 feet 3 inches (283 centimeters) tall and the tallest man that ever lived. But as we know, Daniel Cajanus was only 7 feet 4 inches in height when he was measured by the Royal Society dignitaries in 1742. Since Cajanus, just like the other eighteenth-century giants on show, was very adept at exaggerating his height, this is the only figure that deserves credence. A huge painting of Cajanus used to hang in Brewer's Chapel in the Sint Bavo church, but has been removed to another museum. Thus the pillar with the inscription about Cajanus's height is the only memorial of him, not counting the stone slab from under which his remains were taken away. This column "like a tall bully, lifts its head and lies," however, and in a way Cajanus has had the last laugh after all.

What has confused some commentators is that Daniel Cajanus actually shrank during the last ten years of his life. A study of his skeleton revealed the cause for this. In pituitary gigantism, all tissues of the body are affected by the overproduction of growth hormone; this includes the joint cartilage, which becomes diffusely thickened. This abnormal, thickened cartilage is prone to early degradation, however, leading to a disease similar to osteoarthritis. Study of Daniel Cajanus's skeleton clearly showed the outer condyles of both thighbones to be severely destroyed. This deformation of the joint would lead to the development of extreme bandy-leggedness, and thus a loss in height, which would explain why the Reverend Dr. Pearse at the Royal Society was puzzled that Cajanus had become a good deal shorter since he last saw the giant in 1734. It may well be that Cajanus had actually been 7 feet 7 or 8 inches tall in 1734, taking into account the deformity of his knees and the degeneration of the intervertebral substance with age; this figure would tally with the most credible accounts of him. That a person with advanced knee joint disease of this kind would be unwilling to stand up for very long is quite understandable; indeed, considering the state of the knee joints, it is remarkable that Cajanus was at all capable of locomotion during his declining years. A certain Dr. Carl Langer of Vienna University, who was active in the 1870s, used anthropometric techniques to estimate from the length of Cajanus's thighbone that he was actually just over 7 feet 3 inches tall, but the deformity of the thighbone makes this estimate less reliable.

As giants come, Daniel Cajanus was by no means one of the extremes. The tallest man in the world, Robert Pershing Wadlow, was more than 8 feet 11 inches tall. He suffered from pituitary gigantism just like Daniel Cajanus, but represented the most extreme case of this disorder on record in the medical literature. Wadlow died in 1940, at just twenty-two years old, from an infection in one of his enormous feet. Even among eighteenth-century giants on exhibition, Cajanus was by no means an extreme, and his great success was probably as much due to clever marketing—he always claimed to be taller than some other giant recently exhibited and freely exaggerated his height. Furthermore, all records agree that he was a sociable, amusing character, with an impressive flair for languages. The German giant Maximilian Miller was nearly 8 feet tall when he was on show in London in 1733, and the "English Giant" Henry Blacker was 7 feet 4 inches in height. The famous "Irish Giant" Charles Byrne, who was active in the 1780s, claimed to be 8 feet 4 inches tall, just like Daniel Cajanus, but his skeleton, still kept at the Hunterian Museum in London, shows that in reality he was 7 feet 10 inches.

It is only in fairy tales that giants are stupid; overproduction of growth hormone does not cause any slowing of the intellect, in spite of its deleterious effect on many other organ systems. It is true that the aforementioned Irish Giant seems almost to have been an imbecile, but his habit, formed since his early teens, of drinking at least one large bottle of gin or whisky every day cannot have benefited the development of his intellect. In contrast to this sottish fellow, Daniel Cajanus was a prudent, intelligent man. Although it would have been "politically correct" to pay lip service to him as a poor freak condemned to earn his living by exhibiting himself, it would be more realistic to point out that he really made the best of his extreme condition. Rather than have to fight against poverty in the cold, unpleasant Finnish countryside, Daniel Cajanus saw large parts of Europe, met interesting people, was introduced to the king of France and the president of the Royal Society, and accumulated enough wealth to spend his declining years in relative comfort.

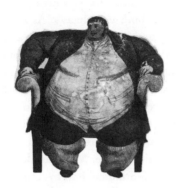

Daniel Lambert,
the Human Colossus

TO BECOME RENOWNED AS THE MOST CORPULENT man of whom authentic records exist is not the kind of celebrity any one would wish for, but this was the fate of the enormous Daniel Lambert, who lived between 1770 and 1809. Six men of normal build could be buttoned into Lambert's waistcoat, and his stockings were the size of linen sacks. Daniel Lambert's contemporaries were fascinated with this prodigy of nature, and in nineteenth-century Britain, his name became synonymous with extreme bulk and heaviness. Although he is no longer considered the heaviest man in the world, Daniel Lambert is still remembered, particularly in the Midlands of England, where several inns and public houses are named after him.

❧

Daniel Lambert was born on March 13, 1770, at Blue Boar Lane in Leicester, as the eldest son of the keeper of the Bridewell prison in that town. He had two healthy sisters and a brother who died young. Neither his parents nor his siblings were overweight, according to local sources, which noted, however, that his paternal aunt and uncle were both very heavy. As a boy and a young man, Daniel Lambert was strong and healthy. He was heavily built, with a good appetite, but by no means corpulent. At the age of fourteen, he was apprenticed to Mr. Benjamin Patricks's die-casting and engraving business in Birmingham. This business was a flourishing one in the early 1780s, but the buttons and buckles manufactured there rapidly went out of fashion, and hardly any person wanted to buy them. According to another version, Daniel stayed in Birmingham until Mr. Patricks's firm was completely demolished during the riots in 1791. In either case, Mr. Patricks despaired of ever being able to resurrect the firm, and Daniel had to return to Leicester, where he became assistant keeper of the prison, serving under his own father. As he reached the age of twenty, he began to suspect that he would one day become very heavy and took pains to exercise regularly and to keep up his muscular power, which was extraordinary. He could lift a heavy cartwheel and carry five hundredweight (560 pounds) with ease.

Like his father and uncle, Daniel Lambert was greatly addicted to country pursuits and particularly fond of otter hunting, horse racing, shooting, and fishing. For quite a few years, he regularly taught the Leicester children to swim in the river Soar. Already in his teens, Daniel Lambert took a keen interest in the breeding of sporting dogs, mainly spaniels, setters, terriers, and pointers. One day, Daniel was standing outside his father's house on Blue Boar Lane, watching a party of itinerant Savoyards who were performing in the street with their dancing bears. Suddenly, one of Daniel Lambert's dogs flew at a large bear and bit it viciously in the rear quarters. The bear was muzzled, but when the dog attacked again, the bear dexterously knocked it on the head and crushed it to the ground. The Savoyards were annoyed at this untoward interruption of their performance and prepared to take the muzzle off the bear, in order for it to finish off the poor dog. Daniel Lambert came up and prevailed on them to allow him to remove his dog, but a Savoyard ignored him and instead loosened the muzzle. Daniel snatched a pole from this man and called out that he would kill the bear if it lay in his power. The moment the bear's muzzle was removed, Daniel struck it a tremendous blow. The bear was stunned for a moment, and the dog managed to escape. The bear attacked Daniel instead, and he had to fight for his life. The weather was frosty, and he fell heavily just in front of the infuriated animal, but rose again just in time to strike the bear a resounding blow with his left hand. The bear was nearly knocked out cold and declined further contest. The performers complained to the authorities that Daniel Lambert had interrupted their performance and beaten one of their animals severely, but the local magistrate was no friend of these foreign jugglers and merely ridiculed them.

In the early 1790s, Daniel Lambert's father retired as keeper of the prison, and Daniel succeeded him. For many years, this huge, rotund figure became a familiar sight to the Leicester people, as he sat outside the prison gates smoking his pipe. The sedentary life at the prison did not agree with him at all, and as the years went by, Daniel's weight steadily increased. In 1793, he weighed 448 pounds but was still strong and active. He once walked from Woolwich to London without showing signs of fatigue, and during the swimming lessons in the river Soar, his powers of floating enabled him to swim with two men of ordinary size sitting on his back. It was a source of grief to him when, in 1801, he had to give up hunting, since both he and the poor horse he rode were too out of breath to keep up with the rest of the hunt.

All sources agree that Daniel Lambert was a competent keeper of the prison. His attitude toward the prisoners was more humane than was expected at the time. Far from establishing a regime of terror at the Bridewell prison, he often gained friends among the prisoners and made every exertion to help them when they went up for trial. It was said that few criminals left the prison without expressing their gratitude to him and that many shed tears when the time came for them to leave their cells! In the early 1800s, Daniel's weight had increased to about 560 pounds and there was apparently some concern whether he was still capable of being in charge of the prison. He was certainly fortunate that the contented prisoners in his charge did not try to escape; any attempt to pursue them would have been futile due to his extreme bulk. A certain James Neale, who visited the Bridewell prison in 1803, ironically wrote, "Had this fat man studied a thousand years, he would not have thought on a *profession* better calculated to suit his constitutional propensity to ease." Although Daniel Lambert had a very good reputation locally, Neale thought him a very improper person to be the keeper of a prison.

❧

At Easter 1805, the Bridewell prison was closed, since the magistrates had decided to move the prisoners to a new institution for forced labor. Daniel Lambert liked his work at the prison and would probably have preferred to stay on, but the magistrates were firm in their decision. They granted him an annuity of fifty pounds for life, as a declaration of the universal satisfaction

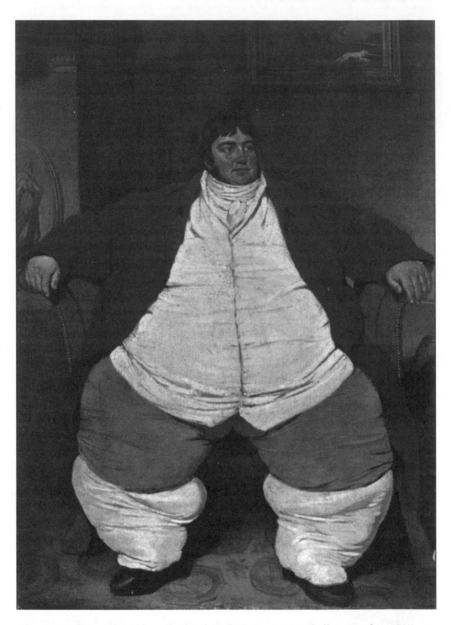

A portrait of Daniel Lambert, by his friend Benjamin Marshall, painted in 1806 during his first season in London. Reproduced by permission of the Newarkes House Museum, Leicester.

he had given in the discharge of his duties. After he left the prison, Daniel became little more than a recluse in his own house. He could not visit horse races or cocking matches any more, due to the interest in his person from the impudent populace. The reputation of this prodigiously fat man had spread throughout England, and many travelers wanted to see him as a curiosity. Lambert was quite sensitive about his grotesque appearance, and he detested such visits. Once, a gentleman from Nottingham who knew Lambert's interest in horses was admitted into his house under the pretense of asking his advise about the pedigree of a certain mare. Daniel Lambert, who was shrewd enough to perceive from his manner the real nature of his errand, brusquely told him that the mare in question "was by *Impertinence* out of *Curiosity*." Another stranger tried to entice the great man from his house by pretending to ask him about some fighting cocks. Daniel Lambert's servant knew that his master never saw strangers, but the man persisted. Lambert overheard their conversation, opened a window, and instructed his servant to "tell the gentleman that I am a *shy-cock*."

Daniel Lambert was not only very averse to putting himself on show; he also steadfastly refused to weigh himself, although jocose and unfeeling friends offered to let him have the use of one of their weighing machines for cattle. Finally, these same friends took him to a cocking match in Loughborough. Poor Daniel had to climb into the carriage sideways, but finally managed to squeeze through the door. While they were on the way to the match, the others left the carriage under some pretense or other, and the carriage was driven over a large weighing machine. After they subtracted the weight of the carriage, which had previously been ascertained, they could tell Daniel Lambert, to his great mortification, that his weight was now nearly 700 pounds (50 stone). His extreme corpulence prevented him from doing any work, and in spite of the annuity from the Leicester magistrates, he was soon facing dire financial straits. With the greatest reluctance, he decided to travel to London and exhibit himself for money there. Several friends had previously suggested this ignominious way of earning his living, but he had always refused. In March 1806, he chose to profit from his extreme obesity, which previously had caused him only misery.

On April 4, 1806, Daniel Lambert left Leicester in a purposely constructed carriage and took up residence in the heart of London, at no. 53 Piccadilly. He was widely advertised in the newspapers and on handbills, and when he began to see visitors on April 7, numerous spectators paid a shilling to see this human colossus, the heaviest man in Britain. This unenviable title had previously belonged to the grocer Edward Bright, known as "the Fat

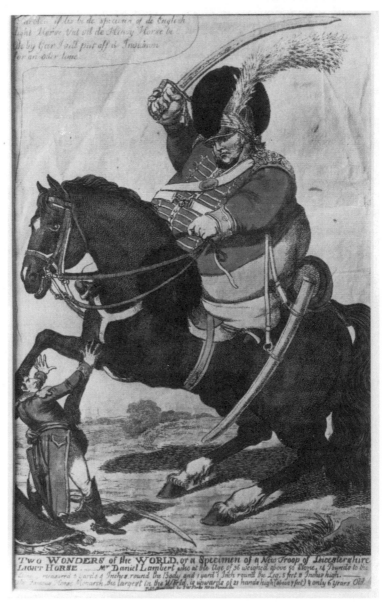

Daniel Lambert attacks Napoleon Bonaparte, in the caricature "The two Wonders of the World." Reproduced by permission of the Newarkes House Museum, Leicester.

Man of Essex," who was well known for his appetite and who drank a gallon of beer a day. He weighed 616 pounds at the time of his death in 1750. Among the runners-up were the 340-pound bookseller John Love and the enormous Dr. Stafford, on whose gravestone the following words were inscribed:

> *Take heed, O good traveller! and do not tread hard,*
> *For here lies Doctor Stafford, in all this churchyard.*

A reporter from the *Times* newspaper wrote:

> The concourse of fashionable visitors to the house of Mr Lambert . . . has been very great, during the last two days. To find a man of his uncommon dimensions (weighing no less than fifty stone, or 700 lbs) possessing great information, manners the most affable and pleasing, and a perfect ease and facility in conversation, exceeded our expectations, high as they had been raised. The female spectators were greater in proportion than those of the other sex, and not a few of them have been heard to declare, how much they admired his manly and intelligent countenance.

A journalist from the *Morning Post* who visited Daniel Lambert on April 13 was similarly impressed with his intelligence and affable manner, and the politeness with which he answered the numerous questions from the audience. Not less than four hundred people came to see this "prodigy of human dimensions," from twelve until five o'clock.

There was immediate interest also from the medical profession, and the *Medical and Physical Journal* published an article giving "the correct particulars" of this human phenomenon. Daniel Lambert was 5 feet 11 inches high and weighed upward of 700 pounds. In spite of his extraordinary bulk, he enjoyed perfect health: his breathing was free, his sleep undisturbed, and all functions of his body in excellent order. Daniel Lambert ate ordinary food, he told the doctor, and drank only water and no alcoholic beverages. On examination, the doctor found that there was immense accumulation of fat within the abdomen, and enormous tumefaction of the thighs, legs, and feet. Daniel Lambert never felt pain or discomfort from the stretching of the skin, but he had had four or five attacks of erysipelatous inflammation of the legs, which had caused a permanent scaliness and thickening of the skin. This account agreed with the local sources that Daniel's weight had gradually increased from the age of twenty, but disagreed in stating that both his father and his uncle had been heavy men, although the weight of either had not exceeded 420 pounds. Many people were amazed that Daniel Lambert's habits of life were very far removed from those usually associated with great corpulence: he ate only one course at meals (he claimed), drank no ale, and slept no more than eight hours per night, always with the window open. He was never heard to snore. He was mentally alert and active, read widely, and sang in a strong tenor voice.

Once he had conquered his habitual shyness and aversion to putting himself on show, Daniel Lambert had a gregarious, extroverted personality and the manners of a gentleman. At least at the beginning, this gave his apartments the air of a fashionable resort rather than a sordid freak show. Early nineteenth-century people did not share the present-day obsession with leanness, and Daniel was considered as a "prodigy" or a wonder of nature, rather than a repulsive monstrosity. Among the Londoners, it became highly fashionable to visit him, and even more fashionable to be his friend. His interests coincided with those of the upper and middle classes of society, and he could spend hours discussing horses and hounds with them. He had brought seven setters and two pointers with him to London, and sold these animals to Mr. Mellish and Lord Kinnaird for not less than 218 guineas in all, a sum showing the high regard for his breeding among fanciers of sporting dogs. Daniel Lambert insisted on being treated with civility, and every man who entered his rooms, even Quakers, had to remove their hats. Once, a French impresario tried to persuade Lambert to accompany him back to tour France, but although the man assured him that Napoleon Bonaparte would make his fortune when they entered Paris, "Lambert, who had too much good sense to be the dupe of a designing Monsieur, declined in the most emphatic style of a true son of John Bull," as expressed in an anti-French newspaper. Daniel Lambert's greatest triumph during his season in London was when he was presented to King George III; unfortunately, the king's reaction was not recorded.

One day Daniel Lambert was visited by a party of eight ladies and six gentlemen from the channel island of Guernsey, who had traveled to London to see this prodigy, after he had been eloquently described to them by a neighbor. Lambert suggested that they remain in London for a few days and see the remaining sights of the town, but they declared that since they had achieved the sole purpose of their journey, they had no desire to visit any other attractions. After Daniel Lambert had stayed in London a few months, he was visited by the famous midget "Count" Joseph Boruwlaski, poor Bébé's former adversary, who had later made a fortune touring Europe. He was by now seventy-four years old and lived in comfortable retirement in Durham. Boruwlaski was renowned for his excellent memory, and he could actually recollect that Daniel Lambert had come to see *him* several times in Birmingham, at the time Daniel was working as an apprentice at the die-sinker's business. As poor Daniel's weight had increased at least threefold since that time, the witty Boruwlaski exclaimed, "Ah mine Got, I have seen dis face twenty years before at Birmingham, but certainly it be anoder body!" Daniel Lambert inquired whether the count's wife was still living, but the count replied that she was not, and that he was not very sorry because this lady, who was of normal stature, used to put him on the mantel-piece, from whence he did not dare to jump down, during their domestic arguments. One of Lambert's sleeves would have provided enough cloth for Boruwlaski's coat. The elderly count then felt one of Lambert's legs, exclaiming, "Ah mine Got! pure flesh and blood—I feel de warm. No deception! I am pleased, for I did hear it was deception." Those present when these two personages met were envied by all London's innumerable lovers of curiosities: as eloquently expressed in a newspaper, ". . . it was *Sir John Falstaff* and *Tom Thumb*, which must have afforded a *double* treat to the curious."

A somewhat less appealing and probably more trustworthy, description of Daniel Lambert on show is provided by the *Memoirs of Charles Mathews* written by his wife Anne. Charles Mathews was a popular actor who visited Daniel Lambert many times and found him a pleasant and intelligent man. Mrs. Mathews wrote that Lambert, who was evidently becoming somewhat bored with being on show, received his visitors in a "half-courteous, half-sullen manner." It was distressing to Charles Mathews and his wife to hear the coarse observations made by some of the visitors, and they pitied Lambert's plight before a host of unfeeling individuals who asked rude questions about his appetite. Another pet subject for these hecklers was the size and cost of Daniel Lambert's coat. One woman was particularly solicitous to find out the cost of this garment, but Lambert replied sullenly that if she made him a present of a new coat, she would then find out exactly what it cost. An obnoxious fellow was equally persistent in his attempts to have the same question elucidated, and rudely remarked that since he had contributed a shilling toward the cost of Lambert's next coat, he had the right to demand any information about it. "Sir," rejoined Lambert, "if I knew what part of my coat your shilling would pay for, I can assure you I would cut out the piece."

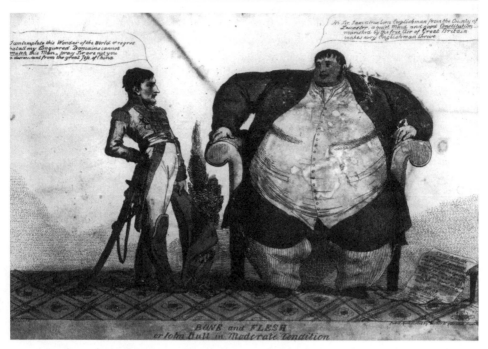

"Bone and Flesh," a caricature published in 1806. Reproduced by permission of the Newarkes House Museum, Leicester.

Daniel Lambert's wit made him a formidable foe to these hecklers, and when a young snob, who had walked around the great man for some time scrutinizing his appearance through his quizzing glass, finally asked Lambert whether it was true that he liked dogs, he received the deserved retort, "Yes, Sir, all kinds of dogs, except *puppies*!"

The production of caricature prints was particularly prolific in the late eighteenth and early nineteenth centuries. In Daniel Lambert's time, the most popular topics for caricatures were the war with France, the controversial politician Charles James Fox and his proposals for peace, and the unpopular measures of taxation on tobacco and other commodities. The early nineteenth-century buyers of prints were easily amused, and in the caricatures, John Bull was depicted beating Napoleon with a cudgel, refusing the crafty Fox's offers of peace, and objecting against the novel taxes, often using violence against the persons of the ministers involved. The traditional figure of John Bull was that of a stout, well-nourished countryman, and it took little inspiration for the draftsman to put Daniel Lambert in his place.

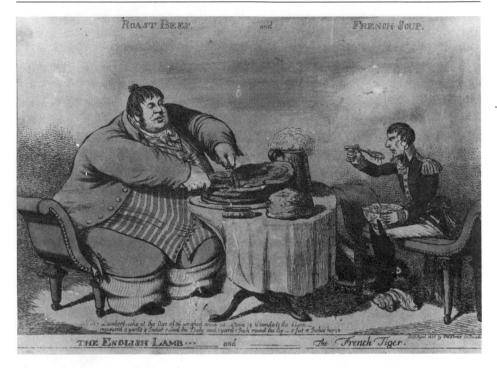

Daniel Lambert and Napoleon take luncheon, in the caricature "The English Lamb and the French Tiger." Reproduced by permission of the Newarkes House Museum, Leicester.

Charles James Fox was also quite fat, and in one caricature, "The two greatest Men in England," he is depicted as being the same size as Lambert, with a projecting paunch. Another caricature was entitled "Fox feeding Daniel Lambert with Peace from a Barrel."

In "Bone and Flesh, or John Bull in Moderate Condition," Daniel Lambert received Napoleon Bonaparte as one of his visitors. Astonished by the sight of Lambert, the emperor says, "I contemplate this Wonder of the World, and regret that my conquered Domains cannot match this Man, pray Sir, are you not a descendant of the great Joss of China?" Daniel Lambert replies, "No Sir, I am a true born Englishman from the County of Leicester, a quiet Mind and good Constitution nourished by the free Air of Great Britain makes evry [sic] Englishman thrive."

In "The English Lamb and the French Tiger," Daniel Lambert and Napoleon I are sitting at a dining table. Lambert completely fills his chair,

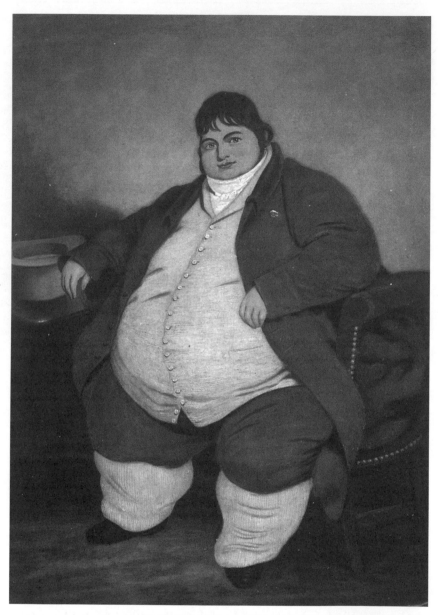

Another portrait of Daniel Lambert, owned by the Stamford Town Council.
Reproduced by permission.

but the emperor sits in the middle of his too-high seat. Daniel Lambert placidly carves a round of beef, with a tankard of brown stout in front of him. Napoleon eats only a bowl of soup, regarding Lambert's roast beef with a sinister stare, just like a present-day Frenchman in a London restaurant, fearful of mad cow disease. In the caricature "Two Wonders of the World, or a Specimen of a New Troop of Leicestershire Light Horse,' Lambert is dressed in a militia uniform and seated on the horse Monarch, the largest in the world and about 7 feet high. He attacks the tiny Napoleon, who drops his hat and sword and holds up his hands in terror, exclaiming, "Parbleu! If dis be de specimen of de English Light Horse vat vil de Heavy Horse be? Oh, by Gar, I vill put off de Invasion for an oder time!"

❧

Daniel Lambert's great success in London exaggerated his most sanguine expectations, and he returned to Leicester a wealthy man. Like Daniel Cajanus sixty-two years earlier, he had been wise enough to remain his own master and never became the dupe of some cunning showman who wanted to "manage" him and exploit his fame. In Leicester, he resumed his earlier occupations: visits to race meetings and cockpits, and the breeding of sporting dogs and fighting cocks. The *Leicester Journal* of September 19, 1806, reported that at the Leicester Races, "among the distinguished characters upon the turf we were glad to see our old friend, Mr Daniel Lambert, in apparent high health and spirits." After his lucrative season in London, he was now able to build up a fine pack of coursing greyhounds; although he was unable to follow them on horseback, he enjoyed watching them from his carriage as they pursued a hare through the open landscape. In December 1806, Lambert went on tour to Birmingham, Hickley, and Coventry, among other cities; a newspaper marveled that in spite of all his attention to regimen, his bulk still increased steadily. In early 1807, he returned to London and took rooms in Leicester Square. Unfortunately, he fell ill after a few months in the metropolis, and his physician Dr. Heaviside suspected that the London air did not agree with his constitution. Daniel Lambert was advised to return to Leicester, but later the same year, he recovered enough to make a series of tours in the provinces. In the summer of 1808, he again came to London for a shorter period and sold a brace of spaniel puppies at Tattersall's for seventy-five guineas. Daniel Lambert received an offer of one hundred guineas for a small terrier bitch, said to be the finest in England, but he refused to sell his favorite pet. This little terrier always slept by his bed and remained his loyal companion until the day of his death.

Throughout the years when he exhibited himself in London, Daniel Lambert was one of the sights of the town, and not a few foreign tourists visited this prodigy. One of those who saw "the Human Colossus" was the Swedish artillery captain Johan Didrik af Wingård, who had been sent to London in 1808 to purchase a large quantity of English rifles for the Swedish militia. According to his memoirs, one of af Wingård's ambitions was to explore "the filthy side of English street life"; his acquaintance with a man named Mathews, who may have been some kind of pimp, ensured that the Swede soon made giant strides toward achieving this purpose. Captain af Wingård's more edifying pursuits included visits to music halls, museums, and exhibitions of natural curiosities. He saw a panorama of a recent battle between the British and French fleets, and went to Guy's Hospital to visit an American albiness. She demonstrated an automaton that could reply to questions and tell fortunes using a large glass ball, but the Swede exposed a conjurer skulking behind a screen, maneuvering this "automaton." Johan Didrik af Wingård was much more impressed by Daniel Lambert, the sight of whom he eloquently described in his memoirs:

> This enormously fat man sat in a sofa wide enough for three or four people, and filled it well. He had a really quite handsome, small head, at least compared with his ungainly body. Had he been able to stand up, a feat that really must have been impossible for him to perform, he would have been quite a tall man. His wide cheekbones and huge double chin did not disfigure him very much, but his belly, dressed in a striped waistcoat, resembled a huge featherbed, and his legs, dressed in similarly colored stockings, were the size of two large butter kernels. This unfortunate man, who was not destined to live long, had permitted his relatives to make a show of him for profit, since no company could be prevailed upon to insure his life. Maybe Count Carl de Geer still keeps a portrait of this hideous mass of flesh, since this noble gentleman certainly purchased one when we saw Lambert together.

In October 1808, the *Times* newspaper reported that Daniel Lambert was showing himself in York, probably during the course of another tour of the provinces. In June 1809, he traveled to Cambridge and then to Huntingdon and Stamford. He often mixed business with pleasure during his tours, and his visit to Stamford coincided with the Stamford Races. One account actually stated that Stamford was the last town where he intended to show himself for money, probably since he was now financially independent. On June 20, he occupied an apartment on the ground floor of the Waggon and Horses inn (he could no longer walk up stairs). He was tired after his journey but still in good spirits. In the evening, he sent a message to the *Stamford Mercury* newspaper to order some handbills and advertisements. With the words "as the Mountain could not wait upon Mahomet, Mahomet would go to the Mountain," he requested the printer to call on him to receive the particulars about these handbills. In the evening, the printer came to see him. Daniel Lambert was still in bed and admitted to feeling fatigued, but he was as business-minded as ever and anxious that his handbills be delivered in time. The following morning, he rose as usual and seemed to be in good health. Just as he was about to start shaving, he suddenly complained of a great difficulty in breathing, and ten minutes later died. As quoted from his obituary in the *Stamford Mercury*:

> Nature had endured all the trespass she could admit; the poor man's corpulence had constantly increased until, at the time we had mentioned, the clogged machinery stood still, and this prodigy of mankind was numbered with the dead!

Just a few days before the death of Daniel Lambert, he had been weighed with Mr. King's famous Caledonian Balance in Ipswich, where he turned the scales at 739 pounds (52 stone, 11 pounds). Since the putrefaction of this huge corpse was extreme, a coffin of suitable size was constructed with the greatest expedition, and an immense grave dug at the back of St. Martin's Church in Stamford. The coffin consisted of 112 superficial feet of elm and was built on two axle trees and four clog wheels, thus enabling the mourners to wheel Daniel Lambert to his final place of rest. It was 6 feet 4 inches long and 4 feet 4 inches wide, and in shape almost resembled a square box. On the day after Daniel Lambert's death, the corpse was put into this huge coffin with the greatest difficulty, and the window and wall of the room were pulled down to allow his exit. On the morning of June 23, the coffin was wheeled toward the churchyard. A regular sloping descent had been constructed from the grave, but it still took twenty men nearly half an hour to maneuver the coffin into the grave. Although this rather tragic-comical ceremony could by no means be compared with the grandiose funeral of

Daniel Cajanus sixty years earlier, a huge crowd of people of all ages, many of whom had seen Daniel Lambert while he was alive, gathered to pay the great man their last respects. His friends in Leicester paid for a handsome gravestone, with the inscription:

> *In Remembrance of*
> *that PRODIGY in NATURE*
> *DANIEL LAMBERT*
> *a Native of LEICESTER*
> *who was possessed of*
> *an exalted and convivial Mind*
> *and, in personal Greatness*
> *had no COMPETITOR:*
> *He measured three Feet one Inch round the LEG*
> *nine FEET four INCHES round the BODY*
> *and weighed*
> *FIFTY TWO STONE ELEVEN POUNDS*
> *He departed this life*
> *on the 21st of June*
> *1809*
> *AGED 39 YEARS*
> *As a Testimony of Respect*
> *this Stone is erected*
> *by his Friends*
> *in Leicester.*

❧

Shortly after Daniel Lambert's death, Mr. J. Drakard of Stamford published his biography: *The Life of that Wonderful and Extraordinary Heavy Man, the late Daniel Lambert*. This was by no means the first account of Lambert's life that appeared before the reading public. In 1808, a short biography of him had been incorporated into *Granger's Wonderful Museum and Magazine Extraordinary*. This amazing collection is one of several early-nineteenth-century anthologies of curious biographies: large, well-illustrated, multivolume compilations of "wonderful Occurrences, singular Events, heroic Adventures, absurd Characters, remarkable for eating, drinking, fasting, walking &c., memorable Exploits, amazing Deliverances from Death and various other Dangers, strange Accidents, extraordinary Memoirs &c." Daniel Lambert shares the three thousand pages of this wonderful publication with characters like "Peter the Wild Boy," "the Hairy Girl," "Foolish Sam,"

"Frederich III King of Prussia," and "the Kangaroo"; he is the only one of them to be honored by having his portrait as the frontispiece of one of the volumes. *Granger's Wonderful Museum* and other works of a similar nature easily found readers; none of these dictionaries of curious biography, with names like Smeeton's *Biographia Curiosa*, Kirby's *Wonderful Museum*, and the *Eccentric Magazine*, could do without an illustrated account of the life and death of Daniel Lambert.

Not long after his death, Daniel Lambert became something of a cult figure, particularly in the Midlands. Everything connected with him was preserved as a curiosity, and there were quite a few stories, real and invented, about his exploits. The tale of his encounter with the bear is one of them, and it is curious to note that an earlier version, dating from the time Lambert was still alive, actually stated that the bear was the victor and that poor Daniel was completely shattered by his narrow escape from the furious beast. Daniel Lambert's friends arranged several auctions to sell his clothes and other effects, including his specially made carriage; many of these items went into the hands of collectors and lovers of curiosities and have been preserved to this day. The Victorians actually started a secondary production of Daniel Lambert memorabilia: his figure in china or as a glazed inkwell, a metal inkstand showing him in the act of carving up a goose, and a ceramic teapot that is opened by taking Lambert's head and shoulders off.

In 1806, a huge statue, or perhaps rather bust, of Daniel Lambert was made in wax. It later found its way to the United States and was exhibited at Mix's Museum in New Haven, Connecticut, in 1813. In 1828, this statue, or a similar one, was at the Vauxhall Gardens in Boston, whose proprietor was proud to announce that he had acquired, through contacts in Leicester, a complete set of Lambert's clothes to dress it in. This huge wax statue later came into the ownership of none less than P. T. Barnum and was exhibited at his American Museum in New York. When the American Museum was ravaged by fire in 1865, some workmen made a valiant attempt to save the Lambert statue. Staggering under its weight, they tried to carry it downstairs, but it started to melt from the heat and had to be left behind in the flaming inferno.

Throughout England, particularly around Leicester and Stamford, many inns and public houses were named after Daniel Lambert, and had his portrait on their signs. Lambert's name seemed to imply that good food was provided in extremely generous helpings, with ale in proportion. Even in London, public houses were named after him, and in particular, the Daniel Lambert tavern on Ludgate Hill propagated the great man's fame for many

254 years. A fine portrait of Lambert, by Mr. Singleton, R.A., and a showcase containing his stout walking stick are found in the lobby. Mr. James Dixon, proprietor of the Ram Jam Jam inn, Stamford, went one better in 1826. He actually bought the suit of clothes that Daniel Lambert wore at the time of his death and exhibited it at his tavern, which was renamed the Daniel Lambert inn. Once, six stout laborers were buttoned up in Lambert's enormous waistcoat. In 1846, Daniel Lambert's clothes were seen by P. T. Barnum and his tiny protégé, the fourteen-year-old midget Charles Stratton, otherwise known as General Tom Thumb. Barnum donated one of Tom Thumb's own costumes to Mr. Dixon, to be exhibited next to that of Daniel Lambert. General Tom Thumb was apparently quite fascinated by Lambert's wearing apparel. He again visited Stamford in 1859, when twenty-seven years old, and was tied up like a parcel in one of the great man's stockings. In 1866, Tom Thumb, in company with his equally diminutive wife Lavinia Warren, his sister-in-law Minnie Warren, and the competing midget Commodore Nutt, again saw Lambert's clothes; all four midgets could pass through the knee of Daniel Lambert's breeches at one time. Later in 1866, the clothes of Daniel Lambert and General Tom Thumb were purchased by Mr. Thomas Tasker Wells, owner of the Old London tavern in Stamford. This gentleman continued to exhibit them for many years. In 1892, Mr. Wells produced a thirty-two-page pamphlet, consisting of Drakard's biography of Daniel Lambert, along with some newspaper cuttings, portraits of Daniel Lambert and Tom Thumb, and copies of letters proving that the clothes were the genuine article and not a fraud.

Several famous nineteenth-century authors mentioned Daniel Lambert and his extraordinary career. In William Makepiece Thackeray's *Barry Lyndon*, an old servant named Tim, who had stayed in Ireland during Barry's prolonged travels on the continent, "had managed to grow monstrously fat in my absence, and would have fitted almost into Daniel Lambert's coat." In the early chapters of his famous *Vanity Fair*, the corpulent "Jos" Sedley, the brother of Amelia Sedley and once the suitor of Becky Sharp, recklessly drinks a huge punch bowl when he and his friends visit Vauxhall. He gets exceedingly drunk and finally begins to sing and dance in front of the astonished guests: "'Brayvo, Fat un!' said one 'Angcore, Daniel Lambert!' said another; 'What a figure for the tight-rope!' exclaimed another wag, to the inexpressible alarm of the ladies, and the great anger of Mr Osborne." There are no hints in Thackeray's letters or notebooks that he actually sought information about Lambert, but stories about the great man from Leicester were probably still circulating when the young Thackeray was amusing himself in London during the 1830s. Many other nineteenth-century writers used the well-known name of Daniel Lambert as a synonym for hugeness. Charles Dickens delivered his thoughts on Daniel Lambert, and also the "armless and legless wonder" Miss Biffin, in *Nicholas Nickleby*. The absentminded Mrs. Nickleby describes a neighbor with the following words: "'The Prince Regent was proud of his legs, and so was Daniel Lambert, who was also a fat man; he was proud of his legs. So was Miss Biffin: she was—no', added Mrs. Nickleby, correcting herself, 'I think she had only toes, but the principle is the same.'" In his magazine *Household Words*, Dickens later added that after Daniel Lambert had become a wealthy man from putting himself on show, he had devoted his life to sporting pursuits: he had kept thirty terriers, and his only literature had been the *Racing Calendar*. Thomas Carlyle's trenchant criticism of Hudson's proposed statue of Oliver Cromwell contained the words: "This big swollen and gluttonous 'spiritual Daniel Lambert' deserved a coalshaft from his brother mortals: let at least his column be ugly!" A florist's catalogue, printed in 1834, speaks of the "Daniel Lambert" carnation, apparently a giant of its species. Herman Melville's *Mardi* describes a breach in a palisade with the words that it was "wide enough to admit six Daniel Lamberts abreast." Herbert Spencer speaks of a "Daniel Lambert of learning" in his *Study of Sociology*, and in George Meredith's *One of our Conquerors*, London is described as the "Daniel Lambert of cities." Lord Macaulay also alluded to the great man from Leicester in one of his essays: "To paint Daniel Lambert or the living skeleton, the pig faced lady or the Siamese twins, so that nobody can mistake them, is an exploit within the reach of the signpainter." The poet Thomas Moore ridiculed the corpulent prince regent by pretending to write a letter from the prince's tailor, who begs his master's pardon for making a too small coat:

> *. . . my Wife, who's the Queen of all Slatterns*
> *Neglected to put up the Book of new Patterns*
> *She sent the wrong Measures too—shamefully wrong—*
> *They're the same us'd for poor Mr Lambert when young;*
> *But bless you! they wouldn't go half round the R*g—t—*
> *So, hope you'll excuse yours till death, most obedient . . .*

Daniel Lambert is no longer the most corpulent man of whom authentic records exist. The free access to calory-rich food for the overconsuming people of the industrialized world, particularly in the United States, has led to obesity becoming something of the "national disease" of that country. The

256   fact that 20 percent of Americans are obese, many of them grossly so, is soon apparent to any visitor to that country. In certain individuals with a psychological or physical predisposition to corpulence, the abundance of "junk food" can lead to disaster. The highest undisputed weight for a human being remains 1,069 pounds for the American Robert Earl Hughes, born in 1926 and buried in a pianoforte-sized coffin in 1958. For most of his adult life, Hughes was on exhibition in various fairs and sideshows in the Midwest. There have been several later pretenders to the unappealing title of the human heavyweight of all times, but some of them appear to have been "doctored" by unscrupulous dieting experts, who have exaggerated the initial weights of their patients to draw attention to their own prowess; others rely on sensation newspaper evidence alone. The hippie Francis John Lang weighed 1,187 pounds, according to the newspapers, and could not be admitted for treatment of gallbladder inflammation at the Veterans Administration Hospital in Houston, because of the impossibility of getting him through the doors. He was instead treated inside the caravan, parked in the hospital car park, in which he lived, like a large fish in a rather small aquarium. In 1988, another American, Walter Hudson, claimed that he had weighed 1,400 pounds (100 stone), thus nearly twice Lambert's weight, before he started dieting. He was a prisoner in his own house because he could not squeeze through the doorway. After being put on a starvation diet, he claimed to have lost 900 pounds; the 500-pound Hudson emerged through the doorway of his house for the first time in eighteen years and instantly became an American media celebrity. It was later claimed that Hudson was exploited by the company fabricating the diet nutrients he took, and that the whole thing was a scam: Hudson did not weigh more than 800 or 900 pounds to begin with, and lost at most 150 pounds. In a 1988 newspaper article, an American nutritionist claimed that Hudson had slimmed down from 1,204 pounds to 518. Another of his success stories, Mike Partelano, had once weighed 1,022 pounds, but lost 280 of them with the help of a diet consisting of vitamin and mineral drinks and small helpings of raw fruit and vegetables. Another newspaper story told the sad tale of the American Michael Hebranko, who had weighed 994 pounds, but lost 798 of them with help from a nutritionist. He had a relapse, however, ate five hot dogs at the airport, and again became a food addict. He rapidly increased in weight to 798 pounds, but after a lengthy treatment in hospital managed to lose 290 of them. In 1999, this same individual was again in the newspapers, after it became necessary for the New York emergency services to demolish a wall in order to forklift the 1,100-pound Hebranko to an ambulance.

In the British Isles, only one man, the publican William Campbell, has exceeded Daniel Lambert's weight. He was the landlord of the Duke of Wellington public house in Newcastle, and weighed 750 pounds at the time of his death in 1878. Like Daniel Lambert, he once exhibited himself in London, at the Egyptian Hall; also like his distinguished predecessor, he was said to have been a man of considerable wit and intelligence. When the heaviest woman in Britain, Nellie Lambert Ensall, exhibited herself in Birmingham in 1910, she claimed to be Daniel Lambert's great-granddaughter. This is probably untrue, however, since Lambert never married and is unlikely to have had any children, but she may still have been related to him in some way. Daniel Lambert still has relatives living in Leicester, and in 1970, they met to dine on the two-hundredth anniversary of his birth.

During Daniel Lambert's lifetime, it was frequently observed that since he did not eat to excess, and never drank ale, his extreme corpulence could only be due to some unknown, obscure disease. Several later commentators suggested that there must have been something seriously wrong with his "glands," although they did not detail exactly what. Modern biology would not agree, however. Obesity can be separated into a primary form, which occurs without other disease being present, and a secondary form, where the corpulence has some external endocrine or genetic cause. For example, myxedema (severe lack of thyroid hormone) may cause obesity, as may Cushing's syndrome of hyperproduction of corticotropic hormone. More uncommon causes include Fröhlich's syndrome of hypothalamic insufficiency and certain rare genetic syndromes like the Laurence-Moon-Biedl syndrome and the Prader-Willi syndrome. Daniel Lambert had no symptoms of either hypothyroidism or hypothalamic insufficiency, nor had he the typical moon face of a patient with Cushing's syndrome. Patients with the Prader-Willi or Laurence-Moon-Biedl syndromes may become extremely corpulent, but are often quite feeble both bodily and mentally, with a tendency toward diabetes and severe eye disease that can lead to blindness. Sources agree that in spite of his extreme corpulence, Daniel Lambert was a strong, powerful man, and that until 1806, he had no complaints about disease, except for erysipelas and venous insufficiency in both legs. His intelligence was clearly above average. Thus, it is very likely that Daniel Lambert suffered from primary obesity. Indeed, the popular belief that very obese individuals have something wrong with their "glands" is very ill-founded; in fact, only a small minority of them have an endocrine cause for their obesity. The above-mentioned Robert Hughes used to blame his corpulence on a singular accident: when three years old, he suffered from whooping cough and "ruptured his thyroid gland." This explanation, eagerly swallowed by the journalists, deserves a place among the "true greats" of medical cock-and-bull stories, along with the tale of the Irishman who tried to convince the doctor that he had caught venereal disease from borrowing another man's trousers.

Several of the grossly obese Americans discussed here seem to have had troubled life stories, and to have been far from mentally sound, with an addiction to food that can be likened to that of an alcoholic for strong drink. If the contemporary accounts are to be believed, Lambert did not overeat and never touched a pint of beer in his life. It is true that some individuals with what is known as morbid obesity have an abnormal tendency to gain weight. Their weight certainly increases more than that of a normal person when eating the same calory-rich diet. It has been speculated that some obese people have a persistent upregulation of the lipoprotein lipase enzyme, which regulates the liberation of triglycerides from lipoproteins; these triglycerides are incorporated into the fatty tissue. This hypothesis is supported by the fact that obese individuals have an upregulated lipoprotein lipase activity even after dieting to a normal body weight; this is one of the very few metabolic abnormalities in a person with primary obesity that actually persists when the individual loses weight. Nevertheless, the main causes of primary obesity are overeating of calory-rich food, in combination with a sedentary lifestyle. When a senior registrar in endocrinology five years ago, I had occasion to see several obese patients who vehemently claimed that no matter how they tried to lose weight by various diets, they still steadily gained weight. This was investigated by means of treating them as inpatients for a week and feeding them a very strict low-calory diet. The patients were far from fond of this regimen, and the nurses sometimes had to stand guard to prevent expeditions to the hospital snack shop! In every single case, however, the patients lost weight during these trials, an experience (often, alas, vainly) intended to increase their enthusiasm for changing their diets in a more permanent way. Nearly all overweight people have a tendency to understate their intake of calories, and it is by no means unlikely that Lambert was one of them. He would indeed almost have been unique in Leicestershire sporting circles if he had never had a second helping of roast beef and never tasted a tankard of brown ale. It is also very instructive that Daniel Lambert managed to keep his weight within reasonable limits as long as he led an active life, but that his corpulence increased very rapidly as soon as he sat down permanently in the prison-keeper's chair. If Daniel Lambert had lived today, he would probably have been surgically treated with either a gastroplasty or a gastric bypass. Briefly described, these operations remove or bypass the major part of the stomach pouch, and the remaining small gastric reservoir leads to the feeling of fullness even after quite a small meal. I have seen both operations performed with good effect, and they certainly seem to provide a more lasting benefit than the various fads of dieting, which may well be of benefit on a short-term basis, but allow the individual to regain the lost weight as soon he or she cannot stand the meager, low-calorie helpings of diet food any more.

Another unsolved problem is Daniel Lambert's cause of death. None less an authority than the *Dictionary of National Biography* proposed that he died of "fatty degeneration of the heart," but this does not appear likely. In extremely corpulent individuals, there is a gradual development of cardiac failure, for the reason that the peripheral resistance increases due to the immense mass of well-vascularized fatty tissue. The circumstances of his death again speak against cardiac insufficiency as the direct cause of death, however, as it was reported that he felt well that fatal morning, before *suddenly* complaining of acute difficulties in breathing. A letter from Elizabeth Gilbert to her sister Ann, written in Stamford just after Lambert's death, which is kept in the Cambridge University Library, also points out that Daniel Lambert did not have a clue about his impending, sudden death. A more likely hypothesis is that Daniel Lambert died from a massive pulmonary embolism. It is certain that he suffered from venous insufficiency of the legs, with repeated erysipeloid infections. One of the best accounts of Lambert's life, that in the *Beau Monde and Monthly Register* magazine, mentioned that in his later years, he suffered very much from pain in his legs. Venous insufficiency of the legs predisposes for venous thrombosis, as does his corpulence and the fact that he had spent the entire day before his death in a recumbent position. Daniel Lambert's corpse was not autopsied, however, and thus the exact cause of death will never be known.

The morbidly obese twentieth-century Americans described earlier have all had tough lives. They have been regarded as repulsive "losers," ridiculed by strangers in the street, and treated with disgust by all and sundry. Finally, their choice was either to become a recluse in their own house or to join the sideshow, just like Daniel Lambert in 1806. The public's expectations of the fat man on show were somewhat different in 1806, however, and the attitude toward him more forgiving than today. When reading contemporary accounts of Daniel Lambert, one is struck by the fact that he was viewed like a "curiosity" and a "human wonder" rather than a repulsive, deformed freak.

260   Even though Daniel Lambert was forced by circumstance to join the rank of the early-nineteenth-century "freaks," his exhibition was a very superior one. To many people, he personified the true Englishman, the stouthearted John Bull, in figure as well as in his rural and sporting interests. Otherwise, Lambert's time was not one noted for kindness to deformed individuals. An example is the massively steatopygous "Hottentot Venus" Saartje Baartman, who was exhibited like an animal in front of a gawking audience, who made rude jokes and prodded her prodigious behind with their umbrellas to make sure there was no imposture. This happened in 1810, just after Lambert breathed his last; his old friend Charles Mathews was not the only educated Londoner to find the exploitation of her too pitiful to bear in silence. But then she had the added disadvantages of being black (from the Cape Colony), female, and hardly able to speak the English language, while Lambert was an affable, middle-class man.

    The twentieth-century negative attitude to fat people has also struck the story and life of Daniel Lambert. Just a few years ago, his gravestone was vandalized and the word "FATTY" inscribed across it in huge letters. This disgraceful vandal represents a tiny minority, however, and Daniel Lambert remains a well-known and respected figure throughout the Midlands, particularly in Leicester and Stamford. His armchair, riding crop, prayer book, walking stick, waistcoat, breeches, shirt, gloves, and stockings are at the Newarke Museum in Leicester. The complete set of his clothes formerly exhibited at the Old London inn are now at the Stamford Museum, where a full-scale model of Daniel Lambert has been dressed in his coat, breeches, hat, and stockings. The portrait and walking stick from the Daniel Lambert tavern at Ludgate Hill are now exhibited at the George Hotel in Stamford, where I saw them in 1998. Lambert memorabilia are valuable: in 1990, a pair of his socks was sold at auction for 270 pounds. Many people consider Daniel Lambert as a symbol for the city of Leicester, and in 1981, a play called *The Ghost of Daniel Lambert* chronicled the history of the town. Many visitors to the Leicester Museum, particularly the schoolchildren, are fascinated by the permanent exhibition about Lambert's life and death. Not long ago, there was an advertisement in the *Leicester Mercury* newspaper, with a large portrait of Daniel Lambert and the text, "Think big! Leicestershire the location for the successful business!"

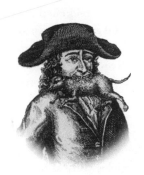

Cat-eating Englishmen
and French
Frog Swallowers

A MONG THE VAST MANUSCRIPT COLLECTIONS OF
the British Library are seven large folio volumes full of press cuttings, handbills, and advertisements, collected by the Reverend
Daniel Lysons in the late eighteenth century. Lysons was a distinguished
scholar and clergyman, but he was also a habitué of London low life. In the
gloomy back streets of the metropolis, he hobnobbed with quacks, mounte-
banks, jugglers, and exhibitors of animals and human freaks; in his huge
scrapbooks, he collected all the information he could procure about them.
Antiquaries and historians recognize Lysons's *Collecteana* as valuable source
material on cultural history. When studying these immense scrapbooks, one
is constantly impressed with the wealth of interesting material, which constantly tempts the mind to stray toward novel attractions, and the eccentric-
ity of intellect required to form such a bizarre and multifarious collection. In
one of the volumes, a startling newspaper cutting from the *World*, of March
13, 1788, has been pasted in:

Amongst the curious Betts of the day, may be reckoned the following: The *Duke* of *Bedford* has betted 1000 guineas with *Lord Barrymore*, that he does not—*eat a live Cat*! It is said his Lordship grounds his chances upon having already made the experiment upon a Kitten. The Cat is to be fed as *Lord Barrymore* may chose.

⁀♥

The Londoners greeted this bizarre report from the upper-class sporting circles with immediate interest. Several letters and articles were submitted to the editor of the *World*, and published under the headline *Cat Eating*. An authority on blood sports pointed out that "the bet of his Grace of Bedford, that Lord Barrymore will not eat a live Cat, is not without precedents in the annals of sporting." He had himself, at a racecourse near Kildare, witnessed an imbecile Irishman devouring five fox cubs, after fifty pounds had been wagered by the spectators. Another correspondent had seen a Yorkshire shepherd eat a live black tom cat, which had been carefully selected for its size and tenacity. This had happened in 1777, and it was remarked that the callous snobs responsible for this outrage had rewarded the wretched shepherd with the princely sum of two guineas. Lord Barrymore seems to have become rather worried when he saw his bizarre wager being much publicized in the papers, and he sent an official disclaimer to the editor of the *World*:

> In the Bett that was stated in this Paper, we understand that there was a mistake—as *Lord Barrymore* only betted, that *he found a man* who would eat a Cat.

Richard Barry, the seventh earl of Barrymore, was established as one of the leading rakes of London when he was hardly out of his teens: in a contemporary peerage, he was stated to have "wasted his fortune and his health among gamblers, pimps, and players." He raced horses, bet on pugilists, and roamed about the streets of London with his cronies, drinking, fighting, whoring, and spending recklessly out of the family fortune. The earl was nicknamed "Hellgate" for his rakehellish ways; his clubfooted, evil brother the Honorable Henry Barry was called "Cripplegate"; his other brother the Honorable Augustus Barry was nicknamed "Newgate" since this was the only prison with which this learned cleric, who shared Lord Barrymore's

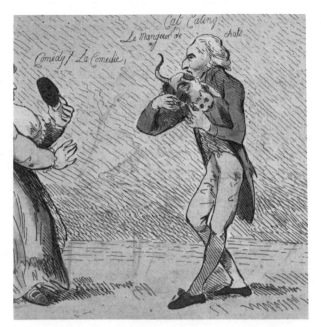

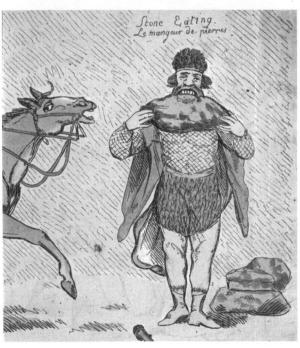

A cat eater and a stone eater, from the English caricature "Fashionable Follies," published in London 1788. From the author's collection.

264   taste for low life to no little extent, had not yet made a personal acquaintance; their sister, Lady Caroline Barry, was nicknamed "Billingsgate" (after
the foul-mouthed fishwives who congregated at this old London gate) for
her coarse language. The Barrymore siblings had the run of London until
1793, when the earl was shot by accident. By this time, he had spent the
major part of the family fortune on his amusements and various harebrained
schemes of his own invention.

Francis Russell, the fifth duke of Bedford, was a wealthy magnate who
was often seen at the racecourse and in the gambling parlors; he bragged
that at the age of twenty-four, he had scarcely opened a book. He was a
crony of Lord Barrymore, of long-standing. The two noblemen, both of
whom courtiers to the extravagant Prince of Wales, had bet five hundred
guineas against four hundred, a sum exceeding the life earnings of a day laborer. The duke's comments on hearing of Lord Barrymore's unsporting
volte-face have, perhaps unfortunately, not been recorded to posterity, nor is it
known whether Lord Barrymore managed to recruit a man willing to eat a
cat. According to Mr. J. F. Robinson's well-informed book *The Last Earls of
Barrymore*, the wager was put at the first spring meeting at the racecourse, on
March 12, 1788, and the earl did, from the beginning, point out that *he would
procure* a man willing to eat a live cat.

But although Lord Barrymore was never to sink his teeth into a cat's
body, it is certain that a similar wager was made in January 1790, and that a
live cat was eaten at a public house in Windsor. One of the correspondents of
Sporting Magazine was there to witness the disgusting proceedings. A 9-
pound cat had been selected as the victim, and "the Man-monster . . . made
a formidable attack on the head of his antagonist, and with repeated bites,
soon deprived it of existence." He then devoured his prey without even strip-
ping off the skin, leaving only the bones "as memorials of a most astonishing
instance of the exercise of a brutal appetite, and the degradation of human
nature." According to the *Public Advertiser* of February 3, 1790, the notorious
cat eater of Windsor had later "given another proof of the brutality of his dis-
position—an instance too ferocious and sanguinary, almost to admit of public representation." At a public house, perhaps the same one where he had
eaten the cat, he suddenly, and without reason, hacked off one of his hands
with a billhook. He gave no reason for this depraved action, except "his total
disinclination for work" and that he hoped that this desperate deed would induce the overseers of his parish to provide for him during the remainder of
his life. For many years thereafter, lurid newspaper stories about men eating
live cats abounded. In 1820, the philanthropist Mr. Henry Crowe, M.A.,

who was an early champion of animal's rights, held this up as one of the worst outrages of all in his book *Zoophilos*: "Is it conceivable that the wretch who could EAT A LIVE CAT for a wager, or that another, who could do the same to *amuse* the populace as a mountebank (anecdotes said to be well attested), should either of them feel qualms or compunction at adding even cannibalism to murder?"

The scholars of olden times have supplied many more or less trustworthy accounts of the great eaters, or polyphagi, of olden times. According to the learned Vospicius, the Emperor Aurelius once amused himself by watching a peasant devouring in turn a roast suckling-pig, a roast sheep, and a roast wild boar, all served with a generous supply of bread and wine; the man coped with this formidable task within one day's time. In the year 1511, another gluttonous peasant performed before the court of the Emperor Maximilian: he ate a fatted calf raw and started tearing a sheep's carcass with his powerful jaws, before the courtiers interrupted this somewhat monotonous amusement, at the emperor's request. The Danish anatomist Caspar Bartholin once saw a student who could drink copious amounts of wine; at autopsy, the stomach of this individual was observed to be of enormous size. Helwigius claimed to have seen a man who could devour 90 pounds of food for his dinner, and Professor Martyn, of Cambridge University, observed a boy who could consume 370 pounds of food in a week's time. A pig was fattened on the vomits of this boy and sold at the market for a good price, although one would rather suspect that this porker's unusual diet was not disclosed to the unsuspecting buyer.

In early-seventeenth-century England, a glutton named Nicholas Wood, who was known as "the Great Eater of Kent," performed at many country fairs and festivals. He was a native of the village of Harrietsham near Maidstone in Kent. In his youth, Nicholas Wood was employed as a servant of a local gentleman, but the rumor of his prodigious appetite was soon widespread, and he became a local hero. It was said that he had once eaten a whole hog, and that although he was a strong, stoutly built laborer, he had to spend all his estate to provide food for his insatiable belly. Once, when invited by Sir Warham St. Leger to his Kentish seat at Leeds Castle, Nicholas Wood won a bet by eating a dinner intended for eight people. Another local gentleman, Sir William Sedley, laid an even more magnificent table for the Great Eater; this was the first time this celebrated glutton had been defeated. After a valiant effort, Nicholas Wood fell to the floor in a deathlike trance.

266   His stomach was distended like a huge balloon. Fearing that the glutton would die, Sedley's servants laid him down near the fireplace and smeared his belly with fat to make it more readily distensible; the insensible man was then carried up to bed, many spectators fearing for his life. The day after, the Great Eater revived, but his fickle benefactor decided to mock the once-famous performer. Sir William Sedley's stewards dragged him outside, and he was put in the stocks to be jeered by the populace. At the castle of Lord Wotton in Boughton Malherbe, Nicholas Wood got his own back; he won a bet by eating seven dozen rabbits and was again celebrated by his friends for using his unique talents to score off those above him in society. Nicholas Wood's greatest misfortune occurred at the market of Lenham, where a cunning trickster named John Dale made a bet that he could fill the Great Eater's belly at the price of a mere two shillings. He accomplished this feat by soaking twelve one-penny loaves of bread in six pots of very strong ale; Nicholas Wood fell asleep and remained insensible for nine hours, after finishing only half of this strongly alcoholic meal.

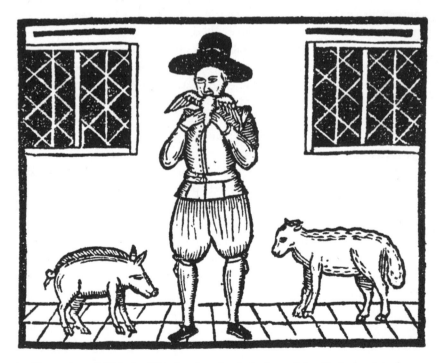

An illustration of Nicholas Wood eating the duck, from John Taylor's original pamphlet.

In 1630, Nicholas Wood met the poet John Taylor, who was visiting a country inn in Kent. Here, the poet saw the Great Eater win a bet by devouring a breakfast consisting of a leg of mutton, sixty eggs, three large pies, and an enormous black pudding. This was all the food in the inn's larder, but Nicholas Wood was still hungry. The waiter ran out to fetch a large duck, which the Great Eater tore to pieces and ate, leaving only the beak and quills.

John Taylor was deeply impressed by this exhibition of a brutal appetite: with his poetic imagination, he could envisage that the duck, which, a mere minute ago, had been peacefully swimming in the pond of the tavern, now "swomme in the whirlepole or pond of his mawe." John Taylor paid Wood twenty shillings to visit him in London some time later. In the meantime, the shrewd lyricist had made up a cunning plan to cash in on his new acquaintance. Nicholas Wood had never performed in London, and his gluttonous orgies would be a novelty even for the blasé citizens of the metropolis. After a grandiose advertisement campaign, the Great Eater was to make his bow to the London audience at the Bankside bear garden. At the first show, he would wolf down a wheelbarrow full of tripe; at the second, devour "as many puddings as would reach over the Thames." At the subsequent shows, he would eat a fat calf worth twenty shillings, and then twenty sets of sheeps' innards. Initially, Nicholas Wood felt disposed to accept this plan, hoping, perhaps, to become a superstar of gourmandising. His literate agent wrote a pamphlet to celebrate "the Admirable Teeth and Stomachs Exploits of Nicholas Wood"; it was widely spread among the Londoners, who were soon curious about this novel attraction. John Taylor spared no superlatives to describe his artist's enormous powers of digestion. His intestinal tract was a stall for oxen, a sty for hogs, a park for deer, a warren for rabbits, a pond for fishes, a storehouse for apples, and a dairy for milk and honey. His jaws were a mill of perpetual motion, and his capacious stomach the "rendez-vous or meeting place for the Beasts of the Fields, the Fowles of the Ayre, and Fishes of the Sea." But when the day of the grand opening was imminent, the Great Eater's mind became increasingly worried: he suffered from stage fright, and remembered, with horror and apprehension, the many distasteful and dangerous practical jokes he had encountered during his long and perilous career. The embarrassing anesthesia in Lenham had not been forgotten, and shortly before he left for London, he had lost all but one of his teeth at the market of Ashford, after being tricked into eating a shoulder of mutton *with bones and all*. One day, Nicholas Wood escaped from his lodgings in London, never to be heard of again. His manager-in-spe, John Taylor, had to be content with his long complimentary poem to "the Great Eater of Kent," containing the lines:

> *Thou that putst down the malt below the wheat,*
> *That dost not eat to live, but live to eat,*
> *Thou that the sea-whale and land-wolf excells,*
> *A foe to Bacchus, champion of god Bael's:*
> *I wish if any foreign foes intend*
> *Our famous isle of Britain to offend,*
> *That each of them had stomachs like to thee,*
> *That of each others they devoured might be.*
> *Though Maximus, Rome's great emperor*
> *Did forty pounds of flesh each day devour,*
> *Albinus the emperor did him surpass:*
> *Five hundred figs by him down swallowed was,*
> *Of peaches he consumed one hundred more,*
> *Of great muskmellons also half a score,*
> *One hundred birds, all at one meal he cast*
> *Into his paunch, at breaking of his fast.*

In the early 1700s, a Bohemian countryman became famous for his capacity to eat great amounts of raw meat. He performed widely in Germany and Austria. Once, he breakfasted on a calf roasted whole and he was able to devour a leg of mutton in a matter of minutes. In 1709, this Bohemian glutton was advertised in a handbill, which depicted him seizing a puppy between his powerful jaws. He holds a large ham and a goblet of ale in his hands. At his feet lies a cat, happily unaware of the fate he had in store for it. Another feat of this disgusting performer was that he could crush a large stone between his powerful jaws.

An imbecile Irishman named Thomas Eclin performed similar wonders in London of the 1740s and 1750s. According to the newspapers, he was "remarkable for his Vivacity and Drollery in the low Way." His feats included eating live dogs and cats and leaping head first into the Thames when the weather was freezing cold. Thomas Eclin was fond of drinking copious amounts of gin, and after his death from vomiting blood, the *Daily Advertiser* announced the sale of a drawing in his honor, depicting the cat eater "with the just Emblems of his Ambition: a Decanter and a Glass at his Elbow, and a Pipe in his right Hand." There were numerous other performers in the same vein. The *Annual Register* of 1765 reported that a brewer's servant

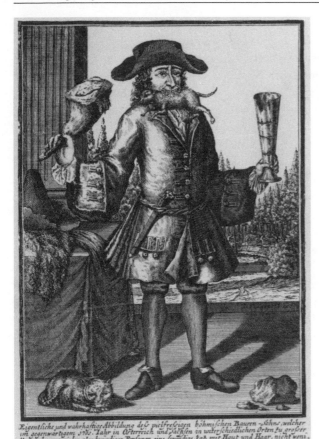

The Bohemian cat-
eating countryman,
from a contemporary
handbill.

named Walter Willey ate a roasted goose of 6 pounds and a quartern loaf, and drank three quarts of porter; he accomplished this feat in little more than an hour, and won a bet of two guineas. According to the *Cambridge Chronicle* of September 13, 1770, a young country lad won a wager through eating an 8-pound leg of mutton, with a quantity of bread and carrots. The next day, he ate "a whole cat, smothered with onions." Another glutton, Charles Tyle, of Stoke Abbott in Dorset, ate 133 eggs within one hour, with a large piece of bacon and a quantity of bread. According to the *Bristol Gazette* of March 13, 1788, afterward he complained that there had not been enough eggs and that he had not yet had a full supper.

There are many other instances of British gluttons making wagers to consume prodigious amounts of food and drink; this unsavory amusement seems to have been relished both in London and in the countryside, and survived well into the nineteenth century. According to the *World* newspaper of March 11, 1790, a man at Stillington in Lancashire drank five quarts of ale and then masticated and swallowed the earthen mug; he did not have long to delight at winning his bet, as he died two days later, probably of intestinal obstruction caused by the fragments of the mug. The *London Packet* of March 2, 1804, told that one glutton had just eaten his length in pork sausages, 2 pounds of new bread, and drunk a quart of porter and two glasses of brandy, all in twenty-two minutes. Another voracious eater, who obviously had a strong predilection for greasy food, ate a pound of butter and a 1½-pound dumpling. The *Observer* newspaper of March 24, 1811, reported that a countryman had just eaten sixty-five raw eggs in eight minutes, for a trifling wager. Another man had eaten a pint of periwinkles, with shells and all, in ten minutes. Encouraged to repeat the performance, he did so, but fell violently ill after accomplishing his feat, and was not expected to recover. The *Times* of August 26, 1824, reported another melancholy event. A man from Jersey ate six raw eggs mixed with half a pint of gin. As the wager was renewed, at a higher amount each time, he repeated this performance three times. With two pints of gin within him, he tore into a quantity of raw bacon and drank two large glasses of brandy. Then he "felt indisposed," went home, and died. Another glutton, William Webber, undertook to eat a roast pig of 10 pounds, served with two quartern loaves and a quantity of potatoes. Having "cleared" an 8-pound pig on Christmas Eve the year before, he began in a capital manner, and drank beer and smoked his pipe in between the generous helpings, but had to give up, according to the *Times* of March 3, 1840, with a pound and a half of meat still on the table before him.

Some years after Nicolas Wood withdrew from show business, an Irish soldier named Francis Battalia appeared in London. This individual had a unique talent: he could chew and swallow large plates full of stone and gravel. After his meal, he shook his body violently, making the stones rustle from the depths of his stomach.

The advertisements claimed that as an infant, Battalia had refused all kinds of food until the wet nurse mixed his gruel with small pebbles. He subsequently relied on the productions of the mineral kingdom for his daily nourishment, growing up to be a vigorous and active fellow, although of short stature. Francis Battalia's performances were described in John Bulwer's *Anthropometamorphosis*, and his portrait, by Hollar, was engraved and

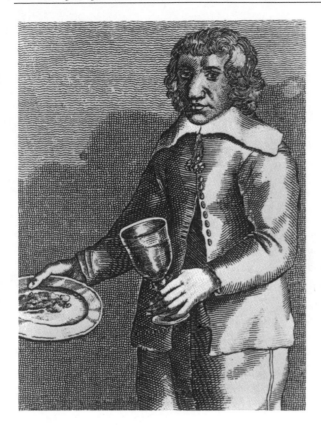

An eighteenth-century engraving of a portrait of Francis Battalia's. From the author's collection.

widely distributed. An artist rather resembling Francis Battalia was performing in the late 1770s, under the short but self-explanatory stage name "The Stone Eater." This time, his partiality for hard-to-chew food was explained by his having been shipwrecked outside the Norwegian coast in 1761. Sitting on an uninhabited, rocky islet, he munched gravel for thirteen years before being saved by a ship passing by. He claimed that his intestinal tract had become used to minerals as the principal source of nourishment. Those who doubted this were invited to his shows, where he ground stones and pebbles between his powerful jaws, with a horrible crunching sound. The Stone Eater was much noticed by the medical establishment: the advertisements bragged that Sir Joseph Banks and the great John Hunter were attracted by his unique accomplishments, but neither of these gentlemen described him in print. It is true, however, that Dr. Munro wrote a short article about the Stone Eater in his *Medical Commentaries*.

Soon, a rival stone eater appeared in London: this fellow called himself Siderophagus and munched iron as well as chewed pebbles. His wife was in the same line of business: under the stage name Sarah Salamander, she drank aquafortis and oil of vitriol like it had been small beer. Another stone eater, either the original one or a usurper of that title, surfaced in 1788 and was still active in the early 1790s; he was immortalized by the comic poet Mr. O'Keefe:

> *Make room for a jolly Stone-eater,*
> *For Stones of all kind I can crunch;*
> *A nice bit of Marble is sweeter*
> *To me than a Turtle or Haunch.*
> *A Street that's well pav'd is my larder—*
> *A Stone you will say is hard meat,*
> *But, neighbors, I think 'tis much harder*
> *Where I can get nothing to eat!*
> *With my crackeldy mash, ha! ha!*
>
> London Bridge *shall just serve for a luncheon—*
> *Don't fear—I would make it a job:*
> The Monument *next I will munch on,*
> *For fear it would fall on my nob:*
> Ye Strand *folks, as I am a sinner,*
> *Two nuisances I will eat up;*
> Temple-Bar *will make me a good dinner,*
> *Because on* St. Clement's *I'll sup!*

One of the contemporaries of the English stone eater was a French glutton named M. Dufour. At one of his shows, in 1792, he ate a specially composed banquet before a large and admiring house. As hors d'oeuvres, he had soup of asps boiled in simmering oil, with thistles and burdocks as a salad. Then, he ate dishes of tortoise, bat, rat, and mole; the main course was a roast owl served in a sauce of glowing brimstone. For dessert, he supped on toads decorated with flies, crickets, spiders, and caterpillars. As an encore, M. Dufour swallowed the still-burning candles on the table and washed them down with a flaming glass of brandy. Finally, he swallowed the oil lamp, and the flames glowed from his wide mouth when he made his bow to the enraptured audience.

In February 1799, the French ship *Hoche* was captured by the Royal

Navy off the coast of Ireland. One of the soldiers on board was named Charles Domery. In the military prison, the English guards were amazed by the Frenchman's voracious appetite. Although he received double rations, he kept begging for food from the other prisoners and did not refuse dead cats and rats delivered to him as presents by the curious turnkeys. The other French soldiers said that Charles Domery had always eaten a prodigious amount of food: he had eight brothers, all of them soldiers, with similar voracious appetites. While at an army camp outside Paris, Charles Domery had eaten 174 cats in a year's time. Dogs and rats equally suffered from his merciless jaws, and he also ate 4 or 5 pounds of grass each day, if bread and meat were scarce. He liked raw meat better than cooked or boiled meat, and a raw bullock's liver was his favorite dish. When, in action on board a ship of the line, another sailor's leg was shot off by a cannon ball, Domery grasped it and began feeding heartily, until another mariner tore it away from him in disgust and threw it into the sea. In spite of his gluttonous habits, Charles Domery was of normal build and stature; although he was completely illiterate, the prison doctors considered him to be at least of average intelligence. In September 1799, Dr. Johnston, the commissioner of sick and wounded seamen, decided to perform an experiment to test the Frenchman's preternatural appetite. At four o'clock in the morning, Charles Domery breakfasted on 4 pounds of raw cow's udder, and at half past nine, Dr. Johnston and Admiral Child had prepared a suitable luncheon for him, consisting of 5 pounds of raw beef, twelve large tallow candles, and a bottle of porter. At one o'clock, the glutton again devoured 5 pounds of raw beef, 1 pound of candles, and three large bottles of porter. At five o'clock, he returned to the prison; it was recorded that he was of particularly good cheer after his great feast: he danced, smoked his pipe, and drank another bottle of porter. The following morning, he awoke at four o'clock, eager for his breakfast. None less than Charles Dickens had read an account of Domery's voracious gluttony, and in his *Household Words*, he wrote that Charles Domery "dining in public on the Stage of Drury Lane, would draw much better than a mere tragedian, who chews unsubstantial words instead of wholesome beef."

Another celebrated French glutton, M. Bijoux, was a porter at the zoological garden of the Jardin des Plantes in Paris. He believed himself to be a great naturalist, and even called himself the French Linnaeus, since he had made up an elaborate system of classifying all animals from the appearance of their excrement. To support his studies, he kept a large collection of fecal matter in his private museum. M. Bijoux ate the most disgusting objects without hesitation: he even consumed the body of an old lion that had died of

274   disease in its cage. Once, a sporting nobleman made a bet with Bijoux that he could not devour 9 pounds of hot bread within two minutes. After a frenzied performance, the glutton won his bet, but to the prize of his life: immediately after swallowing the last morsel, he dropped dead. The intestinal tract capable of digesting the King of Beasts thus had to capitulate before a mere *pain riche!*

    In the early 1820s, a glutton named Jacques de Falaise performed at M. Comte's theater in Paris. A native of the Montmartre district, he was a time-honored attraction at various sleazy taverns. His careers apparently had its ups and downs: at least twice, he rose from obscurity to be widely advertised by his managers. He reached some fame among the Parisians, and was interviewed several times by curious members of the medical profession. During his shows, Jacques swallowed eggs and walnuts whole and ate live

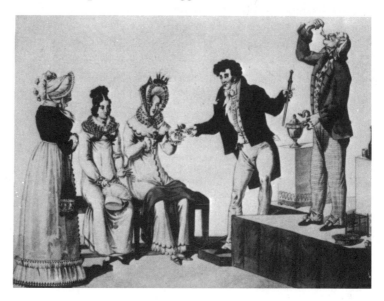

A contemporary print of Jacques de Falaise performing. From the author's collection.

sparrows, crawfish, mice, adders, and eels. Once, after a wager had been entered into, he swallowed fifty-five franc pieces, which nearly killed him, as these coins were as large as half-crowns. Some years later, poor Jacques killed himself by hanging; at autopsy, it was noted that his stomach had many scars of older injuries from the sharp and corrosive substances he had swallowed.

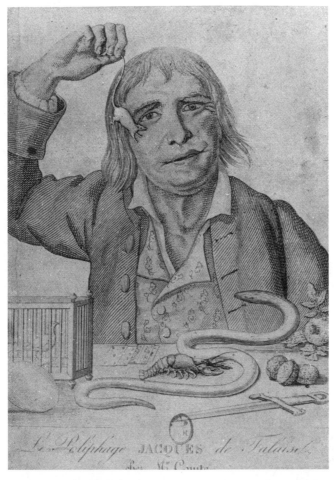

One of Jacques de Falaise's advertisements. From the author's collection.

These unsavory tales from the annals of polyphagy would perchance have seemed exaggerated had they not been surpassed by the foremost glutton of all times, a Frenchman known to his contemporaries as Tararre. It is not known whether Tarrare was his real name or a nickname bestowed on him at some time during his astounding career. The expression "Bom-bom tarare!" was used at this time to describe powerful explosions or fanfares, and it may be speculated that the name Tarrare was bestowed on him to ridicule his prodigious flatulence. Tarrare was born in the French countryside, just outside the city of Lyon. Already as a child, he had an enormous appetite. When he was in his teens, his parents could not feed this monster any more and turned him out of the house. For several years, he scoured the French provinces, in the company of robbers, whores, and vagabonds. Later, he was employed as a clown by an itinerant quack: by swallowing stones, corks, and live animals, he attracted the attention of the curious populace toward the mountebank's spiel about his nostrums and wonder drugs. Tarrare could devour a whole basketful of apples, by swallowing them one by one. In 1788, he left his employer and moved to Paris, to earn a perilous living by means of similar performances in the streets of the French capital. Once, he was struck by acute intestinal obstruction after one of the shows. In agony, Tarrare was carried away to the Hôtel Dieu hospital, where he was treated with a powerful purgative, which had the desired effect. This experience did not induce him to give up his perilous career. Just after he recovered, he volunteered to swallow the surgeon M. Giraud's watch and chain to demonstrate his talents, but the gruff surgeon replied that in that case, he would cut Tarrare's belly open with his sword to recover his valuable timepiece.

At the advent of the revolutionary wars in France, Tarrare joined the army as a recruit, but the frugal diet of the troops did not suffice to quench his insatiable hunger. He was again taken into a hospital, this time in a state of extreme exhaustion. At the doctor's orders, he was given quadruple rations, but to little avail: Tarrare still lurked about, looking for food in the gutters and dustbins. The military surgeons were amazed by Tarrare's immense appetite. They ordered that he was to remain in the hospital to take part in some physiological experiments designed by M. Courville, surgeon to the ninth regiment of Hussars, and Professor Percy, the surgeon-in-chief of the hospital. Many years later, Baron Percy summarized the results in a scientific treatise. Once, during Tarrare's residence in the hospital, a table had been laid for fifteen German laborers just outside the hospital gates. The porters had great difficulties to keep Tarrare at bay, but Dr. Courville, who had observed the glutton lurking nearby, decided to put his digestion to the test. The luncheon of the German laboring men, who were apparently not consulted when the disposal of their food was decided upon, consisted of two enormous meat pies, served with huge plates full of grease and salt, and a pair of two-gallon jugs full of milk and soured milk. The voracious Tarrare ate everything on the table, not leaving even a bread crumb or a drop of milk. After this orgy, he immediately fell asleep. Dr. Courville noted that the skin of his paunch, which was normally lax and flabby in texture, had become widely distended like a huge balloon. In another experiment, Tarrare was given a live cat, which he devoured after tearing its abdomen with his teeth and drinking its blood. He later vomited the fur and the skin. The doctors also fed him live puppies, snakes, lizards, and other animals, and Tarrare did not refuse any of their offerings.

Tarrare's appearance did not betray his canine appetite: he was pale, thin, and of medium height, and his temperament was apathetic. His fair hair was uncommonly thin and soft. His mouth was enormously wide, and the enamel of the teeth much stained. He sweated profusely and was constantly surrounded by a malodorous stench. When Tarrare was starving, the abdominal skin hung like a huge leather bag, which he could wrap round his waist, but when he had eaten a hearty meal, his paunch could distend in a remarkable manner. After one of his feasts, he smelled worse than ever, and his eyes and cheeks became bloodshot. Professor Percy wrote that the methods utilized by "this filthy glutton" to make his rations last were too disgusting to be described in detail. All creatures great and small were in constant danger from his ravenous jaws: "The dogs and cats fled in terror at his aspect, like if they had anticipated the kind of fate he was preparing for them."

⁓❧

After the unsavory experiments at the military hospital had been going on for several months, the French military board inquired how soon Tarrare would be fit for active duty again. The doctors were quite unwilling to lose touch with their valuable "guinea pig," however, and Dr. Courville came up with a bizarre idea. He persuaded Tarrare to swallow a wooden box with a document inside; it turned out that two days later, after a visit to the hospital latrines, the glutton delivered the box with the document in good condition. Dr. Courville went before the army commander, General de Beauharnais, to suggest that Tarrare be recruited into the French secret service as a master spy. Using the wooden box, he could smuggle top secret documents through enemy territory without getting caught! Vicomte de Beauharnais was apparently quite intrigued by this plan, as he ordered Tarrare to perform before several top-ranking officers at the headquarters of the French army at the Rhine; it is unlikely, but by no means impossible, that Napoleon Bonaparte was one of those present. After swallowing the wooden box with ease, Tarrare was rewarded with a wheelbarrow full of raw bull's liver and lungs, which he devoured on the spot, to the consternation of the generals.

After this performance, Tarrare was officially employed as a spy. His first assignment was to deliver a secret letter to a French colonel held captive by the Prussians in a fortress near Neustadt. General de Beauharnais was much less impressed with Tarrare's mental abilities than with his powers of digestion, however, and he did not want to entrust him with any documents of real importance. Although the glutton was tricked into believing that he carried papers of vital importance for the outcome of the war, the general ordered that just a note telling the imprisoned French colonel to send back, by the same messenger, all possible information about Prussian movements of troops, was to be put into the box swallowed by Tarrare.

In the middle of the night, Tarrare was sent off from the French entrenchment, disguised as a German peasant. He did not know a word of German, however, and his manner soon attracted attention. Outside the city of Landau, he was arrested by a patrol of soldiers, who had been called by some watchful countrymen. After the Frenchman was strip-searched and interrogated, the soldiers gave him a sound whipping, but Tarrare did not betray a word about his mission. He was then taken before General Zoegli, the Prussian military commandant, but Tarrare again gave nothing away, although the sinister Germans assured him that once he was installed in their prison, they had ways of making him talk.

Tarrare was not cut out to be a war hero, and after twenty-four hours in the hands of the Prussian counterintelligence, he confessed about the bizarre scheme concocted by the doctors and General de Beauharnais. He was chained to a bog-house, and his tormentors were overjoyed when, at last, he delivered the wooden box. They expected the box to contain top-secret files, as Tarrare had promised them, and were furious when General de Beauharnais's curt letter was read out. Their disappointment was taken out on the wretched Tarrare, who was put on a scaffold with a noose around his neck, and asked to make his peace with the Almighty. At the last minute, General Zoegli, who had had a good laugh at the Frenchman's expense, ordered his life to be spared. Before he was ignominiously driven off near the French lines, Tarrare was given another brutal thrashing, in order to put him off secret-service work for all time.

◆

After his brief and disastrous career as a secret agent, Tarrare was willing to do anything to evade being conscripted into military service. After he was readmitted into the military hospital, he told Professor Percy that he was ready to try any possible cure to rid him of his gluttony. The professor first tried tincture of opium, but without success; he then fed Tarrare sour wine and tobacco pills, but without affecting his preternatural appetite. Professor

Percy had read a case report stating that large amounts of Levantine soft-boiled eggs were a powerful appetite suppressant, but Tarrare was resistant even to this exotic cure. All attempts to make him keep a controlled diet were fruitless: Tarrare sneaked clandestinely out of the hospital to lurk outside the butcher's shops; in the dark back alleys of Paris, he fought the street mongrels for the possession of disgusting carrion found in the gutters and refuse heaps. Within the hospital, he sometimes skulked into the wards to drink the blood from patients treated with venesection. Several times, he was kicked out of the morgue after having taken liberties with the corpses. Some of the doctors requested that Tarrare be committed to a lunatic asylum, but Professor Percy had grown, in some strange way, attached to his former "guinea pig," and still wanted to keep him under observation at the hospital. Some time later, however, a fourteen-month-old infant suddenly disappeared from its hospital bed. Everyone suspected Tarrare of being responsible, and this time, not even the professor could save him; the enraged doctors and porters chased Tarrare away, and he was never seen at the hospital again.

Subsequently, Professor Percy lost sight of his patient for several years. One can only speculate how this monstrous glutton managed to keep alive in a France ravaged by war and revolution. Four years later, Professor Percy heard from M. Tessier, the chief surgeon of the hospital in Versailles, that Tarrare had been admitted to one of his wards. The once-celebrated glutton was in a miserable state of feebleness, and he could hardly rise from his hospital bed. Tararre himself asked to see the professor, for the reason that two years earlier, he had swallowed a stolen gold fork, which he was sure still resided within his intestinal canal; now, he wanted to hear if the knowledgeable physiologist knew of some way to dislodge it from its lair within him, by means of some powerful emetic or laxative! It was apparent to Professor Percy that Tarrare was badly ill, in the last stage of tuberculosis; he was a mere shadow of the vigorous glutton he had been just a few years ago. A month later, Tarrare was struck by a continuous, purulent diarrhea and died within a couple of days. The corpse putrefied uncommonly quickly, and even the surgeons of the hospital, who were used to dealing with rotting corpses, were unwilling to dissect him. M. Tessier had heard of Tarrare's former glory, and he decided to find out what this monster looked like inside, and also to determine whether he really had a golden fork within him as he claimed. At the autopsy, the rotting entrails were bathing in pus. The liver was very large, and the gallbladder distended. The stomach was enormous and filled the major part of the abdominal cavity. No gold fork was found inside Tarrare's intestinal tract. The gullet was uncommonly wide, and when the huge jaws were forced open, the surgeons could see a broad canal down to the stomach.

One would have thought that a ghoul like Tarrare would be absolutely unique in history, but less than thirty years later, a veritable soul mate of his was arrested by the Paris police. His name was Antoine Langulet, and an account of his career was drawn up by a certain Dr. Berthollet in 1825, after Langulet was committed to an asylum for the criminally insane. Antoine Langulet lived in a hovel near the Avenue de l'Opera, not far from the opera house itself. It is stated that he was not a vagabond, but he did no work, and it is not known how he supported himself. At the time of his arrest, he was 5 feet 10 inches tall and weighed a little under 170 pounds. Since an early age, Antoine Langulet had been in the habit of eating the most disgusting substances. He liked putrid meat from a fly-blown cadaver better than a fresh beef steak. He spent the daytime lurking inside his humble abode, but after dusk, he ventured out to scavenge the streets, collecting offal and rotten meat from the gutters and stuffing his pockets with his foul-smelling treasures. Normally, he liked to cook his meat over an open fire and was proud of his ability to tell the difference between different animals. He was a friend of the Paris horse knackers, and they sometimes allowed him to feed on the sick old horses they had killed. He was sure to seek out the most inflamed, livid tissues, or those most altered by disease.

Had Antoine Langulet been content with rotten horse flesh for dinner, he would never have come into contact with Dr. Berthollet and his fellow alienists at the Bicêtre prison. But he had discovered another source for his favorite food: an old cemetery near the Rue de Clichy. After midnight, he left his house and climbed the cemetery gates under the cover of darkness; he brought with him a spade, a maul, and a sledge hammer. With these implements, he unearthed and broke open the coffins of recently buried people and feasted on the rotting corpses. He ate the intestines in preference to anything else. After some months of these outrages, there were rumors that grave robbers were at large in the cemetery, but a doctor who had examined the contents of the unearthed coffins and what remained of their occupants said that this was definitely the work of a human ghoul. The cemetery was guarded in the hope of catching this monster, but the voluntary policemen who were posted to stand guard over the eerie graves were probably just as pleased that their quest was unsuccessful. Finally, a verger saw a creature pulling the body of a young girl from her grave and bravely pursued it. The ghoul outran his pursuers, and still carrying the corpse, climbed the cemetery gates with great agility. He would have been safe had not someone noted some pieces of female apparel outside Langulet's house. As the police burst in, they discovered him eating the corpse, and he was arrested. Dr. Berthollet had expected to find a raving lunatic, but Langulet turned out to be a sensible, rational man, except for his depraved appetite. Antoine Langulet did not consider that he had committed any crime. He freely admitted that ever since his childhood, he had been in the habit of eating what others termed disgusting food, but this taste was perfectly natural to him. More sinisterly, Langulet also admitted that he often wanted to eat the bodies of young children, but he had never been able to summon courage enough to kill them, he said. Bearing this ill-judged remark in mind, Dr. Berthollet recommended that he should be imprisoned indefinitely.

The tales of Tarrare and Langulet will raise a frisson of horror even in the most devoted students of the macabre: the bizarre antics of the French gluttons are almost unbelievable, and one would at first be tempted to suspect that their biographers were guilty of exaggeration. This does not seem to be the case, however. Dr. Berthollet's report is brief and matter-of-fact, and in his book, *The Flesh Eaters*, Mr. Peter Haining claims to have discovered independent evidence of Langulet's career, particularly an account in *Le Figaro*. George Didier, Baron Percy, was one of the leading military surgeons of his time; in his list of publications, the case report about Tarrare seems out of place among his many valuable surgical articles and monographs. Tararre was widely famous among the Parisians, who delighted in the demented glutton's macabre display of his powers of deglutition. It would even seem that a theatrical play was inspired by his singular career.

The gluttons Charles Domery, Tarrare, and Antoine Langulet not only share their French nationality, but also have several other characteristics in common. Neither, in spite of their singular behavior, seemed apparently insane to their contemporaries. Domery's gluttony began at the age of thirteen, and the disgusting habits of Tarrare and Langulet were established at an even earlier age. Although they could eat enormous amounts of food, they never vomited it and did not gain weight. They had a particular preference for raw, or even rotten, meat, and preferred it to meat cooked or fried. Their gluttony enabled them to devour the most disgusting food with alacrity. Both Tarrare and Charles Domery sweated profusely, particularly after a feast, and were continuously surrounded by a nauseating odor. At autopsy, it was noted that Tarrare's habit of swallowing huge chunks of meat, apples, and buns whole had caused a considerable widening of the gullet and stomach. The cause of death is likely to have been intestinal tuberculosis, resulting in intestinal perforation and peritonitis.

The similarity between these three cases would tempt one to suggest that they suffered from a similar abnormality in the cerebral centers regulating the appetite and intake of food. It is known that appetite is primarily regulated by two hypothalamic centers in the brain: a "satiety center" in the ventromedial nucleus and a "feeding center" in the lateral part of the hypothalamus. In experiments with animals whose satiety centers have been destroyed, the animals eat copiously, but only until they reach a certain body weight. It is notable, however, that animals with an injury in another region of the brain, the amygdaloid nuclei, develop a veritable omniphagia, eating even adulterated and tainted food. No case even moderately resembling Domery, Tarrare, or Langulet has been published in the annals of modern medicine, however, and it is thus impossible to determine their correct diagnosis.

Several other historical polyphagi, like Jacques de Falaise and Bijoux, showed distinct signs of mental illness even according to the criteria of their contemporaries. Others, like Thomas Eclin, were simple-minded fools who were forced to perform their disgusting and dangerous feats before the cruel populace. "Human ostriches" have performed at nineteenth- and twentieth-century circuses, swallowing corks, glass, lemons, and paraffin. One of the most famous was English Jack, the Live Frog Eater, who was depicted in a poster, standing beside an aquarium containing his hapless partners. A step down the social ladder were the street performers who swallowed swords, stones, coal, and live animals—indeed, anything that would attract an audience. A specialty of the American sideshow well into modern times was "the geek," a purported wild man who bit the heads off live rats and chickens to drink their blood. Watching the dying animals run or writhe around on the stage was another part of the "fun." The traditional geek was a rundown alcoholic: using a bottle of cheap whisky as a lure, the impresario could persuade them to perform the most degrading feats. It might be a relief for animal lovers to find out that some humanitarian geeks of the 1990s have started to use rubber chickens in their shows.

An artist with much more talent and panache was the Frenchman Louis Claude Delair, who performed as Mac Norton, the Human Aquarium. This stocky, tail-coated gentleman never changed his one act, but it was singular

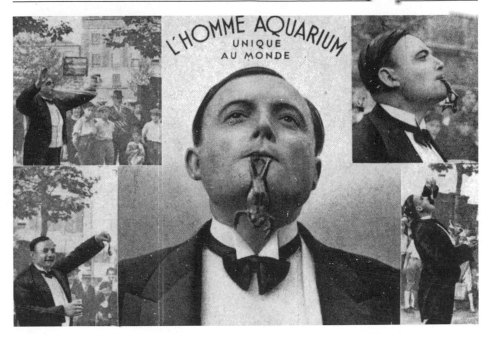

Louis Claude Delair in action.

enough for him to make a comfortable living out of it. After rapidly drinking a large amount of water, Delair swallowed a number of goldfishes and frogs. To the astonishment of the audience, he then vomited them, one by one, until they had all been transferred from their human aquarium within his stomach to their usual glass bowl. Delair bragged that during his forty-year career in show business, he had never lost a single pet. At his final show, held in 1949 four years before his death, Delair resurrected his partners, six fishes and twelve green frogs, from their human aquarium; when the trick was done, he took his bow before the audience, calling out, "All alive and kicking!"

Notes on Sources

The Two Inseparable Brothers; and a Preface

For specific sources on Lazarus-Joannes Baptista Colloredo, see *Historiarum Anatomicarum Rariorum, Centuria I–II* by T. Bartholin (Amsterdam, 1654), 117; *De monstris* by F. Liceti (Amsterdam, 1665), 114, 117, 346; *Questionum Medico-Legalium,* Vol. 2, by P. Zacchias (Frankfurt am Main, 1688), 601; *Histoire et antiquités de la ville de Paris,* Vol. 2, by H. Sauval (Paris, 1724), 564–65; the article by J. Greene (*Gentleman's Magazine 47* [1777], 482–83); and *Memorialls of the Trubles in Scotland and in England,* Vol. 2, by J. Spalding (Aberdeen, 1850), 125–26. A valuable secondary source is the work of H. E. Rollins (*Modern Philology* 16 [1919], 113–38) and *Pack of Autolycus* (Cambridge, Mass., 1926), 7–14.

To write a complete bibliography of the history of teratology is a difficult task, but here I list some of the outstanding sources from the last 150 years. The German teratologists were the leaders in their field in the late-nineteenth century, and books like Friedrich Ahlfeld's *Die Missbildungen des Menschen* (Leipzig, 1880) and Ernst Schwalbe's *Die Morphologie der Missbildungen* (Jena, 1906) still command respect. Another, unrecognized work in the same tradition is the long article by Hans Hübner (*Ergebnisse der Allgemeine Pathologie und Pathologische Anatomie* 15(2) [1911], 1–348). The modern German sources are equally valuable, although often overlooked by foreign writers. Eugen Holländer's *Wunder, Wundergeburt und Wundergestalt* (Jena, 1921) is a classic: well written, with many curious illustrations, and abounding in valuable source material, but somewhat lacking in its scholarly apparatus. This has been put right by later writers, like M. Zoller in *Untersuchungen zu teratologisch-historischen Aussagen kulturhistorischer Dokumente* (thesis, University of Rostock, 1976) and A. Ewinkel in *De Monstris* (Tübingen, 1995). Hans Schleugel's *Showfreaks & Monster* (Köln, 1975) is lacking in historical sophistication, but it is based on the great collection of Felix Adanos, which means that much new material is presented. Two other worthy German sources are A. Sonderegger's *Missgeburten und Wundergestalten* (Zürich, 1927) and J. Kunze and I. Nippert's *Genetik und Kunst* (Berlin, 1986). The French sources begin with Isidore Geoffroy Saint-Hilaire's classic *Histoire générale et particulière des anomalies de l'organisation* (Paris, 1832–1836). Later sources include *His toire des monstres* by E. Martin (Paris, 1880) and *Précis de tératologie* by L. Guinard (Paris, 1893). The more recent French literature is less worthy: M. Monestier's *Human Oddities* (Secaucus, N.J., 1987) has been (badly) translated into English, but although this book contains some interesting facts and curious illustrations, it perpetuates many old errors and creates some new ones. An interesting Dutch book is *De Tentoongestelde Mens* by B. C. Sliggers and A. A. Wertheim (Eds.) (Haarlem, 1993). As for English-language sources, G. M. Gould and W. L. Pyle's *Anomalies and Curiosities of Medicine* (Philadelphia, 1897) is a classic account. A curiously overlooked source is the very thoroughly researched *Diploteratology* by G. J. Fisher, originally published in the *Transactions of the Medical Society of the State of New York* of 1865–1868. C. J. S. Thompson's *The Mystery and Lore of Monsters* (London, 1930) is somewhat dependent on Gould and Pyle's book, but adds much valuable material based on Thompson's research in the British Library and in the archives of the Royal College of Surgeons of London; unfortunately, it is not annotated and lacks a comprehensive list of sources. *Bizarre* by B. Humphries (London, 1965) is a confused account with many errors, and *Victorian Grotesque* by M. Howard (London, 1977) depends much on Gould and Pyle's book; D. Todd's *Imagining Monsters* (Chicago, 1995) does not add much of interest. Two more valuable sources are Frederick Drimmer's *Very Special People* (New York, 1973) and *Born Different* (New York, 1988), which are largely based on original research. A curious "picture supplement" to the former book is *Sideshow* by M. Rusid (New York, 1975). The articles by J. F. D. Shrewsbury (*Journal of Obstetrics and Gynaecology of the British Empire* 56 [1949], 67–87 and 60 [1953], 417–20) and K. Park and L. M. Daston (*Past and Present* 92 [1981], 20–54) deserve particular mention. The brilliant *The Shows of London* by Professor Richard Altick (Cambridge, Mass., 1978) is an encyclopedic source on all kinds of exhibitions in the metropolis, and A. H. Saxon's *P. T. Barnum: The Legend and the Man* (New York, 1989) and *Barnumiana* (Fairfield, Conn., 1995) are similarly valuable sources on all matters relating to Barnum and his career in show business. Among the recent books on the American sideshow are *Freak Show* by R. Bodgan (Chicago, 1988) and *Freakery* edited by R. G. Thomson (New York, 1996); the former is reasonably well researched, but the latter lacks historical perspective and medical knowledge alike. The valuable book *Wonder and the Order of Nature 1150–1750* by L. Daston and K. Park (New York, 1998) is a wide-ranging overview of various aspects of the quest for natural curiosities during the period in question, including a chapter on "monsters."

The Hairy Maid at the Harpsichord

General reviews of older cases of hypertrichosis include the valuable papers by M. Bartels (*Zeitschrift für Ethnologie* 8 [1876], 110–29; 11 [1879], 145–94; 13 [1881], 213–33); A. F. Le Double and F. Houssay's *Les velus* (Paris, 1912); F. Drimmer's *Very Special People* (New York, 1973), 141–47, 311–19; and the papers by A. Ecker (*Globus* 33 [1878], 177–87, 221–24), J. Boullet (*Aesculape* 44 [1961], 3–39), W.-R. Felgenhauer (*Journal de genetique humaine 17* [1969], 1–44), and T. K. Nowakowski and A. Scholz (*Der Hautarzt* 28 [1977], 593–99).

Barbara Urslerin was described by Th. Bartholin (*Historiarum Anatomicarum Rariorum* Cent 1 Hist 42, 1654), H. Jacobsen (*Acta Medica et Philosophica Hafnensis* 1 [1671–72] 274–75), G. Seger (*Miscellania Curiosa* Dec 1 Ann 9 [1680], 246), J. H. Degner (*Miscellania Curiosa* 6 [1742], 35–42), W. Stricker (*Virchows Archiv* 71 [1877], 111–13), V. A. Ecker (*Archiv für Anthropologie* 11 [1879], 176–78), and E. Brackenhoffer in *Voyage de Paris en Italie* (Paris, 1927), 70.

The Gonzales family was further described by C. Th. von Siebold (*Archiv für Anthropologie* 10 [1878], 253–60), F. Kenner (*Jahrbuch der Kunsthistorischen Sammlungen der Allerhöchsten Kaiserbauses* 15 [1894], 250–53), J. G. Ravin and G. P. Hodge (*Journal of the American Medical Association* 207 [1969], 533–35), A. Zanca (*Physis* 25 [1983], 41–66), R. Zapperi (*Annales économies, sociétés, civilisations* 40 [1985], 307–27), and L. Hendrix (*Word & Image* 11 [1995], 373–90) and C. Hertel (*Journal of the History of Collections* 13 [2001], 1–22).

The earliest accounts of the hairy Burmese are in the books *Journal of an Embassy from the Governor-General of India to the Court of Ava, in the year 1827*, Vol. 1, by J. Crawfurd (London, 1834), 318, and *A Narrative of the Mission sent by the Governor-General of India to the court of Ava in 1855* by H. Yule (London, 1858), 193–95. Later articles include those by H. Beigel (*Virchows Archiv* 44 [1868], 418–27), an anonymous author (*La nature* 3 [1875], 121–23), M. E. T. Hamy (*Bulletin de la Société d'Anthropologie de Paris* (Sér. 2) 10 [1875], 78–79), J. J. Weir (*Nature* 34 [1886], 223–24), and M. Guyot-Daubès (*La nature* 15 [1887], 41–43, 86–87). The paper by J. Bondeson and A. E. W. Miles (*Journal of the Royal Society of Medicine* 89 [1996], 403–8) has a complete list of references.

Andrian and Fedor Jeftichejev were described by R. Virchow (*Berliner Klinische Wochenschrift* 10 [1873], 337–39), C. Royer (*Bulletin de la Société d'Anthropologie de Paris* (Sér. 2) 8 [1873], 719–25), E.-R. Perrin (*Bulletin de la Société d'Anthropologie de Paris* (Sér. 2) 8 [1873], 741–50), C. S. Tomes and O. Coles (*British Medical Journal* 1 [1874], 413), an anonymous author (*Popular Science Monthly* 4 [1874], 448–51), M. Bartels (*Zeitschrift für Ethnologie* 16 [1884], 106–13), and J. Parreidt (*Deutsche Monatschrift für Zahnbeilkunde* 4 [1886], 41–54). D. Snigurowicz (*Canadian Journal of History* 34 [1999], 51–82) adds some interesting details about them and other hairy individuals exhibited in Paris.

On Julia Pastrana, see J. Bondeson's *A Cabinet of Medical Curiosities* (Ithaca, N.Y., 1997), 216–44, and its references. On Krao, see the articles by A. H. Keane (*Nature* 27 [1883], 245–46), A. B. Meyer (*Zeitschrift für Ethnologie* 17 [1885], 241–66), Dr. Fauvelle (*Bulletin de la Société d'Anthropologie de Paris* (Sér. 3) 9 [1886], 439–48), and Hr. Maas (*Zeitschrift für Ethnologie* 39 [1907], 425–29), P. Sarasin (*Zoologische Jahrbücher* Suppl. 15, Vol. 2 [1912], 289–328), and P. Mense (*Beiträge zur Pathologische Anatomie und zur Allgemeine Pathologie* 68 [1921], 486–95). Percilla's biography is told by James Taylor (*Shocked and Amazed* 6 [2002], 8–21).

Contributions to the modern scientific discussion of congenital hypertrichosis include articles by M. A. Macias-Flores et al. (*Human Genetics* 66 [1984], 66–70), F. A. M. Burmeister et al. (*Clinical Genetics* 44 [1993], 121-28), J. Bondeson and A. E. W. Miles (*American Journal of Medical Genetics* 47 [1993], 198–212), L. E. Figuera et al. (*Nature Genetics* 10 [1995], 202–7), and R. Balducci et al. (*Clinical Genetics* 53 [1998], 466–68).

The Stone-child

The original treatise of Jean d'Ailleboust, *Portentosum Lithopaedion, sive Embryum Petrificatum Urbis Senonensis* (Sens, 1582), was translated into French as *Le prodigieux enfant petrefié de la ville de Sens*. Ambroise Paré described the stone-child in his *Des monstres et prodiges* (Ed. J Céard, Geneva, 1971), xxii–xxxii, 42–43, 166, 205. The valuable original documents are in the Royal Library of Copenhagen (Gl. kgl. Saml. Nr 1641). Thomas Bartholin mentioned the lithopedion in his treatise *De Unicornu* (Patavii, 1645), 279, and later in his *Historiarum Anatomicarum Rariorum, Centuria I– II* (Amsterdam, 1654), 353–60. The other main sources about the stone-child's stay in Copenhagen are the 1696 and 1710 editions of Holger Jacobsen's *Musaeum Regium*. Later sources include *Kunstkammeret* by H. C. Bering Liisberg (Copenhagen, 1897), 56–59; *The Origins of Museums* edited by O. Impey and A. MacGregor (Oxford, 1985); and *The Royal Danish Kunstkammer 1737*, Vol. I–II, edited by B. Gundestrup (Copenhagen, 1991). Worthwhile later material on historical and medical aspects of lithopedions include the thesis *Das Steinkind von Leinzell* by W. Kieser (University of Stuttgart, 1854), and the articles by F. Küchenmeister (*Archiv für Gynaekologie* 17 [1881], 153–252), W. S. Bainbridge (*American Journal of Obstetrics* 65 [1912], 31–52), E. Stübler (*Archiv für Geschichte der Medizin* 18 [1926], 103–6), D. S. P. Tien (*Chinese Medical Journal* 67 [1949], 451–60), L. A. Chase (*Canadian Medical Association Journal* 99 [1968], 226–30), C. J. Fagan et al. (*Archives of Surgery* 115 [1980], 764–66), H. Stofft (*Histoire des sciences médicales* 20 [1986], 267–85), and J. Bondeson (*Journal of the Royal Society of Medicine* 89 [1996], 13–18). On Jean d'Ailleboust, see *La famille d'Ailleboust* by D. Fauteux (Montréal, 1917), 8–14, and the article on him by J. Balteau in the *Dictionnaire de biographie Française*, Vol. 1 (Paris, 1933), 934.

The Woman Who Laid an Egg

Two excellent Danish biographies of Olaus Wormius are H. D. Schleperen's *Museum Wormianum* (Copenhagen, 1971) and E. Hovesen's *Lægen Ole Worm* (Aarhus, 1987). Wormius's original description of the magical egg was in his *Museum Wormianum* (Amsterdam, 1655), 311–12, and Thomas Bartholin's account in his *Historiarum Anatomicarum Rariorum, Centuria I–II* (Amsterdam, 1654), 10–13; an English translation of the latter, with some errors, was published in the *Bulletin of the New York Academy of Medicine* (47 [1971], 431–32). The German observations by Jungius and Virdung were published in the first series of the *Miscellania Curiosa* (Ann. 2, Obs.

250, and Ann. 3, Obs. 68). The original documents cited concerning the transfer of
the egg are in the Nationalmuseum, Copenhagen (I, 14), in the Rigsarkivet, Copenhagen (Seddelreg. 12–13), and in the.Zoological Museum of Copenhagen. Brief
modern discussions of egg-laying women in fable and myth are provided by C. J. S.
Thompson in *The Mystery and Lore of Monsters* (London, 1931), 59–60; V. Newall in
An Egg at Easter (London, 1970), 40–44; and A.-B. Hellbom (*Ethnos* 28 [1963], 63–
105).

The Strangest Miracle in the World

The most thorough work on this subject is the book *The Prolific Countess* by Jan
Bondeson and Arie Molenkamp (Loosduinen, 1996; available from Stichting oud
Loosduinen, Museum de Korenschuur, Margaretha de Hennebergweg 2a, 2552 BA
Loosduinen, Holland), which is fully annotated throughout and contains a complete
list of references. The book (in Danish) entitled *Grevinden med de 365 børn* by K. Nyrop
(*Fortids Sagn og Sange* 5, Copenhagen, 1909) contains a worthy review of the literature, but has found few readers throughout the years. Quotations from some old
Dutch manuscripts are from the valuable *Oorkondenboekvan Holland en Zeeland*, Vol. I.
(Amsterdam, 1865) edited by L. P. C. van den Bergh; other manuscripts have been
inspected at the British Library Department of Manuscripts (Cotton Vit. E. V. and
F. XV., and Tib. C. XI.; and Sloane MSS. 1710. 5 ff), the Bodleian Library (MS
Rawlinson D. 1191, ff 21–22), the Royal Library (The Hague), and the Gemeentearchief of Naaldwijk. Articles directly dealing with the Loosduinen legend include
those by H. E. Rollins (*Notes and Queries* 12S. 11 [1922], 351–53), L. van Acker
(*Biekorf-West-vlaams Archief* 92 [1993], 113–34), and J. Bondeson and A. Molenkamp
(*Journal of the Royal Society of Medicine* 89 [1996], 711–16). Local history aspects are
discussed in the various chapters of the book *Zeven en een Halve Eeuw Abdijkerk Loosduinen* edited by V. Hildebrandt (Loosduinen, 1981). On the hydatidiform mole hypothesis, see the articles by A. Brews (*Journal of Obstetrics and Gynaecology of the British
Empire* 46 [1939], 813–35), L. J. Rather (*Bulletin of the New NEw York Academy of
Medicine* 47 [1971], 508–15), and A. Östör (*Anatomic Pathology* 1 [1996], 165–78).
Medical and historical aspects on multiple births are dealt with by A. Bastin (*Aesculape* 19 [1929] 289–98), in two valuable articles by C. F. Mayer (*Acta Geneticae
Medicae et Gemellolgiae* 1 [1952] 118–35, 242–75), and in the modern reviews of M. M.
Clay (*Clinics in Developmental Medicine* 107 [1989], 11–29) and S. Vaksmann et al.
(*Journal de gynécologie, obstetrique et de biologie reproductif* 19 [1990], 261–67). The main
sources on Bishop Hatto are S. Baring-Gould's *Curious Myths of the Middle Ages* (London, 1888), 447–70, and the German treatise on this subject by M. Beheim-
Schwarzbach, *Die Mäusethurmsage von Popiel and Hatto* (Posen, 1888).

290   Some Words about Hog-faced Gentlewomen

The oldest sources are the pamphlet *A certaine Relation of the Hog-Faced Gentlewoman* (London, 1640) in the British Library, and the poems in II. E. Rollins's *A Pepysian Garland* (Cambridge, 1922), 449–54. James paris du Plessis's account is in his *History of Prodigies*, kept in the British Library Department of Manuscripts (Sloane MSS 5246). The Grenville volume on hog-faced gentlewomen is in the British Library (G. 2188). The original 1815 newspaper articles were in the *Times* (16/2 3d and 17/2 3b) and the *Morning Chronicle* (17/2 3b). Other sources include T. Prest's *Magazine of Curiosity of Wonder* (1(22) [1836], 168–69); anonymous articles in *Chambers's Edinburgh Journal* (14 [1850], 106–7), *Notes and Queries* (2s. 11[1861], 266, 496–97), and *Dublin Medical Press* (51 [1864], 313); H. Wilson and J. Caulfield's *The Book of Wonderful Characters* (London, 1869), xi–xix; J. Ashton's *Humour, Wit, and Satire of the Seventeenth Century* (London, 1883), 49–55; R. Chambers's *The Book of Days*, Vol. 2 (London, 1888), 255–57; and J. Ashton's *Social England under the Regency*, Vol. 1 (London, 1890), 377–84. The Dutch sources are the articles by G. J. Boekenoogen (*Volkskunde* 16 [1904], 1–17, and 20 [1908], 1–8), and A. de Cock's *Volksage, Volksgeloof en Volksgebruik* (Amsterdam, 1918), 19–20. Modern sources include T. P. C. Kirkpatrick's *The History of Doctor Steevens' Hospital* (Dublin, 1924), 112–13; the article by A. C. Posner and M. A. Beer (*American Journal of Obstetrics and Gynecology* 63 [1952], 1157–61); and F. C. Sillar and R. M. Meyler's *The Symbolic Pig* (London, 1961), 35–36; foremost of them is Ricky Jay's eminent book *Learned Pigs and Fireproof Women* (London, 1987), 27–36.

Horned Humans

Thomas Bartholin wrote widely about horned humans in his *Historiarum Anatomicarum Rariorum* (Cent. 1 hist. 78, 128–29; Cent. 5 hist. 27, 44–46) and his *Epistolae Medicinales*; see also his correspondence with Olaus Wormius in *Breve til og fra Ole Worm*, Vol. 1 (Copenhagen, 1965), 338, 356, 452, 460. By far the best collection of stories of horned humans is *Ueber Keratose* by Dr. Hermann Liebert (Breslau, 1864). The earlier thesis *Des cornes* by A. Dauxais (Paris, 1820) adds some French observations. Older medical articles on horned humans include those by W. C. Worthington (*Lancet* 1 [1836], 143–44), E. Wilson (*Medico-Chirurgical Transactions* 27 [1844], 52–69), and W. Giese (*Magazin für die Gesammte Heilkunde* 66 [1848], 474–84). Paul Rodriguez was described in the *Medical Repository* (New York) (NS 5 [1820], 88–90); Mother Horn, in the *American Journal of the Medical Sciences* (NS 21 [1851], 50–51); and the horned Indian boy, by J. M. Richardson in the *Indian Medical Gazette* (70 [1935], 159). Mary Davies and her horn were described in Kirby's *Wonderful and Eccentric Museum* (6 [1820], 164–67), in *Notes and Queries* (159 [1930], 159, 171, 212–13, 249, 282), and by A. MacGregor (*The Ashmolean* 3 [1983], 10–11). Later articles include those by H. L. Nietert and E. A. Babler (*Annals of Surgery* 43 [1906], 907–11), M. Joseph (*Archiv für Dermatologie und Syphilologie* 100 [1910], 343–54), J. Avalon (*Aesculape* 41 [1958], 3–9), B. Lennox and B. R. Sayed (*Journal of Pathology and*

Bacteriology 88 [1964], 575–79), R. C. H. Yu et al. (*British Journal of Dermatology* 124   291
[1991], 449–52), and T. Korkut et al. (*Annals of Plastic Surgery* 39 [1997], 654–55).
My article in the *American Journal of Dermatopathology* (23 [2001], 362–69) reviews
medical aspects of historical cases, and the valuable article by M. Michal et al. (*American Journal of Surgical Pathology* 26 [2002], 789–94) adds some curious modern instances of horned people. Later popular and literary articles include those by J. O.
Wood (*Huntington Library Quarterly* 29 [1966], 295–300, and *Isis* 58 [1967], 239–40),
C. L. Regan (*English Language Notes* 5 [1967], 34–39, and *American Notes and Queries*
12 [1974], 133–34), P. Sieveking (*Fortean Times* 43 [1985], 36–40), J. P. Runden
(*Melville Society Extracts* 71 [1987], 9–11), and R. Mellinkoff (*Journal of Jewish Art* 12
[1987], 184–98). Dr. Arthur MacGregor, of the Ashmolean Museum, Oxford, and
Professor M. H. Kaufman, of the Department of Biomedical Science, University of
Edinburgh, are thanked for valuable help.

The Biddenden Maids
    The older sources are generally referenced in the text. Three important papers
on the Maids are those by J. W. Ballantyne (*Teratologia* 2 [1895], 268–74), G. Clinch
(*The Reliquary and Illustrated Archaeologist* NS 6 [1900], 42–46), Marcel Baudouin (*Revue de chirurgie* 25 [1902], 513–77), and J. Bondeson (*Journal of the Royal Society of
Medicine* 85 [1992], 217–21). The latter has a long list of references. Important historical material on conjoined twins includes the articles by A. P. Chavarria and P. G. Shipley (*Annals of Medical History* 6 [1924], 297–302), A. F. Guttmacher (*Birth Defects* 3
[1967], 10–17), G. H. Schumacher et al. (*Anatomischer Anzeiger* 164 [1987], 225–36,
291–303), J. Bondeson (*Journal of the Royal Society of Medicine* 86 [1993], 13–18), and
S. Geroulanos et al. (*Gesnerus* 50 [1993], 179–200); R. M. F. van der Werden (*Twin
Research* 2 [1999], 30–32) and A. W. Bates (*Twin Research* 5 [2002], 521–28). I was
also fortunate enough to possess an extra-illustrated, bound copy of Dr. G. J. Fisher's
Diploteratology, originally published in the *Transactions of the Medical Society of the State
of New York* of 1865–1868. On Helen and Judith, see the article by J. J. Torkos (*Medical Proceedings* 9 [1963], 271–77); on Millie-Christine, see J. Martell's excellent *Millie-Christine: Fearfully and Wonderfully Made* (New York, 2000); on the Blazek sisters, see
the articles by R. Henneberg (*Berliner Klinische Wochenschrift* 40 [1903], 798–801,
829–33), B. H. Breakstone (*American Medicine* NS 17 [1922], 221–26), and H. Schierhorn (*Anatomischer Anzeiger* 160 [1985], 353–65). Some modern medical articles on
conjoined twins and their surgical separation are those by R. G. Harper et al. (*American Journal of Obstetrics and Gynecology* 137 [1980], 617–29), R. M. Hoyle (*Surgery,
Gynecology and Obstetrics* 170 [1990], 549–62), G. A. Machin (*Birth Defects Original Article Series* 29(1) [1993], 141–79), R. Spencer (*Journal of Pediatric Surgery* 31 [1996],
941–44), and M. L. Hilfiker et al. (*Journal of Pediatric Surgery* 33 [1998], 768–70). Important information has also been derived from the pamphlet *The Story of Biddenden*
and other local history sources. The Trustees of the Chulkhurst charity and the Biddenden Local History Society are thanked for important information.

292   The Tocci Brothers, and Other Dicephali

The main sources on the Fair Maidens of Foscott are *Through Ten English Counties* by J. J. Hissey (London, 1894, 141–44) and an anonymous article in the *British Medical Journal* (1 [1902], 915–16). Other older historical instances of dicephali are described by G. Schwalbe in *Die Morphologie der Missbildungen* (Jena, 1906), 75–79; E. Holländer in *Wunder, Wundergeburt und Wundergestalt* (Jena, 1921), 64–71; and J. F. D. Shrewsbury (*Journal of Obstetrics and Gynaecology of the British Empire* 56 [1949], 67–85). The sad fate of Ritta-Christina was discussed in anonymous articles in *La clinique* (1 [1829], 200, 254–55) and *Bulletin des sciences medicales* (18 [1829], 169–72). Later articles include those by M. Saint-Ange (*Journal hebdomadaire de medécine* 6 [1830], 42–49), H. Danerow (*Litterarischen Annalen der gesammten Heilkunde* 16 [1830], 454–82), E. Serres (*Mémoires de l'academie Royale des Sciences* 11 [1832], 583–895), P. J. S. Whitmore (*French Studies* 21 [1967], 319–22), and S. J. Gould (*Natural History* 91 (11) [1982], 18–22). Articles on the Tocci brothers include those by S. Fubini and A. Mosso (*Giornale della r. Accademia di Medicina di Torino* (Ser. 3) 23 [1878], 13–26), P. Colrat and F. Rebatel (*Lyon Medical* 29 [1878], 274–80), Dr. Grünwald (*Virchows Archiv* 75 [1879], 561), R. Virchow (*Zeitschrift für Ethnologie* 18 [1886], 47–50 and 23 [1891], 245–46), an anonymous author (*Scientific American* 65 [1891], 374), R. P. Harris (*American Journal of Obstetrics* (NY) 25 [1892], 460–73), M. Baudoin (*Gazette medicale de Paris* (Sér. 13) 4 [1904], 200), and L. Gedda (*Acta Genetica Medica e Gemellologica* 5 [1956], 1–13). The influence of the Tocci brothers on Mark Twain was discussed by R. A. Wiggins (*American Literature* 23 [1951], 355–57), N. Fredericks (*Nineteenth-Century Literature* 43 [1989], 484–99), and M. Shell (*Arizona Review* 47 (2) [1991], 29–75). Later articles and reviews on dicephalus twins include those by G. B. Gruber and H. Eymer (*Beiträge zur Pathologische Anatomie und zur allgemeine Pathologie* 77 [1927], 240–76), G. B. Gruber (*Abhandlungen der Gesellschaft der Wissenschaften zu Göttingen*, Math.-Phys. Klasse III. Folge 4, 1931), G. Aschan (*Upsala Läkareförenings Förhandlingar* NF 47 [1941–42], 289–304), H. Scherrer (*Virchows Archiv* 323 [1953], 597–621), P. G. Brewster (*Acta Genetica Medica e Gemellologica* 11 [1962], 450–56), G. Schnesinger (*Anatomischer Anzeiger* 143 [1978], 176–82), E. S. Golladay et al. (*Journal of Pediatric Surgery* 17 [1982], 259–64), and J. R. Siebert et al. (*Teratology* 40 [1989], 305–10). The separation of Katie and Eilish was discussed by C. Myser and D. L. Clark (*Literature and Medicine* 17 [1998], 45–67), and in many newspaper and magazine articles. The information on the Hensel twins is from an article in the Swedish magazine *Exxet* (15 [1996], 6–17), for which the material had been fetched from an article in *Time* and a television documentary. On the recent debate on ethical aspects of surgery on conjoined twins, see the articles by D. C. Thomasma et al. (*Hastings Center Report* 24 [1996], 4–12), J. Raffensperger (*Pediatric Surgery International* 12 [1997], 249–55), and A. Domurat Dreger (*Studies in the History and Philosophy of Science* 29 [1998], 1–29).

The royal museum at Drottningholm Castle was described by the antiquary A. Lindblom in a typewritten volume entitled *Lovisa Ulrikas Museum °a Drottningholm* (Stockholm, 1927); the only copy is kept in the archives of the castle architect's office, the Royal Castle, Stockholm. A much shortened version was printed in the *Nationalmusei °Arsbok* (9 [1927], 85–123). Y. Löwegren, *Naturaliekabinett i Sverige under 1700 — talet* (Lychnos-Bibliotek 13, Lund, 1952), 295–321, provided another, independent account. Further important manuscript material is kept at the Riksarkivet (kungl. ark. [Dr. L. Ulrika] K268 fasc. 11), and the Drottningholm Castle inventories at the Slottsarkivet (DI:9–11, 13–15, 17–19, 28, 32, 37). Two early guidebooks are those by O. Carlén, *Drottningholm, Dess historia och närmaste omgifningar* (Stockholm, 1879), 38–39, and A. Björklund, *Beskrifning öfver Kongl. Lust-Slotten Drottningholm och China* (Stockholm 1796), 50–68.

The four major biographical papers on Nicolas Ferry are those by G. Richard (*Mémoires de l'académie de Stanislas* (Sér. 6) 30 [1933], 97–114), J. Avalon (*Aesculape* 29 [1939], 107–13), A. Benoît (*Bulletin de la Société Philomatique Vosgienne* 9 [1883–84], 111–26), and Dr. Liégey (*Annales de la Société d'Émulation des Vosges* 16 [1889], 135–50). M. Kast's early account was published in the *Histoire de l'academie Royale des Sciences* (1746), 44–45. Anecdotes of Nicolas Ferry's life at Lunéville were told by E. Garnier, *Les nains et les géants* (Paris, 1884), 153–63; by G. Maugras in his books *La cour de Lunéville au XVIIIe siècle* (Paris, 1904), 218–21, and *Dernières années de la cour de Lunéville* (Paris, 1906), 236–39, 396–99; by P. Boyé, *La cour polonaise de Lunéville* (Nancy, 1926), 230–37; and by J. Levron, *Stanislas Leszcynski* (Paris, 1984), 286–91, 338–41, 396, 402. Dr. Morand's lecture was published in the *Histoire de l'académie Royale des Sciences* (1764), 62–71.

Count de Tressan's lecture on Nicolas Ferry was reported to have been privately printed, but no copy has been available to me. At least parts of this lecture, extensively quoted by J. Avalon in the paper referred to earlier, were kept in the archives of the Academie des Sciences in the 1920s. The Princess de Talmont described Nicolas in another rare publication, *Lettre d'une personne de Lunéville à un de ses amis de Paris*, quoted by M. Richard in his aforementioned paper. Apart from the official autopsy report of Dr. Morands, Count de Tressan published an addendum in the obscure collection *Aldovrandus Lotharingiæ de Bucholtz*, quoted by M. Richard. The important account by the surgeon M. Saucerotte was published in the *Journal encyclopédique*, Sept. 1768. An exhaustive account of Nicolas Ferry's skeleton was published by G. L. Buffon et al. in *Histoire naturelle générale et particulière, avec la description du Cabinet du Roy*, Vol. 15 (Amsterdam, 1771), 97–100. Other sources include I. Geoffroy Saint-Hilaire, *Historie générale et particulière des anomalies de l'organisation*, Vol. 2 (Paris, 1832), 148–53; the papers by R. Guérin (*Journal de la Société a'Archéologie Lorraine* 27 [1878], 78–79), Dr. Porak (*Bulletin et mémoires de la Société Obstétricale et Gynécologique de Paris* 6 [1890], 77–78), and L. Manouvrier (*Bulletin de la Société d'Anthropologie de Paris* (Sér. 4) 7 [1897], 264–90); and the books by H. Gilford, *Disorders of Growth and Development* (London, 1911), A. Rischbieth and A. Barrington, *A Treasury of Human Inheritance*, Vol. 15 (London, 1912), 552, 562, 568, and H. P. G. Seckel, *Bird-headed Dwarfs* (New York, 1960), 71–78. More recent articles include those by N. Fitch et al. (*American Journal of Diseases of Children* 114 [1970], 260–64), F. Majewski and T. Goecke (*American Journal of Medical Genetics* 12 [1982], 7–21), E. Thompson and M. Pembrey (*Journal of Medical Genetics* 22 [1985], 192–201), and J. Bondeson (*American Journal of Medical Genetics* 44 [1992], 210–19). M. Pierre Chanel, conservator of the Castle Museum of Lunéville, and Frau Dr. J. Lessmann, Museum für Kunst und Gewerbe, Hamburg, are thanked for important information.

Daniel Cajanus, the Swedish Giant

There are two biographical articles about Daniel Cajanus, written in Finnish and Dutch, respectively, by M. Tamminen (*Suomen Museo* 83 [1976], 93–108) and B. C. Sliggers (*Jaarboek Haerlem* [1978], 9–46). Older material about the early career of Cajanus includes C. Giörwell's *Thet Swenska Bibliotheket* (Stockholm, 1757), 53–54, and T. Carpelan's *Finsk Biografisk Handbok* (Helsinki, 1903), 313–19, as well as the scholarly papers by J. R. Aspelin (*Finskt Museum* 18 [1911], 30–34) and J. Finne and Y. Kajava (*Suomen Tiedakatemian Toimikutsa Sarja A.* 25 [1926], 54–56). On his visits to Britain, see the *Daily Advertiser* of September 23 and 27, 1742; the *Biographical Dictionary of Actors* (Eds. P. H. Highfill et al.), Vol. 3 (Carbondale, 1975), 10–11; and the book *The Gigantick Histories of Thomas Boreman* by W. M. Stone (Portland, 1933). On "Little Cajanus," see the paper by A. Wallgren (*Acta Paediatrica* 46 [1957], 232–37). Many aspects of Daniel Cajanus's life are covered in E. J. Wood's encyclopedic *Giants and Dwarfs* (London, 1868), 142–45. His career in Holland was described by W. Greve in his *Natuur-en Geshiedkundige Verhandeling over de Reuzen en Dwergen* (Amsterdam, 1916), 16, 32–38; by J. Marchant, *Verhaal van Reuzen* (Haarlem, 1751), 109; by Th. Schrewelius, *Harlemias, of Eerste Stichting der Staad Haarlem* (Haarlem, 1754); by J. W. Stuffers, *De Groote of Sint-Bavo Kerk te Haarlem na de Resturatie* (Haarlem, 1915), 25–27, 71–72; and also by J. P. van Lennep (*Notes and Queries* 2s. 9, [1860], 423). A valuable modern source is the book edited by B. C. Sliggers and A. A. Wertheim, *De Tentoongestelde Mens* (Haarlem, 1993), 24–25, 73–76. A short description of Cajanus's skeleton is included in the official guide to the Anatomical Museum of Leiden, edited by W. J. Mulder (Leiden, 1984), 23.

Daniel Lambert, the Human Colossus

Contemporary newspaper accounts of Daniel Lambert include those in the *Leicester Journal* (4/4, 11/7, 19/9, 5/12, 1806; 2/10, 9/10, 1807; 23/6, 30/6, 1809; 13/9, 1811), the *Times* (9/4 3a, 12/4 3a, 1806; 17/10 3a, 1808; 26/6 4b, 1809), and the *Morning Post* (14/4 3d, 1806). Other contemporary accounts were in the *Medical and Physical Journal* (15 [1806], 582–83), in the *Gentleman's Magazine* (79 [1809], 219–

20, 681–83; 80 [1810], 153–54; 88 [1818], 207), and in a short-lived magazine called
the *Beau Monde and Monthly Register* (1(4) [1809], 375–77). Also in Kirby's *Wonderful
Museum*, Vol. 2 (London, 1804), 408–10; Granger's *Wonderful Museum and Magazine
Extraordinary*, Vol. 6 (London, 1808), 2673–79; the *Eccentric Magazine*, Vol. 2 (London,
1812–13), 241–48; Smeeton's *Biographia Curiosa* (London, 1822), 249–53; Prest's
Magazine of Curiosity and Wonder (1(3) [1835], 17–19); and Charles Dickens's *Household Words* (5[1852], 546–48). His biography entitled *The Life of that Wonderful and
Extraordinary Heavy Man, the late Daniel Lambert*, was first published in Stamford in
1809, and reprinted in 1892. On the Daniel Lambert tavern in London, see the
articles in the *Daily Telegraph* of January 9, 1908, and the *World's Fair* of May 12,
1912. Later accounts of Lambert include those by O. Hill. (*Middlesex Hospital Journal*
56 [1956] 74–76), R. B. Davis (*Tally Ho! Journal of the Leicester and Rutland Constab-
ulary* 13(3) [1968], 61–66), and an anonymous pamphlet entitled *Daniel Lambert*,
published by the Leicester Museums, Arts and Records Service, 1993. Valuable original material was at my disposal at the archives of the Newarke House Museum,
Leicester, and the Stamford Museum, Stamford. The manuscript account of Lambert's death is in the Cambridge University Library (MSS Add 7221, pp. 117–18,
section 160).

Cat-eating Englishmen and French Frog Swallowers

Lysons' *Colletanea* contains much valuable data about the English gluttons and
"cat eaters." The polyphagi of olden times were described by E. G. Happel in Vol. 1
of the *Relationes Curiosae* (Hamburg, 1683), 375–79, and D. Biett (*Dictionnaire des
Sciences Medicales* 4 [1813], 197–202). Charles Domery was described by J. Johnston
in the *Medical and Physical Journal* (3 [1800], 209) and Charles Dickens's comments
were in his *Household Words* (5 [1852], 546–48). Jacques de Falaise was described
by J. P. Beaudé in the *Revue médicale Française et etrangère* (3 [1826], 521–26) and in
an anonymous article in the Norwegian journal *Eyr* (3 [1828], 292–96). Professor
Percy's paper on Tarrare originally appeared in the *Journal de médecine, chirurgie, phar-
macie &c* (9 [1805], 87–106). It was commented on by J. G. Millingen in his *Curiosities of Medical Experience* (London, 1839), 196–202, and in an anonymous article in
Aesculape (20 [1930], 292–301). On Antoine Langulet, see M. Berthollet's paper in
the *Archives générales de médecine* ((Sér. 1) 7 [1825], 472–73), and P. Haining's *The
Flesh Eaters* (London, 1994), 125–32. A particularly well-written account of "human
ostriches" and similar performers is that of the American magician Ricky Jay in his
masterly *Learned Pigs and Fireproof Women* (London, 1987), 276–99. Further material
is provided by J. Boullet (*Aesculape* 34 [1953], 164–65) and R. Bogdan, *Freak Show*
(New York, 1988), 263–64.

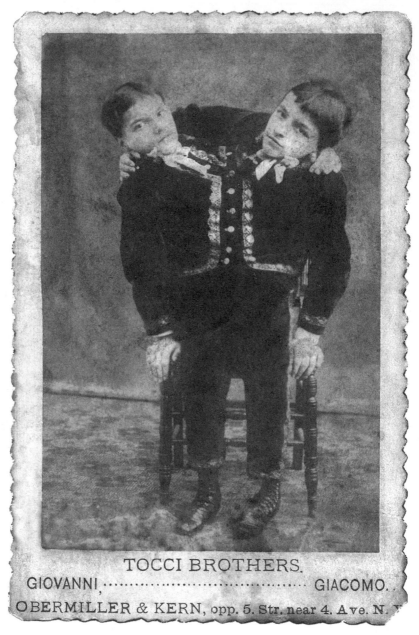

An 1893 New York cabinet card of the Tocci brothers, signed on the back by both twins. From the author's collection.